Nanomedicine-Based Approaches for the Treatment of Dementia

AF843181

Nanomedicine-Based Approaches for the Treatment of Dementia

Edited by

Umesh Gupta
Department fo Pharmacy, Central University of Rajasthan, India

Prashant Kesharwani
Department of Pharmaceutics, School of Pharmaceutical Education and Research, Jamia Hamdard, New Delhi, India

ELSEVIER

ACADEMIC PRESS
An imprint of Elsevier
elsevier.com/books-and-journals

Academic Press is an imprint of Elsevier
125 London Wall, London EC2Y 5AS, United Kingdom
525 B Street, Suite 1650, San Diego, CA 92101, United States
50 Hampshire Street, 5th Floor, Cambridge, MA 02139, United States
The Boulevard, Langford Lane, Kidlington, Oxford OX5 1GB, United Kingdom

Copyright © 2023 Elsevier Inc. All rights reserved.

No part of this publication may be reproduced or transmitted in any form or by any means, electronic or mechanical, including photocopying, recording, or any information storage and retrieval system, without permission in writing from the publisher. Details on how to seek permission, further information about the Publisher's permissions policies and our arrangements with organizations such as the Copyright Clearance Center and the Copyright Licensing Agency, can be found at our website: www.elsevier.com/permissions.

This book and the individual contributions contained in it are protected under copyright by the Publisher (other than as may be noted herein).

Notices
Knowledge and best practice in this field are constantly changing. As new research and experience broaden our understanding, changes in research methods, professional practices, or medical treatment may become necessary.

Practitioners and researchers must always rely on their own experience and knowledge in evaluating and using any information, methods, compounds, or experiments described herein. In using such information or methods they should be mindful of their own safety and the safety of others, including parties for whom they have a professional responsibility.

To the fullest extent of the law, neither the Publisher nor the authors, contributors, or editors, assume any liability for any injury and/or damage to persons or property as a matter of products liability, negligence or otherwise, or from any use or operation of any methods, products, instructions, or ideas contained in the material herein.

ISBN: 978-0-12-824331-2

For Information on all Academic Press publications visit our website at https://www.elsevier.com/books-and-journals

Publisher: Nikki P. Levy
Acquisitions Editor: Joslyn T. Chaiprasert-Paguio
Editorial Project Manager: Timothy J. Bennett
Production Project Manager: Stalin Viswanathan
Cover Designer: Miles Hitchen

Working together to grow libraries in developing countries
www.elsevier.com • www.bookaid.org

Typeset by Aptara, New Delhi, India

Dedication

I would like to dedicate this book to my family and parents who supported me all the way to complete this book. Specially, my mother (Lt. Malti Devi) was an inspiration for me to complete this book. I feel privileged and indebted to my dear wife Namrata (Mini) and my daughters Dhaanya and Maanya who always supported and motivated me to work on this book. I would also like to acknowledge and dedicate this book to my friends, contributors, and research group for their constant and tireless support in the journey of this book.

Umesh Gupta

Contents

Contributors

Mukta Agrawal School of Pharmacy & Technology Management, SVKM's Narsee Monjee Institute of Management Studies (NMIMS), Hyderabad, India

Junia Akhtar Centre for Pharmaceutical Nanotechnology, Department of Pharmaceutics, National Institute of Pharmaceutical Education and Research (NIPER), S.A.S. Nagar, Punjab, India

Amit Alexander Department of Pharmaceutics, National Institute of Pharmaceutical Education and Research (NIPER), Guwahati, Assam, India

Gulin Amasya Department of Pharmaceutical Technology, Faculty of Pharmacy, Ankara University, Ankara, Turkey

Taruna Arora Division of Reproductive Biology, Indian Council of Medical Research, Ansari Nagar, New Delhi, India

Kajal Bagri Department of Pharmaceutical Sciences and Technology, Maharaja Ranjit Singh Punjab Technical University, Bathinda, Punjab, India

Sanya Batheja Department of Pharmacy, School of Chemical Sciences and Pharmacy, Central University of Rajasthan, Bandarsindri, Ajmer, Rajasthan, India

Zerrin Sezgin Bayindir Department of Pharmaceutical Technology, Faculty of Pharmacy, Ankara University, Ankara, Turkey

Jayant Singh Bhardwaj Neuropsychopharmacology Division, Department of Pharmacy, Birla Institute of Technology and Science-Pilani, Pilani, Rajasthan, India

Abhay Bhardwaj KIET School of Pharmacy, Ghaziabad, India

Swapnali Vasant Birajdar Department of Pharmaceutics, National Institute of Pharmaceutical Education and Research (NIPER), Lucknow, Uttar Pradesh, India

Antonio Camins Biomedical Research Networking Centre in Neurodegenerative Diseases (CIBERNED), Madrid, Spain; Department of Pharmacology, Toxicology & Therapeutic Chemistry, Faculty of Pharmacy & Food Sciences, University of Barcelona, Barcelona, Spain

Amanda Cano Department of Pharmacy, Pharmaceutical Technology & Physical Chemistry, Faculty of Pharmacy & Food Sciences, University of Barcelona, Barcelona, Spain; Institute of Nanoscience & Nanotechnology (IN2UB), Barcelona, Spain; Biomedical Research Networking Centre in Neurodegenerative Diseases (CIBERNED), Madrid, Spain; Ace Alzheimer Center Barcelona – International University of Catalunya (UIC), Barcelona, Spain

Akash Chaurasiya Translational Pharmaceutics Research Laboratory, Department of Pharmacy, Birla Institute of Technology and Science, Pilani, Hyderabad, India

Rusham Das Department of Pharmacy, School of Chemical Sciences, & Pharmacy, Central University of Rajasthan

Rahul Deshmukh Department of Pharmaceutical Sciences and Technology, Maharaja Ranjit Singh Punjab Technical University, Bathinda, Punjab, India

Sunil Kumar Dubey Medical Research, R&D Healthcare Division, Emami Ltd, Belgharia, Kolkata, India

Marta Espina Department of Pharmacy, Pharmaceutical Technology & Physical Chemistry, Faculty of Pharmacy & Food Sciences, University of Barcelona, Barcelona, Spain; Institute of Nanoscience & Nanotechnology (IN2UB), Barcelona, Spain

Gerard Esteruelas Department of Pharmacy, Pharmaceutical Technology & Physical Chemistry, Faculty of Pharmacy & Food Sciences, University of Barcelona, Barcelona, Spain; Institute of Nanoscience & Nanotechnology (IN2UB), Barcelona, Spain

Miren Ettcheto Biomedical Research Networking Centre in Neurodegenerative Diseases (CIBERNED), Madrid, Spain; Department of Pharmacology, Toxicology & Therapeutic Chemistry, Faculty of Pharmacy & Food Sciences, University of Barcelona, Barcelona, Spain

Maria Luisa García Department of Pharmacy, Pharmaceutical Technology & Physical Chemistry, Faculty of Pharmacy & Food Sciences, University of Barcelona, Barcelona, Spain; Institute of Nanoscience & Nanotechnology (IN2UB), Barcelona, Spain; Biomedical Research Networking Centre in Neurodegenerative Diseases (CIBERNED), Madrid, Spain

Goutam Ghosh Department of Pharmaceutics, School of Pharmaceutical Sciences, Siksha 'O' Anusandhan (Deemed to be University), Bhubaneswar, Odisha, India

Amit Kumar Goyal Department of Pharmacy, School of Chemical Sciences, & Pharmacy, Central University of Rajasthan

Deepika Grewal Neuropsychopharmacology Division, Department of Pharmacy, Birla Institute of Technology and Science-Pilani, Pilani, Rajasthan, India

Umesh Gupta Department of Pharmacy, School of Chemical Sciences and Pharmacy, Central University of Rajasthan, Bandarsindri, Ajmer, Rajasthan, India

Sanyog Jain Centre for Pharmaceutical Nanotechnology, Department of Pharmaceutics, National Institute of Pharmaceutical Education and Research (NIPER), S.A.S. Nagar, Punjab, India

Biswakanth Kar Department of Pharmaceutics, School of Pharmaceutical Sciences, Siksha 'O' Anusandhan (Deemed to be University), Bhubaneswar, Odisha, India

Oly Katari Centre for Pharmaceutical Nanotechnology, Department of Pharmaceutics, National Institute of Pharmaceutical Education and Research (NIPER), S.A.S. Nagar, Punjab, India

Sumeet Katke Translational Pharmaceutics Research Laboratory, Department of Pharmacy, Birla Institute of Technology and Science, Pilani, Hyderabad, India

Prashant Kesharwani Department of Pharmaceutics, School of Pharmaceutical Education and Research, Jamia Hamdard, New Delhi, India; University Institute of Pharma Sciences, Chandigarh University, Mohali, Punjab, India

Sanskruti Santosh Kharavtekar Neuropsychopharmacology Division, Department of Pharmacy, Birla Institute of Technology and Science-Pilani, Pilani, Rajasthan, India

Vinay Kumar Department of Pharmacy, School of Chemical Sciences and Pharmacy, Central University of Rajasthan, Bandarsindri, Ajmer, Rajasthan, India

Shilpa Kumari Department of Pharmaceutical Sciences and Technology, Maharaja Ranjit Singh Punjab Technical University, Bathinda, Punjab, India

Priyanka Kumari Department of Pharmacy, School of Chemical Sciences, & Pharmacy, Central University of Rajasthan

Shobha Kumari Neuropsychopharmacology Division, Department of Pharmacy, Birla Institute of Technology and Science-Pilani, Pilani, Rajasthan, India

Farhan Mazahir Department of Pharmaceutics, National Institute of Pharmaceutical Education and Research (NIPER), Lucknow, Uttar Pradesh, India

Manisha Mulchandani Department of Pharmaceutics, National Institute of Pharmaceutical Education and Research (NIPER), Lucknow, Uttar Pradesh, India

Jayabalan Nirmal Translational Pharmaceutics Research Laboratory, Department of Pharmacy, Birla Institute of Technology and Science, Pilani, Hyderabad, India

Kanan Panchal Translational Pharmaceutics Research Laboratory, Department of Pharmacy, Birla Institute of Technology and Science, Pilani, Hyderabad, India

Tushar Kanti Rajwar Department of Pharmaceutics, School of Pharmaceutical Sciences, Siksha 'O' Anusandhan (Deemed to be University), Bhubaneswar, Odisha, India

Goutam Rath Department of Pharmaceutics, School of Pharmaceutical Sciences, Siksha 'O' Anusandhan (Deemed to be University), Bhubaneswar, Odisha, India

Shreyasi Ghosh Ray Neuropsychopharmacology Division, Department of Pharmacy, Birla Institute of Technology and Science-Pilani, Pilani, Rajasthan, India

Upal Roy Department of Health and Biomedical Sciences, University of Texas Rio Grande Valley College of Health Affairs One West University Blvd. Brownsville, Texas

Rakesh Kumar Sahoo Department of Pharmacy, School of Chemical Sciences and Pharmacy, Central University of Rajasthan, Bandarsindri, Ajmer, Rajasthan, India

Eliana B. Souto Department of Pharmaceutical Technology, Faculty of Pharmacy, University of Porto, Porto, Portugal; REQUIMTE/UCIBIO, Faculty of Pharmacy, University of Porto, Porto, Portugal

Elena Sánchez-López Department of Pharmacy, Pharmaceutical Technology & Physical Chemistry, Faculty of Pharmacy & Food Sciences, University of Barcelona, Barcelona, Spain; Institute of Nanoscience & Nanotechnology (IN2UB), Barcelona, Spain; Biomedical Research Networking Centre in Neurodegenerative Diseases (CIBERNED), Madrid, Spain; Unit of Synthesis and Biomedical Applications of Peptides, IQAC-CSIC, Barcelona, Spain

Rajeev Taliyan Neuropsychopharmacology Division, Department of Pharmacy, Birla Institute of Technology and Science-Pilani, Pilani, Rajasthan, India

Awesh K. Yadav Department of Pharmaceutics, National Institute of Pharmaceutical Education and Research (NIPER), Lucknow, Uttar Pradesh, India

Sheetal Yadav Centre for Pharmaceutical Nanotechnology, Department of Pharmaceutics, National Institute of Pharmaceutical Education and Research (NIPER), S.A.S. Nagar, Punjab, India

Nilufer Yuksel Department of Pharmaceutical Technology, Faculty of Pharmacy, Ankara University, Ankara, Turkey

Preface

Nanotechnology is progressively gaining interest of scientific fraternity mainly in biological applications for healthcare. However, still there are niche areas, where nanotechnology has limited applicability. The role of nanocarriers in the delivery of drugs has proven to be meritorious than the conventional ways of drug delivery. Particularly in diseases like cancer, diabetes, etc. nanocarriers have resulted into excellent outcome. However, brain disorders like Alzheimer's, Parkinsonism, etc. pose an entirely different challenge as per as drug delivery is concerned. The access of drugs and other bioactives to brain is still a major challenge to deal with. Dementia is a syndrome in which cognitive behavior of a person deteriorates which is difficult to predict beyond aging. This can affect the daily tasks performed by that person including language, learning capacity, memory, comprehension, and ability to carry out simple tasks including judgment. More than 45 million people are affected by dementia worldwide. This chronic disease is reported in almost 10 million new cases every year and hence needs solid treatment strategies. Dementia is the result of several brain disorders which directly or indirectly affects the brain function such as Alzheimer's, brain stroke, etc.

This book entitled *"Nanomedicine-based Approaches for the Treatment of Dementia"* is a fair attempt to report the capability of different nanocarriers such as polymeric nanoparticles, solid lipid nanoparticles (SLNs), dendrimers, liposomes, noninvasive nanocarriers, micelles in treating dementia, and other brain disorders. The complex nature of dementia necessitates the requirement of some of the carrier-mediated drug delivery approaches to mimic the physiological processes of human body for better results. The book is written in context to make readers understand the etiology, possible targets, receptors, and different approaches for the treatment of dementia. Initial chapters of the book emphasize on the understanding of dementia and the remaining chapters deliver the role of the different nanocarriers in treating dementia. Though there are very few products based on nanocarriers, which are there in the market for treating brain ailments; however, this book is also an attempt to accelerate the research in the area of brain targeting of drugs.

The book is comprised of eleven chapters including; Dementia and Neurodegenerative Disorders: An Introduction; Dementia: Etiology, Types, Causes and Prevention; Receptor Attacking Ligands for Active Targeting to Brain; Dendrimer Based Drug Delivery for Dementia; Polymeric Nanoparticles-Based Drug Delivery for Dementia; Solid Lipid Nanoparticles (SLN) Based

Drug Delivery for Dementia; Liposome: A Potential Drug delivery Vector To Treat Dementia; Micelles based Drug Delivery for Dementia; Biologics for the Management Of Dementia; Nanocarrier Based Noninvasive Approaches for Dementia; Futuristic Aspect of Nanocarriers on Targeted Delivery for Dementia. The book is of special interest for the undergraduate, postgraduate, and doctoral students working in the area of dementia and related research. The book can be beneficial to the readers for the understanding the role of nanotechnology in dementia and its critical attributes. Individual chapters are dedicated to one nanocarrier so that the concept and role of each nanocarrier can be understood in more detail. As a final note we believe that the book will be helpful to a reader who is interested or working in the area of treatment of brain disorders including neurodegenerative disorders.

Umesh Gupta and Prashant Kesharwani

Chapter 1

Dementia and neurodegenerative disorder: An introduction

Swapnali Vasant Birajdar[#], Manisha Mulchandani[#], Farhan Mazahir[#], Awesh K. Yadav

Department of Pharmaceutics, National Institute of Pharmaceutical Education and Research (NIPER), Lucknow, Uttar Pradesh, India

[#]Authors contributed equally.

1.1 Introduction

Neurodegenerative disorders are caused due to cognitive decline which leads to neuronal damage in the brain. Impairment in the nerve tissues is the main reason behind these neurological disorders. As neurons cannot reproduce or regenerate. These disorders are incurable and lead to progressive degeneration. Neurons are the cells of the nervous system which helps to perform every function of the body such as moving, thinking, talking, remembering, and thus when the neurons get damage there will be a miscommunication between the nerve cells and results in impairment in these normal functions of the body [1,2]. In the United States, an estimated rate close to 6.2 million or more in peoples who are of age 65 years and elders are standing with dementia nowadays, which is caused due to "Alzheimer's disease" (AD) and additional neurodegenerative disorders. This number strength raises to a value around 13.8 million people through the year 2060 including the advancement of medical developments to prevent, slowdown, or treatment of AD and thus reducing the risk of dementia. AD is a progressed neurodegenerative disease mainly accountable for around 60–80% of all dementia cases. In the current year (2021) for which the numbers have been reported and making the AD more prominent to dementia. In the year 2019 around 121,499 death rates were documented to AD which is subsequent toward dementia.

In the United States, "it is the sixth principal cause of death as reported in the United States which is covering the fifth principal cause for death and it is observed particularly with patients those who are in the stage of 65 years and

Nanomedicine-Based Approaches for the Treatment of Dementia. https://doi.org/10.1016/B978-0-12-824331-2.00007-8
Copyright © 2023 Elsevier Inc. All rights reserved.

elders." In between the year 2000 to the year of 2019, the numerous deaths from heart disease, stroke as well as HIV discovered to be reduced, whereas the reported deaths from AD contributing to dementia were found to be amplified further around 45%. The current COVID-19 pandemic situation in the year 2020 strengthens the rate of deaths from AD proceeding to dementia. In addition, the number adjacent to 11 million households besides other voluntary governesses specified a value of 15.3 billion hours of support and care to the peoples who are misery with AD or additional dementias in 2020 [3].

The brain is the composite organ of the body. It is composed of blood–brain barrier (BBB) Which controls the entry of drugs across the membrane and serves as a guard in the brain. Large molecular weight drugs, hydrophilic drugs cannot cross the BBB. Most 100% of molecules which are larger cannot enter the BBB and the 98% of molecules smaller in size cannot pass easily through the BBB. It does not allow the entry of proteins because the proteins are damaging to the nerve tissues and cause apoptosis. Plasma proteins such as albumin, prothrombin, plasminogen, etc. Their concentration in plasma is higher than the cerebrospinal fluid. This barrier protects the brain from neurotoxins which may be endogenous metabolites of drugs or some supplementary substances which are ingested in the diet [4].

1.2 Dementia

Dementia is neurodegenerative disarray as in this the nerve cells (neurons) mainly get affected and damaged. This leads to loss of neuronal signaling between the nerve cells and creates difficulty in the performance of the daily task, normal routine activities, and functioning of the body. Dementia is a disorder which gets worsens with time and the problem rises more and more as damage to neurons is triggered. The signs and symptoms of dementia are depending on the fact that which part of the brain is mainly affected, if the frontal lobe is affected it will create a problem with the judgment capabilities, intellectual ability of a person, and behavioral changes can occur. If the portion of the temporal lobe of the brain is being affected then it results in memory degeneration. If the parietal lobe gets affected it will distress the language of a person [5,6].

Dementia is chronic, incurable but in some cases, it is reversible such as psychometric disorders, folate deficiency, hypothyroidism, an unpleasant state of mind, abnormal metabolic activities are responsible for such conditions. Dementia is an illness that is characterized by cognitive impairment which leads to disturbance in functions like memory, orientation, language, learning capability but the conscious is not affected in this disease [5,6]. Dementia is the result of rather an interruption to nerve cells primes to improper functioning of the brain, death of brain cells. Symptoms of dementia depend on the location and severity of the damage. Dementia is classified as young-onset before the age of 65 and late-onset which occurs after the age of 65 years. There are several conditions that source to dementia as the main cause of dementia in older people is AD which is responsible for almost 60–70% of all cases and cerebrovascular diseases account for almost 15–20%. In adult's frontotemporal dementia mainly occurs, in this type of dementia the frontal and temporal lobes become shrink and leads to alteration in behavior and problems with language but the memory remains intact. The other causes of dementia are Huntington's disease (HD), Parkinson's disease (PD), Creutzfeldt–Jakob disease is also a cause of progressive dementia. Cerebral contusions in the tissue of the brain can also lead to the loss of cognitive functions which will be another reason for the cause of dementia. Other causes of dementia furthermost to neurodegenerative disorders, which consequences in the polymerization of proteins or mutation in the gene. Alcohol consumption, multiple sclerosis, hypothyroidism, Wilson's disease are correspondingly leading to dementia. There are approximately more than 55 illnesses that are accountable for dementia [5-7].

1.3 Etiology intended for dementia

- Alzheimer's disease (AD)
- Cerebrovascular disease
- Huntington's disease (HD)
- Parkinson's disease (PD)
- Creutzfeldt–Jakob disease (CJD)
- Cerebral contusion
- Hippocampal sclerosis (HS)
- Lewy bodies
- Miscellaneous: alcohol consumption, multiple sclerosis, hypothyroidism, Wilson's disease, etc.

1.3.1 Alzheimer's disease

The worldwide incidence of dementia has been reported approximately across "45 million" people. AD stands as the most popular reason intended for dementia, which is responsible for 60–80% of all dementia instances [8]. AD remains a proceeded neurodegenerative disorder that primarily leads to spare one-half of entirely dementia belongings. The AD is clinically acknowledged with an indication of loss of memory functions and other minor symptoms include cognitive deterioration, poor judgment, distress in decision making, language disorders, temporal loss and it has been correspondingly linked with mood disorders.

AD is escalating relentless neurologic disorder and it is the main cause of dementia and the reason behind the AD is the deposition of abnormal protein in the brain. Amyloid beta (Aβ) is the protein that has 36–43 amino acids in it and this is the main element of the plaques in people with this disease. This mainly occurs in the elderly distinguish between normal aging and AD is usually difficult. In some cases, AD is often misguided as some other mental diseases [8,9].

1.3.2 Cerebrovascular disease

It is mainly consequences when the supply of blood to the brain is affected and this is also a reason to loss of memory and cognitive impairment mainly in elderly patients, which is the main reason for dementia with cerebrovascular disease. The cerebrovascular disease mainly observed in patients who are suffering from AD [10].

1.3.3 Huntington's disease

It is a type of neurological disorder that results in involuntary moments, the escalating loss of memory, and psychological disorders. Loss of memory and impairment in daily activity is the first feature that is seen in this disease. Hence this disease is also contributing to dementia [11,12].

1.3.4 Parkinson's disease

PD results in the damage of nerve cells (neurons) and there is a decrease in the level of dopamine in the brain. The exact cause of this disease is not known but genes and several environmental factors can lead to PD and can cause tremor, slurred speech, rigidity in muscles. Lewy bodies are an important factor when we talk about Parkinson-induced dementia. In this, there is an abnormal deposition of protein which initiates the changes in the brain such as memory loss, cognitive impairment, behavioral and thinking problems [13].

1.3.5 Creutzfeldt–Jakob disease

It is a fatal disease mainly a person can die within the 1 year of onset of the disease. The reason behind this disease is the infection caused by a prion. There is a deposition of prion protein in the brain. This can result in loss of memory, abnormal activities in daily functioning, and results in neuronal damage [14,15].

1.3.6 Cerebral contusion

It is another reason behind dementia as there is damage in the tissues in the cerebrum which is permanent that will increase the amount of anomalous protein in the brain which is responsible for causing AD which will ultimately lead to loss of memory [16].

The rate of dementia depends on various factors:

- Genetic effects
- Age
- Physical activity
- Comorbidity
- Drugs

1.4 Genetic effects

It has a relation with dementia as they can increase the APOE (apolipoprotein-E) gene and this gene is responsible for AD which results in the development of dementia [17].

1.5 Age

It is the major responsible factor for causing dementia as age increases the chances of neuronal damage increase as the various diseases related to the brain which cause degeneration of the brain and this degeneration will lead to cognitive impairment causing dementia [17].

1.6 Physical activity

As we know that a person who has a sedentary lifestyle is more prone to diseases be it any disorder or diseases so physical activities always have a beneficial impact on a person's lifestyle there will be the improvement in cognitive function and the risk of dementia is lower in people those who follow a healthy lifestyle and involve in physical activities [17]

1.7 Comorbidity

As we already discussed the diseases which cause dementia. Hence, we can say that comorbidities can have a great effect on dementia even they can worsen the condition [17].

1.8 Drugs

There are several drugs available in the market and these drugs can cause dementia. Drugs such as benzodiazepines, statins, anti-Parkinson's drugs can lead to dementia[18]. Dementia has a great impact on a person's physical illness and social life. As when we talk about the physical illness, people with dementia will usually suffer a disturbance in their normal routine activities as sleep disturbance, loss of appetite, their attention toward their care is decreased, weight loss thus we can say that people who are suffering from dementia they have to increase the chance of physical illness [18].

Social behavior is also affected due to dementia as difficulty in doing normal activities can bring a person's confidence down thus the person will become socially less active [18]. People with dementia have shown difficulty in managing personal care this can be a severe cause of comorbid conditions as they lose personal care there will be poor hygiene such as poor oral hygiene which is responsible for conditions such as malnutrition [18].

1.9 Psychometric symptoms

These are major types of symptoms in people with dementia this can lead to suicidal thoughts, withdrawal of treatment, mercy killing the chances of depression and delirium increase, and ultimately a person loses the hope to live [19].

- *Apathy*: A behavioral and psychological change that is occurred because of dementia in this lack of enthusiasm. A person loses interest in daily activities [19].
- *Agitation*: It is a type of aggression that can occur in people with dementia as they become irritated with their lifestyle [19].
- *Depression*: It is another symptom that can be observed in people with dementia, it cannot be diagnosed accurately because the memory functions got impaired [19]. In this way, all we can say is dementia has a great impact on a person's life. People with dementia are prone to certain diseases, comorbidities, suicidal thoughts, psychometric disorders, and all of such leads to a physical, social, and economic imbalance in life [19].

1.10 Pathophysiology of neurodegenerative disorder; AD

1.10.1 Amyloid beta peptide

The fabrication of Aβ peptides is mainly responsible for AD, these amyloid plaques are localized extracellular (Fig. 1.1) and as the Aβ production has been enhanced whereas their clearance rate is reduced, it starts to deposit in the brain region involving the orbitofrontal cortex and later developed to the region of the neocortex, hippocampus, basal ganglia, diencephalon as well as amygdala of the brain. The amyloid precursor proteins (APPs) are cleaved by either β-secretase or γ-secretase, resulting in the generation of Aβ peptides, which consequences in the notorious insoluble Aβ fibrils. The APP that has been processed by the

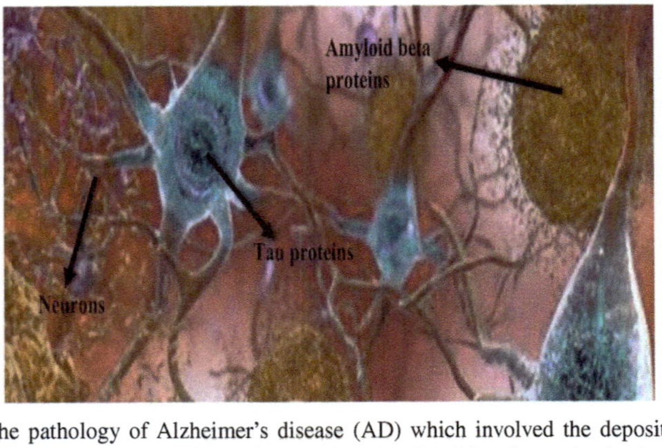

FIG. 1.1 The pathology of Alzheimer's disease (AD) which involved the deposition of "neurofibrillary tangles (NFT)" comprised of hyperphosphorylated "tau" proteins in the neurons and extracellular accumulation of amyloid beta (Aβ) plaques.

α-secretase result in the formation of soluble β-amyloid peptides in the healthy adult, which plays a direct role in neuronal plasticity or its survival, which is found to be protective against excitotoxicity, also it is very significant for the primary development of the central nervous system (CNS). It has been revealed to be vital to uphold synapse formation and transmitting neuronal signals [20].

The amyloid plaques (Aβ) encompass the formation and accumulation of misfolded Aβ tabloids extracellularly. These Aβ tabloid sheets composed of 40–42 amino acids in its misfolded Aβ sheets (Aβ40 and Aβ42). These two Aβ40 and Aβ42 are the main types of Aβ peptides that play a straight, significant role in the pathology of AD. The Aβ40 or Aβ42 sheets then oligomerize, and it relocated to the synaptic clefts, which also hinders the neuronal signaling in the synaptic cleft. These Aβ-peptide sheets further oligomerize toward insoluble Aβ fibrils and these result in the formation of aggregates of Aβ plaques [21,22]. The Aβ40 and Aβ42 responsible for the aggregation of these Aβ peptides and consequently it is central to the development of disorientated plaques. Aβ40 and Aβ42 are two main by-product metabolites of APP. The Aβ42 form is more toxic isoforms of the Aβ finding compared to the Aβ40 isoform.

The existence of Aβ42 in the cerebrospinal fluid certifies the incidence of AD in its preclinical stage, so the Aβ42 peptide is considered to be one of the most frequently accepted biomarkers of AD, which confirm AD over additional neurodegenerative disorders. It is found that the concentration of Aβ40 is 10 times higher than Aβ42 in CSF [23]. The Aβ42 and Aβ40 proportion is generally used as its ratio remains comparable throughout the disease, the ratio of Aβ42:Aβ40 is a potential biomarker in the development of AD, which specifies the Aβ accumulation, fibrillogenesis, and neurotoxicity, as it is consequential to cause dementia. The APP gene is positioned over 21q21 was revealed to be the first contributing gene for AD. The developments in the genetic investigation have been recognized into two different types of ADs which include:

1. "Familial Alzheimer's disease" (FAD)
2. "Sporadic Alzheimer's disease" (SAD)

The significant developments in the year of 1990s and early year of 2000s, it is discovered that the "familial Alzheimer's disease" (FAD) is the consequence of the mutations of autosomal dominant genes in the APP (Fig. 1.2), PSEN-1, and PSEN-2, these are correspondingly positioned over 1, 14, and 21 of chromosomes [24,25]. The genes PSEN-1 and PSEN-2 containing an essential amino acid that breaks the active site through which it catalyzes the γ-secretase enzyme. These alterations triggered to the APP, PSEN-1, and PSEN-2 genes lead to increased production of Aβ peptides that indicate the process of neurodegeneration. The risk involved in the genetic factors for "sporadic Alzheimer's disease" (SAD) was recognized as APOE gene which is a type e4 allele on chromosome number-19 and it is a transporter of "low-density lipoproteins". In AD, the gene APOE exists around 50–60% in all cases of AD suffering patients. Whereas the gene APOE in a healthy adult is contributing about only 20–30% as compared to that of AD patients [8,25].

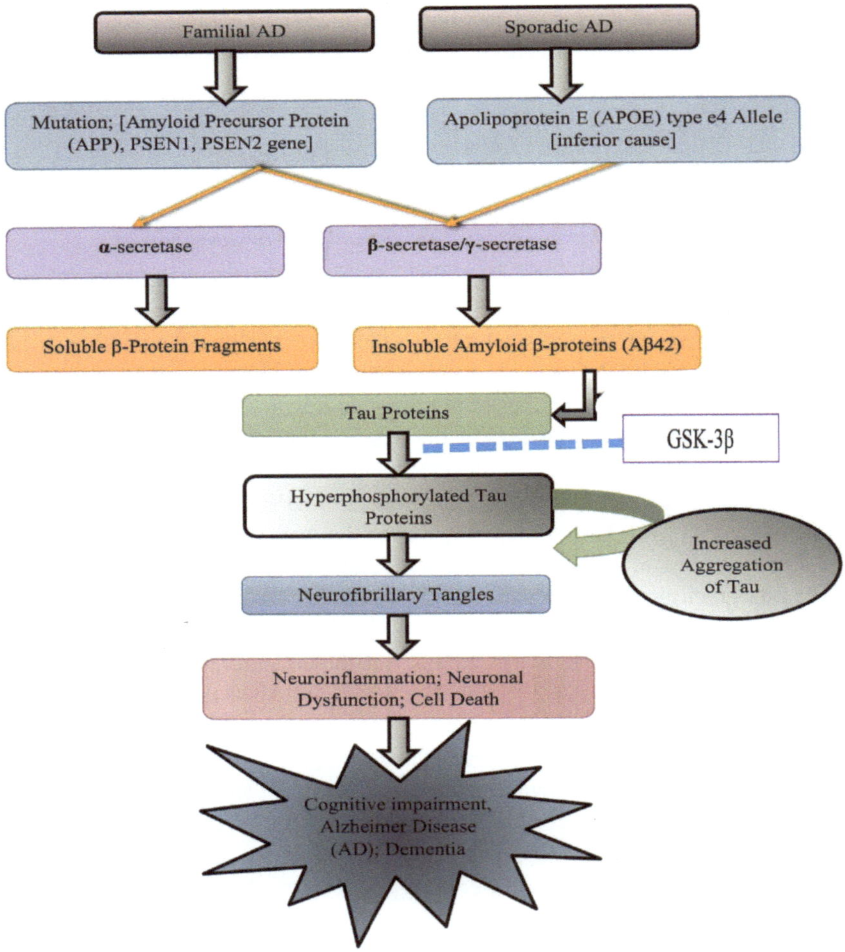

FIG. 1.2 The amyloid beta (Aβ) cascade; tau proteins hypothesis; AD; leading to dementia.

The following genes have been reported to be involved in the pathogenesis of AD [22]

1. Amyloid precursor protein (APP)
2. Complement receptor-1 (CR-1)
3. Apolipoprotein-E (APOE)
4. PSEN-1/PSEN-2 gene
5. Presenile genes
6. Phospholipids linked with clathrin protein
7. Sterol O-acetyltransferase
8. Prostaglandins endoperoxide synthase-2

9. SLC26A38 gene
10. Angiotensin-converting enzyme (ACE)

1.10.2 Tau proteins

The accumulation of these Aβ peptides stimulates the development of "neurofibrillary tangles" (NFT). These NFT principally involved the hyperphosphorylated tau protein. The accumulation of these hyperphosphorylated tau proteins is also a prominent marker for AD protruding toward dementia. In the normal brain, the "three microtubule associated proteins" (MAPs) that are MAP-Tau, MAP1A-Tau/MAP1B-Tau, and MAP2-Tau accomplish the analogous functions, that is, the advancement of microtubule assembly and the stabilization of microtubule. These three MAPs are originating in the normal matured neuron. The biological activity of tau which involved in the promoting assembly and stabilization of microtubules primarily in a neuronal protein is regulated by three main features which are turn out to be decreased by the hyperphosphorylation of tau proteins [26-28]. These are:

- The process of hyperphosphorylation
- Stabilization of microtubule assembly
- Its binding competency to the microtubules

In the normal brain, tau protein (N-Tau) is composed of six proteins and it is resulting from complementary mRNA splicing from a single gene [29,30]. These proteins contrast from tubulin-binding domains whether they comprise three tubulin-binding domains (τ3L, τ3S, or τ3) or four tubulin-binding domains, that is (τ4L, τ4S/τ4) supplements of 31/32 amino acids, respectively. These are located close to the "C" terminal and in each N-terminal portion of the molecule as "the two: τ3L, τ4L, one; τ3S, τ4S, or no; τ3, τ4 supplements of 29 amino acids each." The 1 and 2 amino-terminal supplements have been coded by exon-2 as well as exon-3 correspondingly [28]. In the case of AD and some of the interrelated disorders, it also called tauopathies. The "abnormal tau hyperphosphorylation" leads to its deposition in the exaggerated neurons in AD and the aggregation of strangely hyperphosphorylated "tau" proteins is accompanying with the neurodegeneration and which is the principal cause of dementia. The hyperphosphorylation of tau proteins be situated in the NFT but then again also instigate in the cytosol from the AD brain [29].

The MAP is the major part of tau proteins of well-developed, matured neurons. The MAP-1 and MAP-2 are the two additional neuronal types of MAPs. The MAP functions to interact with tubulin binding, the advancement in the association with microtubule assembly in addition to the stabilization of microtubule. The aberrant hyperphosphorylation of tau proteins in AD cytosol counteracts the binding to tubulin and does not endorse microtubule assembly as well as interrupts the microtubule functioning instead of its binding to the microtubule [31]. The activity of the tau recommends to the microtubule assembly, is controlled via its degree of hyperphosphorylation process.

The normal brain of a human comprises around 2–3 moles of tau proteins and the progression of hyperphosphorylation of tau proteins reduces its biological activity. As compared to the normal brain with AD brain there are about three to fourfolds of supplementary hyperphosphorylated tau than the normal adult brain tau. Further, these tau proteins oligomerize toward Paired Helical Fragment (PHF), which are combined through the Straight Filament (SF) in this hyperphosphorylated state which produces the "NFT" [32]. The uncharacteristic hyperphosphorylation of tau protein (AD P-Tau) in the cytosol yields sedimentable, oligomeric tau proteins, and it is the reason aimed at neurodegeneration by disturbing the microtubules network and requisitioning the normal MAPs [33].

In frontotemporal dementia, the tau mutations are found to produce neurodegeneration over promoting uncharacteristic hyperphosphorylation of tau. The AD P-Tau accumulates into PHF through the SF, establishing NFT. The neurodegeneration of AD P-Tau protein is not only occurring in AD rain but it also seen in other neurodegenerative diseases, for example, frontotemporal dementia through parkinsonism which is associated with chromosome 17, that is (FTDP-17) (Fig. 1.3) provoked by the mutation toward tau, and other reasons may comprise as pick disease, dementia pugilistica, corticobasal degeneration, and the progressive supranuclear palsy [32,34].

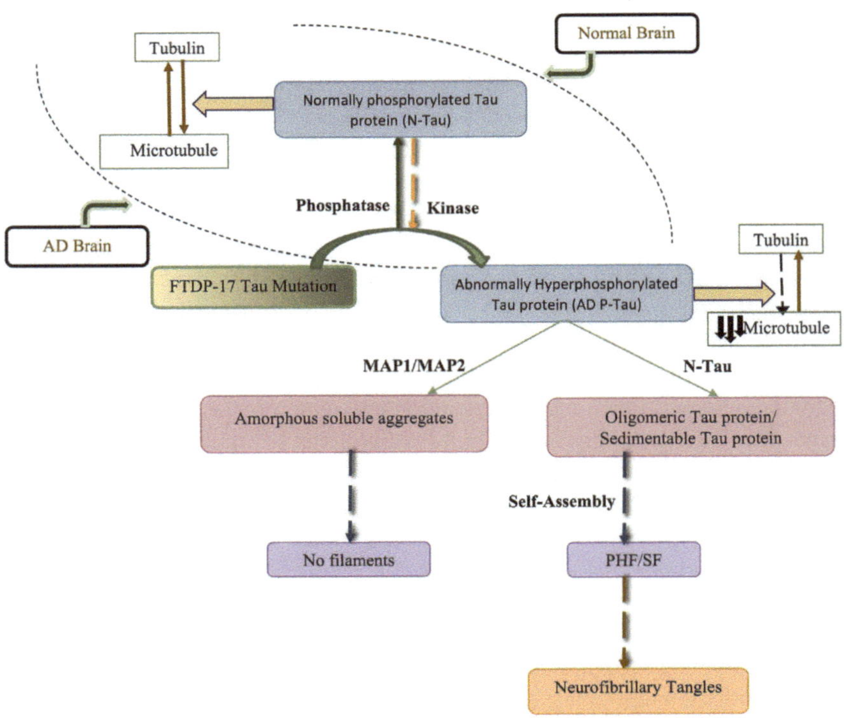

FIG. 1.3 Tauopathies from the normal brain tau and abnormal brain tau.

In the normal brain, the tau proteins in NFT are frequently called ghost tangles, which is known to be ubiquitinated, that is, it has ubiquitin reactivity, however, in AD brain the abnormally hyperphosphorylated tau proteins (AD P-Tau) collected from AD brain cytosol was originate which do not have ubiquitin reactivity. These overall studies recommend that the AD P-Tau proteins prime to its accumulation into NFT [28].

1.10.3 Heat shock protein

The pathological accumulation of abnormal proteins is linked to the alteration in mitochondrial dysfunction and the redox state homeostasis. It is discovered to be the emerging cause of neuronal dysfunction and the cellular death prominent to dementia. The heat shock protein (HSP) is also identified as heat stress protein. These are the intracellular molecules that protect the biological tissue from damage. These proteins enhance the production of cytokines and by the receptor-mediated interface, it gives signals toward the antigen-presenting cell [35]. The HSPs are mostly formed when these proteins are exposed to high temperatures normally higher than the required temperature for the normal development of proteins. The HSPs are also melded by additional reasons which comprise oxidation, external stress, a revelation to toxins, free radicles, and heavy metals, etc. The accumulation of unfolded proteins in the brain results in dementia which is monitored by neuronal dysfunction, neurodegeneration which is associated with diseases like AD, PD, HD, multiple sclerosis, etc.

Chaperone distinguishes the tau proteins which deal with the HSP70/HSP40 complex initially, then after it forms the transitional composite with HSP90 and HSP70-HSP90 establishing protein (HSP) [36]. Subsequently for the development of AD and additional inter-related neurodegenerative disorders the chaperone is also a targeted therapeutic approach because it regulates the stability of tau proteins. The tau proteins promote the assembly and stabilize the microtubules. The levels of the disease-associated tau get reduced intracellularly by the inhibition of the HSP90 adenosine triphosphatase (ATPase) and HSP70's ATPase. Over the elderly patients, the HSP gene forms polymerization owing to an autoimmune disorder, inflammatory response, neurodegenerative diseases, cardiovascular diseases. When these HSPs are exposed to some mechanical stress it becomes activated, which complementarily binds to DNA, so therefore these proteins are also named as "heat shock elements."

1.11 Pathogenesis of Parkinson's disease

PD is primarily characterized by the following rationalizes which subsidize the prominent cause of dementia that involves:

- The progressive degeneration and loss of dopaminergic neurons
- Lewy bodies and aggregation of α-synuclein
- Neuroinflammation

The disease is principally accompanied by the deficiency of striatal dopaminergic neurons (DA) and consequent neuronal loss in the region of substantia nigra pars compacta, which is located in the midbrain. It is the main hallmark of PD, which is a leading cause of dementia.

The PD is contributing around 50–60% cause of all dementia, comprises the symptoms of PD such as mental dysfunction, dyskinesia, memory impairment, poor judgments, etc. Dopamine is a chemical neurotransmitter that transports the signals from one neuronal cell to another nerve cell through the synapse. When it travels to the synapse, it gets metabolize by two enzymes, COMT (catechol-O-methyl transferase) and MAO (monoamine oxidase). The use of MAO inhibitor or COMPT inhibitor is a suitable approach for preventing neuronal destruction from metabolism in PD.

The mitochondrial dysfunction representing the pathogenesis of PD is accompanying by the destruction of dopaminergic neurons in response to neurotoxic 6-hydroxydopamine, that is, it having the chemical structure of "1-methyl-4-phenyl-1,2,3,6-tetrahydropyridine (MPTP)." The neurotoxic "MPTP" gene is responsible for the process disturbance in the degeneration of tyrosine hydroxylase positive (TH+) dopaminergic neurons and it acts as a precursor for the synthesis of levodopa which converts to dopamine [37]. The MPTP triggers the progressive destructions and centrals to death of dopaminergic neurons involved in the region of "substantia nigra pars compacta" and it further decreases the mitochondrial complex-1 neuronal activity. The degradation of dopaminergic neurons in the substantia nigra, supplementarily leads to alterations in the pathway of basal ganglia, which centrals to further alterations in the neurotransmitter activity of GABA, glutamate, and serotonin release.

PD is largely associated with "Lewy bodies," which comprises insoluble α-synuclein aggregates. The deposition of α-synuclein restraints the stimulation of microglia and further centrals to neuroinflammation accelerates the progressive neurodegeneration of dopaminergic neurons in the brain. The process of neuroinflammation produces significant changes in microglia which impair the process of α-synuclein degradation and its uptake from the extracellular cell [38]. The inflammation mediated by immune response is showed to be a significant attribute for the degradation of the dopaminergic neuron. In several studies, it is found that neuroinflammation may also subsidize the aggregation of α-synuclein [39]. This neuroinflammation associated with PD has been demonstrated by several epidemiological studies. Other genetic factors may also contribute to the PD which involves a mutation to the glucocerebrosidase gene principals to "Gaucher's disease." It is accompanying by an autosomal recessive disorder.

1.12 Pathogenesis of vascular dementia

Vascular dementia (VaD) is also the prevalent cause of cognitive impairment indicating around 8–15% of all dementia cases. It is triggered due to vascular lesions or vascular ischemia in the neuronal area of the brain [40]. These produce a discrepancy in the cortical and frontal area of the brain with meddlesome basal ganglia cortical, and in ascending pathways by producing lesions in the subfrontal area, thalamus, white matter, and basal ganglia which affects the memory, cognition, and behavioral functions. The irregularities in the neurotransmitter pathways in the cholinergic system of basal ganglia diffuse the white matter lesions and other vascular lesions that are tangled in the central radiation field of the projection pathway. The dysfunction in this cholinergic pathway might reduce the cerebral blood flow and hypoperfusion which is a major cause of VaD. The Lesions involving in the striatonigral dopaminergic system owing to lacunar infarctions in the white matter and basal ganglia might give rise to "Lewy bodies" and VaD.

1.13 Pathogenesis of Huntington's disease

HD is a genetic disorder, which is an "autosomal dominant disease." It is clinically characterized by psychotic disorders, progressive dementia, behavioral and kinetic disorders, leading to neurodegeneration, atrophy, neuronal loss. HD is triggered by a trinucleotide (CAG), CAG is the codon for glutamine. The repeated extension in the huntingtin (HTT) gene that initiates an elongated polyglutamine recurrence in the huntingtin protein. The abnormal extension of the CAG on the HTT gene results in monogenic, autosomal dominant, a neurodegenerative disorder such as HD [41,42]. The extension in this CAG primes to cognitive impairment. Most of the studies also recommend that along with CAG repeated extension other factors also contribute to the neuropathological variations which are accountable for cognitive impairment, such as environmental factors and genetic variables. The defect in a single gene called HTT assembles to HD which further elucidations for a neurodegenerative disorder resulting in dementia. Several studies suggest that the genetic variability on chromosome-15 which is responsible for the age factor also contributes to motor functioning and cognitive dysfunction [43,44].

The HD contributes to the several pathways that lead to cell death, which include a deficiency of the "brain-derived neurotrophic factor" (BDNF) [45]. These BDNF in HD is reduced, which grounds neuronal cell death. Also, several neurodegenerative cell deaths were found in arrears to oxidative stress. Several studies strongly suggest that oxidative stress mainly contributing to HD which initiates neuronal cell deaths directing to dementia. HD affects basal ganglia which involve the whole brain. In the preliminary stage of HD, it is found that the volume of gray matter decreases, and also there is a reduction in the brain metabolism processes, and cortical thinning was observed which resembles the neuronal dysfunction [43,46].

1.14 Treatment of neurodegenerative disorders

1.14.1 Alzheimer's disease

A. Cholinesterase inhibitor: Donepezil, galantamine, and rivastigmine
B. NMDA blocker: Memantine
C. Combination therapy

A. *Cholinesterase inhibitor*: Donepezil, galantamine, and rivastigmine are the drugs that can be used for the treatment of dementia. This drug can inhibit acetylcholinesterase. This drug should be given when AD is diagnosed and taking into account the history of the patient. When we talk about dosing frequency it should be like

- **Donepezil**: the initial treatment begins with 5 mg QD (once a day) if permits then it can increase up to 10 mg BD (twice a day).
- **Galantamine**: The initial treatment begins with 4 mg BD (twice a day) if permits after a month we can go for 8 mg BD. The maximum dose can be 12 mg BD.
- **Rivastigmine**: The initial treatment begins with 1.5 mg BD if permits increase up to 3 mg within 15 days. The maximum dose which can be tolerated is 12 mg BD.

Treatment should be discontinued if the patient does not respond to therapy as the diseases are incurable so this medication cannot be a cure as well as they cannot work for everyone.

B. *NMDA blocker*: N-methyl-D-aspartate receptor is a glutamate receptor. Memantine is the NMDA antagonist drug that results in decreasing the deterioration of cognitive impairments. The dose of the drug started with 5 mg QD it can be increased up to 10 mg BD. When cholinesterase inhibitors are no longer effective memantine is used [19].

C. *Combination therapy*: When we use a combination of NMDA blocker and cholinesterase inhibitor the combination was well tolerated and effective such as donepezil and memantine combination was found to be effective in treating neurological symptoms and are responsible for increasing the awareness toward daily life activities [19].

1.14.2 Parkinson's disease

A. Dopamine precursor—levodopa
B. Dopamine agonist—bromocriptine, pramipexole
C. DOPA decarboxylase inhibitor—benserazide, carbidopa
D. MAO inhibitors—selegiline, rasagiline
E. COMT inhibitor—tolcapone, entacapone
F. NMDA receptor antagonist—amantadine
G. Anticholinergics—biperiden, benzhexol
H. Antihistamines—orphenadrine, promethazine

A. *Dopamine precursor*: Levodopa can be regarded as the first line of treatment for PD. It is the finest among all other treatments and better than other categories in improving motor functions. The dose of levodopa is 300–400 mg on daily basis. We can elevate the dose up to 600 mg [47,48].

B. *Dopamine agonist*: This can help in improving the symptoms such as the involuntary moment of the body. Pramipexole can bind with the dopamine receptor subtype it does not have any affinity toward the other adrenergic and serotonin receptor. Bromocriptine is an ergot derivative it has an impact on the D2 subtype as well as on the serotonin receptor [47,48].

C. *DOPA decarboxylase inhibitor*: Benserazide and carbidopa are the drugs that can produce dopamine via levodopa as they are given in combination with levodopa and increase the level of dopamine by increasing the efficiency of treatment [47,48].

D. *MAO inhibitors*: Rasagiline and selegiline are monoamine oxidase inhibitor they can help in reducing the symptoms and improving the motor functions given in combination with levodopa. Selegiline can selectively inhibit the MAO B and its action cannot be reversed [47,48].

E. *COMT inhibitors*: Tolcapone and entacapone are catechol O methyl transferase inhibitors. They are given in combination with levodopa and DOPA decarboxylase inhibitor whereas all drugs which come under this category have a short half-life [47,48].

F. *NMDA antagonist*: Amantadine can increase the level of dopamine in the brain but they are not as great as levodopa in terms of efficacy. It helps in improving motor functions [47,48].

G. *Anticholinergics*: This drug can help in reducing the symptoms of tremor and benefits in the symptoms of excessive saliva secretion which occurred during this disease but they are less effective when compared to levodopa [47,48].

H. *Antihistamines*: This drug acts on the H1 receptor and has a similar action to that of anticholinergics but they are not as efficient as them but helps in providing relief in the symptoms of the disease [47,48].

This is therapies and treatment which are used for PD and helps in easing the condition.

1.14.3 Huntington's disease

- *Tetrabenazine*: This drug can reduce and give relief in involuntary movements that are caused by this disease. This drug is the drug that was initially permitted by the FDA for the treatment of this disease [49,50].
- *Antipsychotic drugs*: Drugs such as risperidone, haloperidol, and chlorpromazine are used to lessen the effect of chorea caused by this disease. These drugs can also help in providing relief in psychological symptoms which are caused by this disease [51].
- *Benzodiazepines*: Drugs such as clonazepam and diazepam can help lessen the symptoms of chorea [52].

1.14.4 Creutzfeldt–Jakob disease

This is a rare type of neurodegenerative disorder there is no proper treatment for this disorder but only two drugs clonazepam and sodium valproate used as a palliative therapy [53].

1.14.5 New drug targets for dementia

- *Bapineuzumab*: It is the monoclonal antibody which attached with Aβ and reduces the amount of plaque this will ultimately lead to the betterment of cognitive functions in animal models but it has shown no benefit in phase 3 trials [54].
- *Crenezumab, gantenerumab, solanezumab*: These three are also under their research phase for reducing the amount of beta-amyloid plaque.
- *Anavex 2-73*: It is an S1R (sigma-1 receptor) activator it can decrease oxidative stress, mitochondrial dysfunction, and most importantly it can inhibit the tau hyperphosphorylation, it is under its phase 3 trial for the treatment of AD [54].

1.14.6 Miscellaneous treatment

- *Ginkgo biloba*: This can be used in the treatment of dementia but less effective than cholinesterase inhibitors [19].
- *Vitamin E*: This can help in improving brain functioning in AD but no specific evidence is formed.
- *Selegiline*: This can improve the daily functioning of the brain and helps in easing the cognitive impairment (Table 1.1).

1.15 Blood–brain barrier

The BBB is a restrictive barrier that creates complications for entry of the drug into the brain parenchyma. By considering the anatomical as well as functional sites of the BBB, it is composed of the endothelium cells, capillary endothelial cells, extracellular base-membrane, contiguous pericytes, astrocytes, and microglia cells and it is surrounded by the neurons [77]. The BBB involves the junction of tight epithelial cells. This junction is formed among the cerebral endothelial cells, the choroid plexus, and the arachnoid epithelial cells. These tight junctions (TJs) in the BBB prevent the entry of high molecular weight, polar solutes into the brain [78]. The delivery of drugs to the brain across BBB is very challenging due to its complex structure. The BBB is an immense obstacle in the delivery of drugs for pampering neurological disorders such as AD and other neurological disorders accompanying dementia.

The BBB is highly constrained for the transport of macromolecules or highly polar drugs transversely to the BBB into the brain surrounded by specialized

TABLE 1.1 Drugs used for the treatment of various neurological disorders.

Drug	Brand name	Manu-facturer	Dose	Side effects	Refer-ences
Alzheimer's disease					
Ache's inhibitors					
Donepezil	Concept	Cipla	5 mg and 10 mg oral	Diarrhea, loss of appetite, muscle cramp	[55]
	Donepezil	Ranbaxy	5 mg oral	Insomnia, vomiting, muscle cramps	[55]
Galantamine	Galamer	Sun Pharma	4 mg oral	Drowsiness, shakiness, weakness	[56]
	Razadyne	Janssen	4 mg oral	Weight loss, drowsiness	[56]
Rivastigmine	Rivadem	Torrent Pharma	1.5 mg oral	Indigestion, weakness	[57]
	Rivamer	Sun Pharma	1.5 mg oral	Upset stomach, dizziness	[57]
NMDA antagonist					
Memantine	Namenda XR	Merz Pharma-ceuticals	5 mg oral	Tired feeling, weight loss, or gain	[58]
Parkinson's disease					
Dopamine precursor and DOPA decarboxylase inhibitor					
Carbidopa, levodopa, and combination	Sinemet	Merk Pharma-ceuticals	25 mg of carbidopa and 100 mg of levodopa oral	Delusions, hallucinations, or fits	[59]
Dopamine agonist					
Bromocrip-tine	Parlodel	Novartis	5 mg oral	Low blood pressure, dizziness	[60]
Pramipexole	Mirapex	Boehringer Ingelheim Interna-tional GmbH	0.125 mg oral	Constipation, peripheral edema	[61]

Drug	Brand name	Manu-facturer	Dose	Side effects	Refer-ences
Ropinirole	Requip	GlaxoS-mithKline	2 mg oral	Swelling of legs, hands, or feet	[62]
MAO inhibitor					
Selegiline	EL-DEPRYL	Somerset Pharma-ceuticals	5 mg oral	Stomach pain, difficulty in swallowing	[63]
Rasagiline	Azilect	Teva Pharma-ceuticals	0.5 mg oral	Cough, peripheral edema	[64]
COMT inhibitor					
Entacapone	Comtan	Novartis	200 mg oral	Increased sweating, urine discolor-ation	[65]
NMDA receptor antagonist					
Amantadine	SYMME-TREL	Endo Pharma-ceuticals	200 mg oral	Orthostatic, hypotension, confusion, compulsive behavior	[66]
Huntington's disease					
Tetrabena-zine	Xenazine	Prestwick Pharma-ceuticals	12.5 mg oral	Depression, anxiety, insomnia	[67]
Risperidone	Risperdal	Janssen	0.5 mg oral	Restlessness, weight gain	[68]
Haloperidol	Haldol	Ortho-McNeil Pharma-ceutical, Inc.	5 mg (I.M. injection)	Increases prolactin level in the body, urinary reten-tion	[69]
Chlorproma-zine	Largactil	Sanofi-Aventis	10 mg oral	Agitation, imbalance	[70]
Clonazepam	KLONO-PIN	Genetch	0.5 mg oral	Altered walk-ing, memory impairment	[71]
Diazepam	Valium	Roche	10 mg oral	Memory prob-lems, ataxia	[72]

(Continued)

TABLE 1.1 Cont'd

Drug	Brand name	Manu-facturer	Dose	Side effects	Refer-ences
Tetrabena-zine	Xenazine	Reci-pharm Fontaine SAS	12.5 mg oral	Depression, anxiety, insomnia	[73]
Creutzfeldt–Jakob disease					
Sodium valproate	Epilim	Sanofi-Aventis	100 mg oral	Insomnia, weight gain, hair loss	[74]
Glioblastoma					
Temozolo-mide	Temodar	Merck Pharma-ceuticals	5 mg, 20 mg, 100 mg	Convulsions, pain, irrita-tion, itching	[75]
Bevaci-zumab	Avastin	Genetch south San Francisco	10 mg/kg (I.V.)	Vomiting, voice changes	[76]

endothelial cells. The transports of drugs into the brain are mediated by various cellular transport channels these comprise of:

- Amino acid transporters
- Nucleotide transporters
- Nucleoside transporter
- Glucose transporter-1 (GLUT-1)
- Monocarboxylate transporters (MCT-1 and MC-T2)
- Na+/K+ ATPase pumps (ion transporters)

1.16 Structure of blood–brain barrier

The BBB protects the functioning of the "CNS." This BBB is formed by specialized cells such as the astrocytes and pericytes play a significant role in the development of BBB. The BBB is comprised of blood vessels that are formed by specialized endothelial cells, astrocytes, pericytes, surrounded by the neurons [44].

The astrocytes lay down over the continuous basal lamina and act as a strong rigid preventive barrier [44,79]. In the formation of BBB, the neurons also contribute actively to form the BBB. The pericytes occupy the perivascular space which is sandwiched in between the capillary walls and at the end of astrocytes, the only exception includes is in the large vessels where the smooth muscle cells replace these cells [80]. The pericytes are the types of mesenchymal cells, and these pericyte cells play a significant regulatory role in the stability of BBB, in the process of angiogenesis, repair, and sustaining the vasculature tone. It also found to modify the function of astroglia cells and it forms a tough barrier which restricts the entry of drug into the cells.

1.17 Tight junction involved in BBB

The BBB involves the "TJ" and for the formation of TJ, the adherence junction (AJ) protein plays an important role, which is stabilized by α-cadherin, β-cadherin, and γ-cadherin proteins. These junctional complexes are formed in between the endothelial cells which include the AJs and the TJs. In the case of AJs, the cadherin proteins lengthen in the intercellular split is associated with the cells of cytoplasm through the framework of α-cadherin, β-cadherin, and γ-cadherin proteins [78,81]. The occurrence of these adherence proteins is responsible for holding the cells and it delivers structural support. The formation of the TJ is further dependent on these complex proteins such as "junctional adhesion molecules" (JAM), occludin in addition to claudin proteins. These occludin and claudin proteins are interconnected with a regulatory protein such as "Zonula Ocludence-1, Zonula Ocludence-2, Zonula Ocludence-3" proteins and also interconnected to a cingulin protein.

The claudin proteins are composed of about 1–20 isoforms. The TJ is mainly formed by three types of transmembrane proteins, these are claudin, occludin, and JAM [82]. The structure of claudin encompasses two extracellular loops and two intracytoplasmic ends and it has four transmembrane spinning regions [83]. The occluding is a four transmembrane protein sector. It contains two extracellular loops and three intracytoplasmic domains [84]. The JAM is composed of a single transmembrane domain and it also contains two bulky loops like immunoglobulins. The JAMs are also tangled in the functioning of monocyte extravasation [82,85].

1.18 Features of endothelial and specialized cells forming BBB

The peripheral endothelial cells contrast from the brain endothelial cells (Fig. 1.4). Whereas the brain endothelial cells are composed of "TJ," which restricts the passage of drugs across the BBB through paracellular transport mechanism as it produces high resistance due to the TJs as compared to the peripheral endothelial cells [86]. Comparatively the peripheral endothelial cells contain a greater number of endocytic vesicles as compared to the brain endothelial cells which restrict the transport of drugs through BBB by the transcellular flux mechanism [82]. The endothelial cells in the brains are very close to each other which forms the TJ further complex (Fig. 1.5).

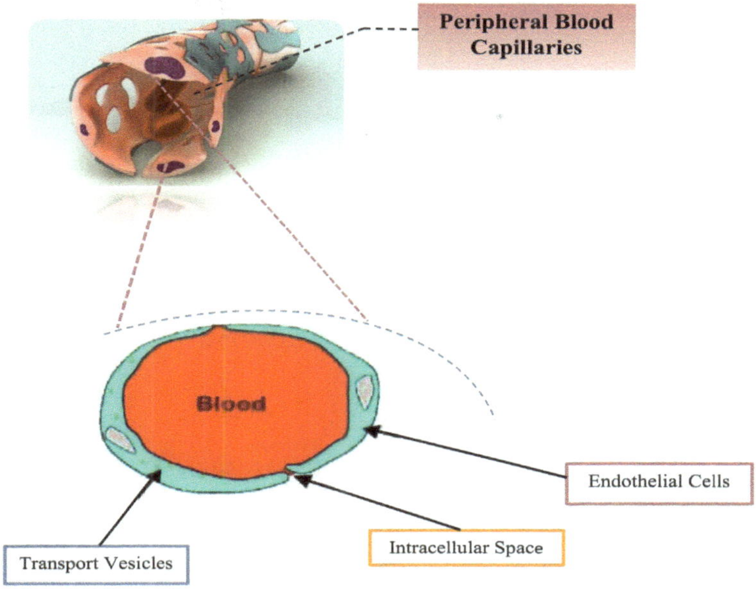

FIG. 1.4 The peripheral blood capillaries which are composed of continuous basal ganglia, endothelial cells containing larger number of transport endocytic vesicles.

The "BBB" primarily composed of four types of cells:

- Endothelial cells
- Pericytes
- Astrocytes
- Microglia

The brain endothelial cells are enveloped by basal ganglia which are produced by pericytes and the external matrix is organized by the collagens, glycoproteins, proteoglycans, laminins, and additional proteins. The astrocytes form a network-like structure around the brain endothelial cells which play a key role in the formation of BBB and it maintains the structure and stability of BBB [87].

The microglia cells facilitate the signaling and the transport of drugs through transcellular pathways. It also sustains the integrity of the BBB. The pericytes in the BBB support the development of endothelial cells [88]. The microglia are not considered as a part of BBB. They are situated just below the BBB. The microglial cells maintain the brain immune system as it can defend against the pathogens which invade the BBB. Some sort of mechanical injury, stroke, or inflammation disturbs the integrity of BBB; this affects the permeability of the dug by disturbing the basal ganglia and endothelial cells [86]. The inflammation contributes to the opening of the TJ to permit the transport of growth factors and antibodies into the brain.

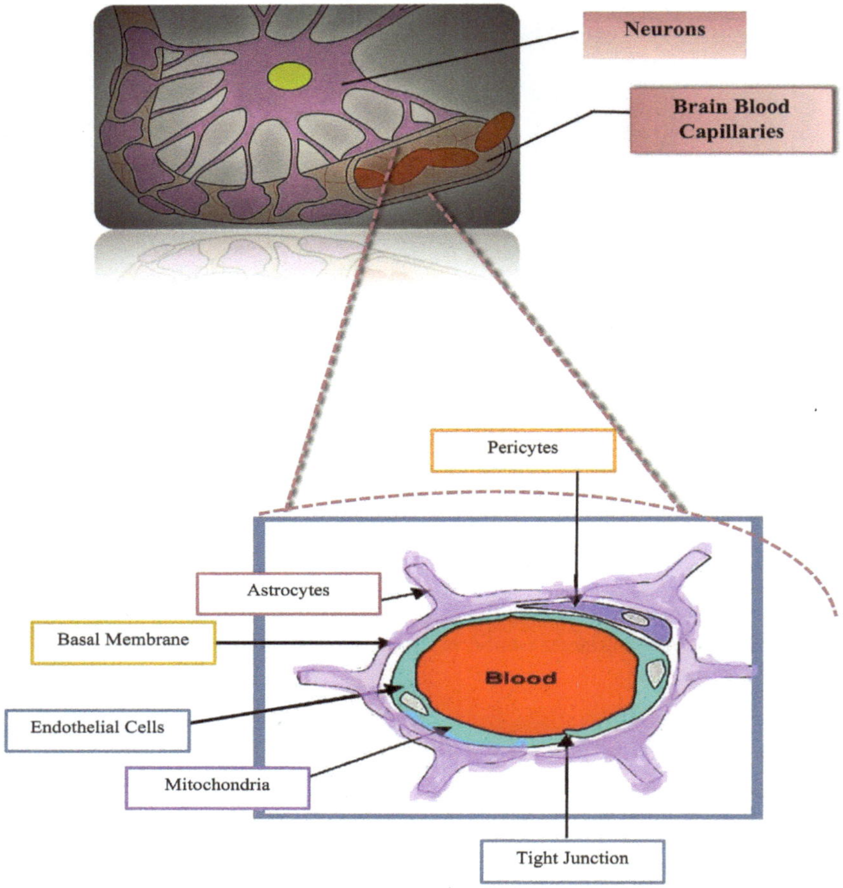

FIG. 1.5 **The blood–brain barrier (BBB) and the cellular components of BBB; which involve the "tight junction," specialized endothelial cells composed of pericytes, astrocytes, microglia, neurons, and endothelial cells containing lower number of transport endocytic vesicles.**

1.19 Mechanisms to permeate the blood–brain barrier

The BBB delivers protection to the CNS from invading the pathogens into the brain. The BBB is impermeable to microorganisms as compared to the peripheral cells. But some microbes can enter the CNS through the transcellular pathway in between the endothelial cells. Most of the ions and nutrients can cross the BBB through the paracellular pathway by the process of diffusion across the junctional endothelial cells. The proteins and hormones involve the transport across the brain endothelial cells by the mechanism of receptor-mediated transport (RMT). Some other transport pathways correspondingly contributing to the transport of drugs through the junctional pathway.

1.19.1 Transcellular pathway

The transcellular pathway involves the transport of drugs into the brain in between the endothelial cells, which is an energy-independent or energy-dependent process. The mechanism involved in this transport system may include ligand-mediated transport or adsorptive-mediated transport mechanism [82]. The ligand-mediated transport consists of the binding of the drug as a ligand to the endothelial cells which act as a receptor. Whereas the process of adsorptive-mediated transcytosis is based on the charge interaction between the drug and the surface of endothelial cells.

1.19.2 Paracellular pathway

The transport of drugs across the BBB includes the process of diffusion through the paracellular pathway. Most of the lipophilic and the low molecular weight solutes cross the BBB by this paracellular pathway. This pathway is more significant for the targeting of the therapeutic agents intended for the treatment of neurodegenerative disorders and with additional dementia, those drugs are having high lipophilicity, these are effectively transported across the BBB to treat neurodegenerative disorders and other dementias. This pathway is based upon the concentration-dependent gradient phenomenon [89]. The concentration gradient or electrochemical gradient drives the moment of the drug through the endothelial cells into the brain.

1.19.3 Clathrin-mediated endocytosis

The clathrin-mediated endocytosis is an important pathway in the transport of nutrients, the large molecular weight proteins, hormones, and most of the drugs for the treatment of neurodegenerative disorders which is an important strategy for the treatment of dementia [90]. In the clathrin-mediated endocytosis process, the drug molecules adsorb over the surface of endothelial cells where it having a high affinity for the receptors and there is a formation of vesicles that are coated by clathrin protein and into which the drug is embedded. These clathrin-coated vesicles form a complex with additional protein molecules such as dynamin, endophilin, amphiphysin [91].

These proteins initiate the movement of these coated vesicles into the cells. Once the clathrin-coated vesicles enter the cells then a coating of clathrin is released and these clathrin proteins further reach the surface for further uptake of other solute molecules into the brain. The clathrin-mediated endocytosis is a saturable process, due to its limited number of receptor proteins at the sight of the endothelial membrane [92]. As compared to other peripheral tissue, the number of clathrin-mediated receptors is huge in the brain. This clathrin-mediated endocytosis is also called receptor-mediated endocytosis or receptor-mediated transcytosis. The cell membrane carries the negative charge over the surface and the drugs which carry positive charge over it is a highly relevant strategy for transport of drug across the BBB by charge interaction through adsorptive-mediated transcytosis [93].

1.19.4 Carrier-mediated pathway

The transport of drugs by this pathway involves the brain parenchyma and systemic circulation. The brain endothelial cells are composed of several carrier transporters such as amino acid carrier transport. Depending upon the physicochemical characteristics of each amino acid the endothelial cells containing different types of carriers. The small, neutral amino acids are transported across the BBB by A-amino acid carrier transport, whereas bulky, neutral, and aromatic amino acid molecules are transported by N/L-type of amino acid carrier systems [82]. This pathway is likewise significant for treating the neurodegenerative diseases contributing to dementia, as many of the therapeutic agents are resulting from amino acids. This carrier-mediated pathway is limited as it is a saturable process when the number of carrier systems is limited in the brain endothelial cells [94].

1.19.5 Receptor-mediated transport

RMT is an extensively used, promising strategy over other transport systems to cross the BBB to treat dementia as one of the CNS disorders. The RMT primarily involves the transport of proteins such as transferrin and most of the lipoprotein molecules into the brain [95]. In this transport the drug molecule binds to a specific receptor over the endothelial cells and the transport across the cell takes place by endocytosis and exocytosis process.

The molecular weight of a therapeutic agent of proteins such as transferrin is up to 80 kDa to large molecular weight lipoproteins varying in size up to 80 nm in diameter can be easily transported across BBB by this RMT mechanism. Currently, the most of strategies involve the pegylated liposomal formulation which is linked to transferrin to target the transferrin receptors and the therapeutic agent is transported across the brain by this RMT to treat neurological disorders corresponding to dementia [96,97].

1.19.6 Blood–brain barrier models

1.19.6.1 In vitro blood–brain barrier models

They help us in depicting the exact environment of the body without the use of any animal. We can take cells from the body, that is, from the natural environment to study the effect of target molecules.

1.19.6.2 Micro blood–brain barrier models

The microfluidic grounded BBB model denotes the BBB more precisely. Almost all the BBB requires covering of alkoxysilane groups and oxygen for the activation of plasma for adsorption and this will help in the growth of endothelial cells (Fig. 1.6). There must be a covalent attachment for permanency as a noncovalent attachment will be affected by environmental factors [98].

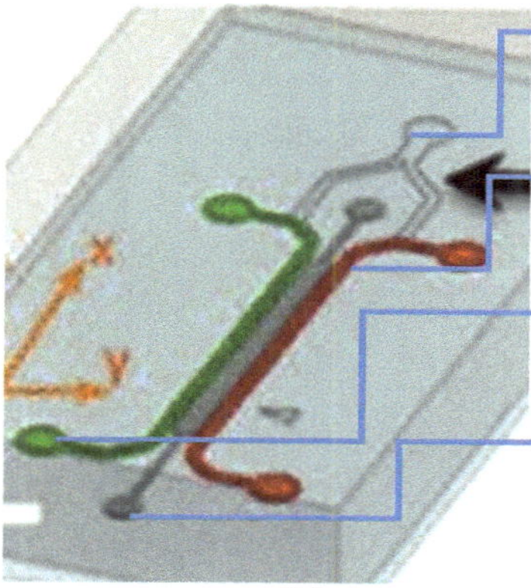

FIG. 1.6 **Microfluidic blood–brain barrier (BBB) structure shows all the components of brain help in the in vitro assessment of drugs for neurodegenerative disorders.**

We can also use collagen instead of silane groups because sometimes their polymerization leads to uneven endothelial cell layer hence leads to instability but this alone cannot depict the exact BBB as the natural one [98].

1.19.6.3 Several advantages of using this model

- They can benefit in coculturing of various cells.
- They assist us in incorporating shear stresses on endothelial cells.
- Allows us in high-resolution assistance.
- Monitoring intracellular and extracellular responses of drugs.
- Neurotoxicity of drugs can be detected.
- Newly targeted drugs for neurodegenerative diseases can be tested accurately.

1.19.6.4 Immortalized rat brain cell lines

These cell lines are primarily mimicking the endothelial cells of the BBB:

- *RBE4*: This cell line helps in depicting the transporters which are used for the entry of drugs but it is not able to depict the barriers of BBB properly [99,100].
- *TR BBB and TM BBB*: These cell lines have transporters such as GLUT1 and P-glycoprotein and this plays a significant role in transporting the drug molecules across the membrane. Cell lines were obtained from the endothelial cells of rats and mice [50,51].
- *HCMEC/D3*: These cell lines are derived from the tumor but they are not able to depict the exact endothelial cell environment [99,100].
- *Human brain microvascular endothelial cell lines*: These cell lines represent the exact physiological environment of the BBB. This includes all the transporters and bond proteins that are part of BBB [99,100].

So, in this way, we can use various cell lines for the new drug targets without the use of any live animal.

1.19.7 In vivo studies

Transgenic mouse models can be used for the studies of neurodegenerative disorders like AD and various other cognitive impairment diseases can be studied by using a mice model.

What does transgenic mean?

In this, we can combine a single or an additional DNA sequence by the means of genetic engineering in a mouse. We are using this because they can depict the exact situation of the disease production of abnormal protein behavioral changes related to this type of this cannot be seen in vitro studies like cell culture (Table 1.2) [101].

1.19.8 Nanomedicine a therapeutic approach for neurodegenerative disorders and corresponding dementia

Nanomedicine is a widely accepted "novel drug delivery technology" for the effective transport of therapeutic agents across the BBB. For several years, the research has been going on to design a new drug delivery technology to overcome the challenges associated with the conventional drug delivery systems.

TABLE 1.2 Types of mice models used in the study of neurodegeneration.

Property	Strain	Speciality	Use	References
Single transgenic APP Tg	PDAPP	Phenotype and loss of neurons can be shown in this model	This model can be used for neuroinflammation, neurotoxicity studies, and beta protein production	[101]
	Tg2576			[101]
	J20			[101]
	APP23			[101]
Double transgenic	APPPS1	Pathophysiology Alzheimer's disease can be studied properly	Beta protein aggregates and drugs targeting it can be detected by using this model	[101]
	5XFAD			[101]
Triple transgenic	3x Tg -AD	Neurofibrillary tangles can be detected which are the sign of Alzheimer's disease	In this, we can also study behavioral change caused by Alzheimer's disease. Cerebrospinal fluid markers can also be detected	[101]

Most of the therapeutic agents for the treatment of neurodegenerative disorders such as AD, PD, and interrelated disorders corresponding toward dementia consist of cholinesterase inhibitors (rivastigmine, donepezil, galantamine), dopaminergic drugs, serotonin, MAO inhibitors, and COMT inhibitors, and many others are formulated by using nanotechnology-based approaches such as prodrug delivery approach, passive targeting by diffusion, by formulating as nanoformulation or by active targeting approaches, etc. [102].

The drug-loaded nanoparticles with dimensions ranging from 1 to 100 nm have a potential approach for targeting and easy uptake through the BBB. The physiology of the brain as it is surrounded by lipid barrier which creates complications for transport of macromolecules and hydrophilic drugs through the brain, to overcome this problem; the solid lipid nanoparticles/nanocarriers (SLNs) are suitably developed for improving the penetration of drug to the target site in the brain. The lipid core of these lipidic nanoformulations by incorporating fatty acids, triglycerides, mineral oils makes the nanocarrier suitable for crossing the BBB through the transcellular pathway [103]. The lipidic nanocarriers such as SLNs, liposomal formulations are highly effective nanotechnology-based approaches for the treatment of several neurodegenerative disorders and interrelated disorders corresponding to dementia.

The nanotechnology-based drug delivery is widely used everywhere, but the main rationale of this chapter is to deliberate the nanomedicines as a beneficial approach to deliver the drug transversely through the BBB to treat the targeted neurodegenerative disorders centrals to dementia. The nanoparticles of nano range size from 3 to 200 nm passing drug across the brain by paracellular pathway [104]. These are developed as polymeric nanoparticles, metallic nanoparticles, SLNs, nanocrystals, etc. providing the targeted delivery of therapeutic agents by encapsulating into the suitable nanocarriers or by ionic interaction with polymers or nanocarriers surface to deliver the drug across the brain for treating most of the neurodegenerative disorders and thereby dementia.

1.19.8.1 Nanomedicine for neurodegenerative diseases

As we discussed that AD is one of the primary causes behind dementia as we can do only treatment of symptoms in neurodegenerative diseases for Alzheimer's, we have anticholinesterase inhibitors and NMDA receptor antagonist.

Rivastigmine is a drug that has low bioavailability and it is highly hydrophilic so for this purpose its entry into the brain is restricted but we can increase the bioavailability by using nanomedicine technology. As several other cholinesterase inhibitors such as donepezil and galantamine are used. It can also allow us to reduce the dose of a drug and minimize the side effects of the drugs.

In Parkinson's, we use many categories of the drug as we talk about L-DOPA its major side effect is dyskinesia when we are trying to prepare a sustained delivery system for L-DOPA by using nanotechnology it will reduce the dose which results in the minimizing the dyskinesia. So many works have going on nano therapies for the treatment of dementia this will help us in creating a targeted drug delivery system (Table 1.3).

TABLE 1.3 Few examples of nanocarriers-mediated delivery of therapeutic agents to the brain.

Drug	Polymer	Study	Results	References
Rivastigmine	Polysorbate 80 and poly butyl cyanoacrylate	In vivo (transgenic rats)	The uptake of the drug has been increased as compared to free rivastigmine	[105]
L-DOPA	Chitosan	In vitro (intranasal in rats)	Delivery in the brain is enhanced and the peripheral degradation is avoided	[106]
L-DOPA	Methyl ester/ benserazide-loaded nanoparticle	In vivo (rats)	The major adverse effect of L-DOPA dyskinesia can be minimized by the use of nanoparticles	[106]
Ropinirole	Poly-lactic-co-glycolic acid	In vitro	98% of the drug can penetrate, hence penetration efficiency is increased	[106]
Ropinirole	Chitosan-coated oil in water nanoemulsion	In vivo (transgenic rats)	Sustained-release preparation. Bioavailability of the drug has been increased	[106]
Bromocriptine	Chitosan	In vivo (mice model)	Brain targeting and adsorption of the nanoparticle-loaded bromocriptine were found to be increased	[106]
Selegiline	Hydrochloride-loaded chitosan nanoparticle	In vitro	In this, the dosing frequency decreased a sustained realize formulation has developed	[106]
Apomorphine	Solid lipid nanoparticles	In vivo (transgenic rats)	Efficacy and bioavailability of drugs have been increased	[106]
Curcumin	Poly n-butyl cyanoacrylate nanospheres	In vitro (cell lines)	Protection of degradation and penetration efficiency has been increased	[105]
Rasagiline	Chitosan-glutamate nanoparticles	In vivo (mice model)	The bioavailability of the preparation has been increased	[106]

1.20 Conclusion

Nowadays, the incidence of dementia is on surge. Dementia associated with severe pathological conditions affect the overall behavioral, social, and economic domains of person. Hence, the dementia as a medical condition needs to be addressed. Although, various FDA-approved therapeutic agents are available, but they have their own side effects and low BBB permeation. Nanocarriers could help to traverse the BBB [107]. Moreover, intriguingly, NPs are also known for easy-going purification, uncomplicated sterilization procedures. As far as delivery of active pharmaceutical agent is concerned, the NPs offer the potential for sustained release, enhanced permeability retention effect, and target-based delivery of active pharmaceutical agents [108–110].

Conflict of interest

Declare no potential conflict of interest.

Consent

All authors have given their consent.

Acknowledgments

Authors are thankful to the National Institute of Pharmaceutical Education and Research, Raebareli (NIPER-R), Department of Pharmaceuticals, Ministry of Chemicals and Fertilizers, Government of India, for providing support in every possible form. The communication no. (NIPER-R/Communication/234) for the submission of this chapter also provided by the NIPER-R.

References

[1] Von Gunten A, Pocnet C, Rossier J. The impact of personality characteristics on the clinical expression in neurodegenerative disorders—a review. Brain Res Bull 2009;80(4-5):179–91. doi:10.1016/j.brainresbull.2009.07.004.

[2] Martin JB. Molecular basis of the neurodegenerative disorders. N Engl J Med 1999; 340(25):1970–80. doi:10.1056/NEJM199906243402507.

[3] Alzheimer's Association Report. Alzheimer's disease facts and figures. Alzheimer's Dement 2021;17(3):327–406. 12328. doi:10.1002/alz.12328. Epub 2021 Mar 23.

[4] Abbott NJ, Patabendige AA, Dolman DE, Yusof SR, Begley DJ. Structure and function of the blood–brain barrier. Neurobiol Dis 2010;37(1):13–25. doi:10.1016/j.nbd.2009.07.030.

[5] Aarsland D, Andersen K, Larsen JP, et al. Prevalence and characteristics of dementia in Parkinson disease: an 8-year prospective study. Arch Neurol 2003;60:387–92. doi:10.1001/archneur.60.3.387.

[6] Geldmacher DS, Whitehouse PJ. Evaluation of dementia. N Engl J Med 1996;335(5):330–6. doi:10.1056/NEJM199608013350507.

[7] Chiu MJ, Chen TF, Yip PK, Hua MS, Tang LY. Behavioural and psychologic symptoms in different types of dementia. J Formos Med Assoc 2006;105(7):556–62. doi:10.1016/S0929-6646(09)60150-9.

[8] David S, Geldmacher MD, Peter J, Whitehouse MD. Evaluation of dementia. N Engl J Med 1996 Aug 1;335(5):330–6. doi:10.1056/NEJM199608013350507.

[9] Khachaturian ZS. Diagnosis of Alzheimer's disease. Arch Neurol 1985;42(11):1097–105. doi:10.1001/archneur.1985.04060100083029.

[10] Goedert M, Spillantini MG. A century of Alzheimer's disease. Science 2006;314(5800):777–81. doi:10.1126/science.1132814.

[11] Knopman DS. Dementia and cerebrovascular disease. Mayo Clin Proc 2006;81(2):223–30. doi:10.4065/81.2.223.

[12] Walker FO. Huntington's disease. Lancet North Am Ed 2007;369(9557):218–28. doi:10.1016/S0140-6736(07)60111-1.

[13] Caine ED, Ebert MH, Weingartner H. An outline for the analysis of dementia: the memory disorder of Huntington's disease. Neurology 1977;27(11):1087. doi:10.1212/wnl.27.11.1087.

[14] Garcia-Ptacek S, Kramberger MG. Parkinson disease and dementia. J Geriatr Psychiatry Neurol 2016;29(5):261–70. doi:10.1177/0891988716654985.

[15] Parchi P, Castellani R, Capellari S, et al. Molecular basis of phenotypic variability in sporadc creudeldt-jakob disease. Ann Neurol 1996;39(6):767–78. doi:10.1002/ana.410390613.

[16] Spencer MD, Knight RS, Will RG. First hundred cases of variant Creutzfeldt-Jakob disease: retrospective case note review of early psychiatric and neurological features. BMJ 2002;324(7352):1479–82. doi:10.1136/bmj.324.7352.1479.

[17] Shams S, Martola J, Granberg T, et al. Cerebral microbleeds: different prevalence, topography, and risk factors depending on dementia diagnosis—the Karolinska Imaging Dementia Study. Am J Neuroradiol 2015;36(4):661–6. doi:10.3174/ajnr.A4176.

[18] Chen JH, Lin KP, Chen YC. Risk factors for dementia. J Formos Med Assoc 2009; 108(10):754–64. doi:10.1016/S0929-6646(09)60402-2.

[19] Ettema TP, Dröes RM, de Lange J, et al. The concept of quality of life in dementia in the different stages of the disease. Int Psychogeriatr 2005 Sep;17(3):353–70. doi:10.1017/s1041610205002073.

[20] Overshott R, Burns A. Treatment of dementia. J Neurol Neurosurg Psychiatry 2005;76(Suppl 5):53–9. doi:10.1136/jnnp.2005.082537.

[21] Priller C, Bauer T, Mitteregger G, et al. Synapse formation and function is modulated by the amyloid precursor protein. J Neurosci 2006 Jul 5;26(27):7212–21. doi:10.1523/JNEUROSCI.1450-06.2006.

[22] McGirr S, Venegas C, Swaminathan A. Alzheimer's disease: A brief review. J Exp Neurol 2020;1(3):89–98.

[23] Tiwari S, Atluri V, Kaushik A, Yndart A, Nair M. Alzheimer's disease: pathogenesis, diagnostics, and therapeutics. Int J Nanomed 2019;14:5541–54. doi:10.2147/IJN.S200490 Jul 19.

[24] Cano A, Turowski P, Ettcheto M, et al. Nanomedicine-based technologies and novel biomarkers for the diagnosis and treatment of Alzheimer's disease: from current to future challenges. J Nanobiotechnol 2021;19:122. https://doi.org/10.1186/s12951-021-00864-x.

[25] Barage SH, Sonawane KD. Amyloid cascade hypothesis: pathogenesis and therapeutic strategies in Alzheimer's disease. Neuropeptides 2015 Aug 1;52:1–18. doi:10.1016/j.npep.2015.06.008 .

[26] Bondi MW, Edmonds EC, Salmon DP. Alzheimer's disease: past, present, and future. J Int Neuropsychol Soc: JINS 2017 Oct; 23(9-10):818–31. doi:10.1017/S135561771700100X.
[27] Nilsberth C, Westlind-Danielsson A, Eckman CB, et al. The 'Arctic' APP mutation (E693G) causes Alzheimer's disease by enhanced Aβ protofibril formation. Nat Neurosci 2001 Sep;4(9):887–93. doi:10.1038/nn0901-887
[28] Lindwall G, Cole RD. Phosphorylation affects the ability of tau protein to promote microtubule assembly. J Biol Chem 1984;259:5301–5.
[29] Himmler DD, Kirschne MW, Martin Jr DW. Tau consists of a set of proteins with repeated C-terminal microtubule binding domains and variable N-terminal domains. Mol Cell Biol 1989;9:1381–8. doi:10.1128/mcb.9.4.1381-1388.1989.
[30] Goedert M, Spillanti MG, Jakes R, Rutherford RA. Crowther multiple isoforms of human microtubule-associated protein tau: sequences and localization in neurofibrillary tangles of Alzheimer's disease. Neuron 1989;3:519–26. doi:10.1016/0896-6273(89)90210-9.
[31] Alonso AC, Zaidi T, Grundke-Iqbal I, Iqbal K. Role of abnormally phosphorylated tau in the breakdown of microtubules in Alzheimer disease. Proc Natl Acad Sci U S A 1994 Jun 7;91(12):5562–6. doi:10.1073/pnas.91.12.5562.
[32] Iqbal K, Alejandradel C, Alonso She Chen M et al. Tau pathology in Alzheimer disease and other tauopathies. Biochim Biophys Acta Mol Basis Dis 2005;1739(2–3):198–210. doi:10.1016/j.bbadis.2004.09.008.
[33] Köpke E, Tung YC, Shaikh S, et al. Microtubule-associated protein tau, abnormal phosphorylation of a non-paired helical filament pool in Alzheimer disease. Biol Chem 1993 Nov 15;268(32):24374–84.
[34] Poorkaj P, Bird TD, Wijsman E, et al. Tau is a candidate gene for chromosome 17 frontotemporal dementia. Ann Neurol 1998;43(6):815–25. doi:10.1002/ana.410430617 Jun.
[35] Graham Pockley A. Heat shock proteins as regulators of the immune response. Lancet North Am Ed2003 August 9;362(9382):469–76.https://doi.org/10.1016/S0140-6736(03)14075-5.
[36] Ponomarenkol M, Kolchanov SN, Proteins HS. Reference Module in Life Sciences Brenner's Encyclopedia of Genetics, 2nd ed.; 2013:402–5.
[37] Simon DK, Tanner CM, Brundin P. Parkinson Disease Epidemiology, Pathology, Genetics, and Pathophysiology. Clin Geriatr Med 2020;36(1):1–12. doi:10.1016/j.cger.2019.08.002.
[38] Zhang G, Wang T, Xia Y, Wan F, Ma K, Guo XF, et al. New perspectives on roles of alpha-synuclein in Parkinson's disease. Front Aging Neurosci 2018;10:370. doi:10.3389/fnagi.2018.00370.
[39] Kannarkat GT, Boss JM, Tansey MG. The role of innate and adaptive immunity in Parkinson's disease. J Parkinsons Dis 2013;3(4):493–514. doi:10.3233/JPD-130250.
[40] Jellinger KA. The pathology of "vascular dementia": a critical update. J Alzheimer's Dis 2008;14:107–23. doi:10.3233/jad-2008-14110.
[41] Tabrizi SJ, Reilmann R, Roos RA, et al. Potential endpoints for clinical trials in premanifest and early Huntington's disease in the TRACK-HD study: analysis of 24-month observational data. Lancet Neurolo 2012;11(1):42–53. https://doi.org/10.1016/S1474-4422(11)70263-0.
[42] Langbehn DR, Stout JC, Gregory S. et al. Association of CAG repeats with long-term progression in Huntington disease JAMA neurology. 2019 Nov 1; 76(11);75–1385. doi:10.1001/jamaneurol.2019.2368.
[43] Horta SM, Sampedro F, Horta-Barba A, et al. Structural brain correlates of dementia in Huntington's disease. Neuroimage 2020;28:102415. https://doi.org/10.1016/j.nicl.2020.10245.

[44] Genetic Modifiers of Huntington's Disease (GeM-HD) Consortium. Identification of genetic factors that modify clinical onset of huntington's disease. Cell 2015;162(3):516–26. doi:10.1016/j.cell.2015.07.003.

[45] Ferrer I, Goutan E, Marin C, et al. Brain-derived neurotrophic factor in Huntington disease. Brain Res 2000;866:257–61. doi:10.1016/s0006-8993(00)02237.

[46] Walker FO. Huntington's disease. Lancet 2007;369(9557):218–28. doi:10.1016/S0140-6736(07)60111-1.

[47] Tripathi KD. Essentials of medical pharmacology, 8th ed. New Delhi, India: Jaypee Brothers Medical; 2018. p. 426–37.

[48] Armstrong MJ, Okun MS. Diagnosis and treatment of Parkinson disease: a review. JAMA 2020;323(6):548–60. doi:10.1001/jama.2019.22360.

[49] Ondo WG, Tintner R, Thomas M, Jankovic J. Tetrabenazine treatment for Huntington's disease-associated chorea. Clin Neuropharmacol 2002;25(6):300–2. doi:10.1097/00002826-200211000-00003.

[50] Hayden MR, Leavitt BR, Yasothan U, Kirkpatrick P. Tetrabenazine. Nat Rev Drug Discov 2009;8(1):17–9. doi:10.1186/1750-1326-5-18.

[51] Unti E, Mazzucchi S, Palermo G, et al. Antipsychotic drugs in Huntington's disease. Expert Rev Neurother 2017;17(3):227–37. doi:10.1080/14737175.2016.1226134.

[52] Walker FO, Young AB, Penney JB, et al. Benzodiazepine and GABA receptors in early Huntington's disease. Neurology 1984;34(9):1237. doi:10.1212/wnl.34.9.1237.

[53] Mc Quain JA, Galicia-Castillo MC, Morris DA. Palliative care issues in Creutzfeldt: Jakob disease. J Palliat Med 2020;23(3):424–6. doi:10.1089/jpm.2019.0652.

[54] Tanaka M, Török N, Vécsei L. Novel pharmaceutical approaches in dementia. NeuroPsychopharmacotherapy 2021:1–18. https://doi.org/10.1007/978-3-319-56015-1_444-1.

[55] Ettema TP, Dröes RM, de Lange J, et al. The concept of quality of life in dementia in the different stages of the disease. Int Psychogeriatr 2005;17(3):353–70. doi:10.1017/s1041610205002073.

[56] Adlimoghaddam A, Neuendorff M, Roy B, Albensi BC. A review of clinical treatment considerations of donepezil in severe Alzheimer's disease. CNS Neurosci Ther 2018;24(10):876–88. https://doi.org/10.1111/cns.13035.

[57] Wood LD, Neumiller JJ, Setter SM. Clinical review of treatment options for select nonmotor symptoms of Parkinson's disease. Am J Geriatr Pharmacother 2020 August ;8(4):294–315. https://doi.org/10.1016/j.amjopharm.2010.08.002.

[58] Williams BR, Nazarians A, Gill MA. A review of rivastigmine: a reversible cholinesterase inhibitor. Clin Ther June 2003;25(6):1634–53 https://doi.org/10.1016/S0149-2918(03)80160-1.

[59] Wirdefeldt K, Odin P, Nyholm D. Levodopa–carbidopa intestinal gel in patients with Parkinson's disease: a systematic review. CNS Drugs 2016;30:381–404 https://doi.org/10.1007/s40263-016-0336-5.

[60] Mahapatra RK, Edwards MJ, Schott JM, Bhatia KP. Corticobasal degeneration. Lancet Neurol 2004 December;3(12):736–43. https://doi.org/10.1016/S1474-4422(04)00936-6.

[61] Alam S, Khan ZI, Mustafa G, et al. Development and evaluation of thymoquinone-encapsulated chitosan nanoparticles for nose-to-brain targeting: a pharmacoscintigraphic study. Int J Nanomed 2012;7:5705–18. doi:10.2147/IJN.S35329.

[62] Rochon PA, Stukel TA, Sykora K, et al. Atypical antipsychotics and parkinsonism. Arch Intern Med 2005;165(16):1882–8. doi:10.1001/archinte.165.16.1882.

[63] Pardeshi CV, Belgamwar VS. Improved brain pharmacokinetics following intranasal administration of N, N, N-trimethyl chitosan tailored mucoadhesive NLCs. Mater Technol 2020;35(5):249–66. doi:10.1080/10667857.2019.1674522.

[64] Sano M, Ernesto C, Thomas RG, et al. A controlled trial of selegiline, alpha-tocopherol or both for the treatment of Alzheimer's disease. N Engl J Med 1997;336:1216–22. doi:10.1056/NEJM199704243361704.

[65] Weinreb O, Mandel S, Bar-Am O, et al. Multifunctional neuroprotective derivatives of rasagiline as anti-Alzheimer's disease drugs. Neurotherapeutics 2009 January;6(1):163–74. https://doi.org/10.1016/j.nurt.2008.10.030.

[66] Olanow CW, Kieburtz K, Stern M, et al. Double-blind, placebo-controlled study of entacapone in levodopa-treated patients with stable Parkinson disease. Arch Neurol 2004;61(10):1563–8. doi:10.1001/archneur.61.10.1563.

[67] Meythaler JM, Brunner RC, Johnson A, et al. Amantadine to improve neurorecovery in traumatic brain injury–associated diffuse axonal injury: a pilot double-blind randomized trial. J Head Trauma Rehabil 2002 August;17(4):300–13 .

[68] Asher SW, Aminoff MJ. Tetrabenazine and movement disorders. Neurology 1981 Aug;31(8):1051–68. doi:10.1212/WNL.31.8.1051 .

[69] Stoppe G, Brandt CA, Staedt JH. Behavioural problems associated with dementia. Drugs Aging 1999;14:41–54. https://doi.org/10.2165/00002512-199914010-00003.

[70] Deyn PP, Rabheru K, Rasmussen A, et al. A randomized trial of risperidone, placebo, and haloperidol for behavioral symptoms of dementia. Neurology 1999 Sep;53(5):946. doi:10.1212/WNL.53.5.946.

[71] Hayden MR, Paul M, Vinik AI, Beighton P. Impaired prolactin release in huntington's chorea: evidence for dopaminergic excess. Lancet North Am Ed 1977;310(8035):423–6.

[72] Edward HP, Carole WC, Mary L, et al. Traumatically induced altered membrane permeability: its relationship to traumatically induced reactive axonal change. J Neurotrauma 1994 Oct;11(5):507–22. http://doi.org/10.1089/neu.1994.11.507.

[73] Calcaterra NE, Barrow JC. Classics in chemical neuroscience: diazepam (valium). ACS Chem Neurosci 2014;5(4):253–60.

[74] Kenney C, Jankovic J. Tetrabenazine in the treatment of hyperkinetic movement disorders. Expert Rev Neurother 2006;6(1):7–17. doi:10.1586/14737175.6.1.7.

[75] Haddad PM, Das A, Ashfaq M, Wieck A. A review of valproate in psychiatric practice. Expert Opin Drug Metab Toxicol 2009;5(5):539–51. doi:10.1517/17425250902911455.

[76] Herrlinger U, Küker W, Platten M, et al. First-line therapy with temozolomide induces regression of primary CNS lymphoma. Neurology 2002 May;58(10):1573–4. doi:10.1212/WNL.58.10.1573.

[77] Friedlander SM, Welch RM. Vanishing disc neovascularization following intravitreal bevacizumab (avastin) injection. Arch Ophthalmol 2006;124(9):1365. doi:10.1001/archopht.124.9.1365.

[78] Langbehn DR, Stout JC, Gregory S, et al. Association of CAG repeats with long-term progression in Huntington disease. JAMA Neurol 2019 Nov 1;76(11):1375–85. doi:10.1001/jamaneurol.2019.2368 .

[79] Joan Abbott N, Patabendige AAK, Diana EM, et al. Structure and function of the blood–brain barrier. Neurobiol Dis 2010;37:13–25. doi:10.1016/j.nbd.2009.07.030.

[80] Wolburg H, Lippoldt A. Tight junctions of the blood–brain barrier: development, composition and regulation. Vascul Pharmacol 2002;38:323–37. doi:10.1016/s1537-1891(02)00200-8.

[81] Kutcher ME, Herman IM. The pericyte: cellular regulator of microvascular blood flow. Microvasc Res 2009;77:235–46. doi:10.1016/j.mvr.2009.01.007.

[82] Tajes M, Ramos-Fernández E, Weng-Jiang X, et al. The blood-brain barrier: structure, function and therapeutic approaches to cross it. Mol Membr Biol 2014;31(5):152–67. doi:10.3109/09687688.2014.937468.

[83] Gonzalez Mariscal L, Betanzos A, AvilaFlores A. MAGUK proteins: structure and role in the tight junction. Semin Cell Dev Biol 2000;11(4):315–24. doi:10.1006/scdb.2000.0178.

[84] Balda MS, FloresMaldonado C, Cereijido M, Matter K. Multiple domains of occludin are involved in the regulation of paracellular permeability. J Cell Biochem 2000;78:85–96.

[85] Palmeri D, van Zante A, Huang CC, et al. Vascular endothelial junction associated molecule, a novel member of the immunoglobulin superfamily, is localized to intercellular boundaries of endothelial cells. J Biol Chem 2000 Jun 23;275(25):19139–45. doi:10.1074/jbc.M003189200.

[86] Abbott NJ, Ronnback L, Hansson E. Astrocyte-endothelial interactions at the blood-brain barrier. Nat Rev Neurosci 2006;7(1):41–53. doi:10.1038/nrn1824.

[87] Wolburg H, Lippoldt A. Tight junctions of the blood-brain barrier: development, composition and regulation. Vascul Pharmacol 2002;38:323–37.

[88] Hellstrom M, Gerhardt H, Kalen M, et al. Lack of pericytes leads to endothelial hyperplasia and abnormal vascular morphogenesis. J Cell Biol 2001 Apr 30;153(3):543–54. doi:10.1083/jcb.153.3.543.

[89] Miller G. Drug targeting. Breaking down barriers. Science 2002 Aug 16;297(5584):1116–8. doi:10.1126/science.297.5584.1116 .

[90] Batchelder EM, Yarar D. Differential requirements for clathrin-dependent endocytosis at sites of cell-substrate adhesion. Mol Biol Cell 2010 Sep 1-9;21(17):3070. doi:10.1091/mbc.E09-12-1044 .

[91] MaldonadoBáez L, Williamson C, Donaldson JG. Clathrin-independent endocytosis: a cargo-centric view. Exp Cell Res 2013 Nov 1;319(18):2759–69. doi:10.1016/j.yexcr.2013.08.008.

[92] Hervé F, Ghinea N, Scherrmann J-M. CNS delivery via adsorptive transcytosis. AAPS J 2008 Sep;10(3):455–72. doi:10.1208/s12248-008-9055-2.

[93] Bickel U, Yoshikawa T, Pardridge W. Delivery of peptides and proteins through the blood-brain barrier. Adv Drug Deliv Rev 2001 Mar 1;46(1-3):247–79. doi:10.1016/s0169-409x(00)00139-3 .

[94] Brasnjevic I, Steinbusch HW, Schmitz C, et al. Delivery of peptide and protein drugs over the blood-brain barrier. Prog Neurobiol 2009 Apr;87(4):212–51. doi:10.1016/j.pneurobio.2008.12.002.

[95] Descamps L, Dehouck MP, Torpier G, Cecchelli R. Receptor-mediated transcytosis of transferrin through blood-brain barrier endothelial cells. Am J Physiol 1996 Apr;270(4 Pt 2 H1149-58). doi:10.1152/ajpheart.1996.270.4.H1149.

[96] Sharma G, Modgil A, Layek B, et al. Cell penetrating peptide tethered bi-ligand liposomes for delivery to brain in vivo: biodistribution and transfection. Control Release 2013 Apr 10;167(1):1–10. doi:10.1016/j.jconrel.2013.01.016.

[97] Lajoie JM, Shusta EV. Targeting receptor mediated transport for delivery of biologics across the blood brain barrier. Annu Rev Pharmacol Toxicol 2015;55:613–31. doi:10.1146/annurev-pharmtox-010814-124852.

[98] Peng B, Tong Z, Tong WY, et al. In situ surface modification of microfluidic blood–brain-barriers for improved screening of small molecules and nanoparticles. ACS Appl Mater Interfaces 2020;12(51):56753–66. doi:10.1021/acsami.0c17102.

[99] Roux F, Couraud PO. Rat brain endothelial cell lines for the study of blood–brain barrier permeability and transport functions. Cell Mol Neurobiol 2005;25(1):41–58. doi:10.1007/s10571-004-1376-9.

[100] Peng Y, Chu S, Yang Y, et al. Neuroinflammatory in vitro cell culture models and the potential applications for neurological disorders. Front Pharmacol 2021;12:671734. doi:10.3389/fphar.2021.671734.

[101] Sasaguri H, Nilsson P, Hashimoto S, et al. APP mouse models for Alzheimer's disease preclinical studies. EMBO J 2017;36(17):2473–87. https://doi.org/10.15252/embj.201797397.

[102] Sharma HS, Castellani RJ, Smith MA, Sharma A. The blood-brain barrier in Alzheimer's disease: novel therapeutic targets and nanodrug delivery. Int Rev Neurobiol 2012;102:47–90. doi:10.1016/B978-0-12-386986-9.00003-X.

[103] Tajes M, Ramos-Fernández E, Weng-jiang X, et al. The blood-brain barrier: structure, function and therapeutic approaches to cross it. Mol Membr Biol 2014;31(5):152–67. doi:10.3109/09687688.2014.937468.

[104] Gregori M, Masserini M, Mancini S. Nanomedicine for the treatment of Alzheimer's disease. Nanomedicine (Lond) 2015;10(7):1203–18. doi:10.2217/nnm.14.206.

[105] Andrieux K, Couvreur P. Nanomedicine as a promising approach for the treatment and diagnosis of brain diseases: the example of Alzheimer's disease. Ann Pharm Franc 2013 July;71(4):225–33. doi:10.1016/j.pharma.2013.04.001.

[106] Hawthorne GH, Bernuci MP, Bortolanza M, et al. Nanomedicine to overcome current Parkinson's treatment liabilities: a systematic review. Neurotox Res 2016;30(4):715–29. doi:10.1007/s12640-016-9663-z.

[107] Sharma N, Bhandari S, Deshmukh R, Yadav AK, Mishra N. Development and characterization of embelin-loaded nanolipid carriers for brain targeting. Artif Cells Nanomed Biotechnol 2017;45(3):409–13. doi:10.3109/21691401.2016.1160407.

[108] Yadav AK, Mishra P, Mishra AK, Mishra P, Jain S, Agrawal GP. Development and characterization of hyaluronic acid-anchored PLGA nanoparticulate carriers of doxorubicin. Nanomed Nanotechnol Biol Med 2007;3(4):246–57. doi:10.1016/j.nano.2007.09.004.

[109] Yadav AK, Mishra P, Jain S, Mishra P, Mishra AK, Agrawal GP. Preparation and characterization of HA-PEG-PCL intelligent core corona nanoparticles for delivery of doxorubicin. J Drug Target 2008;16(6):464–78. doi:10.1080/10611860802095494.

[110] Yadav AK, Agarwal A, Rai G, et al. Development and characterization of hyaluronic acid decorated PLGA nanoparticles for delivery of 5-fluorouracil. Drug Deliv 2010;17(8):561–72. doi:10.3109/10717544.2010.500635.

Chapter 2

Dementia: A journey from cause to cure

Shilpa Kumari#, Kajal Bagri#, Rahul Deshmukh

Department of Pharmaceutical Sciences and Technology, Maharaja Ranjit Singh Punjab Technical University, Bathinda, Punjab, India

#Ms. Shilpa and Ms. Kajal have contributed equally in the preparation of this manuscript and should be considered as first authors.

2.1 Introduction

Increased life expectancy has challenged us with multiple health problems including dementia which can be considered as an outcome of stressful life of 21st century. Dementia is characterized by deficit in memory, attention, judgment, and analytical skills, etc. and become worst as the age grows. According to the WHO, the global number of people living with dementia will rise from 57.4 million today to 82 million in 2030 and 152.8 million in 2050 [1]. The global number of persons living with dementia was estimated to be 57.4 million in 2019, and this number is expected to reach 152.8 million by 2050 [2]. The number and proportion of older persons are quickly increasing in developing countries and dementia is the leading cause of impairment in these regions [3]. The most prevalent type of dementia is Alzheimer's disease (AD) contributes to 60–80% cases, vascular dementia (VaD) with 20% cases, Lewy body dementia (LBD) with 7.5% cases among the various types of dementias and then frontotemporal dementia (FTD).

Dementia is a progressive chronic brain condition or group of symptoms that affects memory, thinking, reasoning, behavior, communication, and other cognitive functions. Pathologically, dementia or cognitive deterioration has been linked with multiple factors such as abnormal accumulation of proteins in the brain, neurotransmitters deficit/imbalance, neuroinflammation, and oxidative stress. Major forms of dementia include AD, LBD, VaD, FTD, and mixed type [4]. The etiology and the symptoms varied among the different types/forms of dementia but sometimes display mixed symptomatology. The pathogenic mechanisms, progression of the disease, and the current available treatment strategies are varied among the different types of dementias [5]. Various researchers are working hard to know the exact pathological mechanisms and

Nanomedicine-Based Approaches for the Treatment of Dementia. https://doi.org/10.1016/B978-0-12-824331-2.00011-X
Copyright © 2023 Elsevier Inc. All rights reserved.

the biomarkers of dementia and the drug targets to introduce the treatment instead of providing the symptomatic relief. Here in this chapter we have discussed the types, neurobiology, disease progressions, their symptomatology, and the treatment details for each type of dementia.

2.2 Types of dementia

Dementia is now a leading field of interest and investigation. Around 1.62 million deaths were reported due to dementia in 2019 worldwide [2]. There are multiple factors responsible for dementia initiation and progression but no exact cause is known till date [6]. Dementia occurrence and progression can be understood via three stages:

Early stage: Forgetfulness, lost in familiar places
Middle stage: Forgetting recent events and people names, change in behavior
Late stage: Difficulty in recognizing family members, relatives and friends, difficulty in performing daily activities and increased need of assistance and care

Moreover dementia has multiple forms depending on the region affected, etiologies and symptoms. Among all AD is the most common form of dementia that accounts for around 60–70% of total dementia cases. Other types of dementia include LBD in which abnormal protein aggregates are found inside neurons, VaD due to impaired blood flow, FTD mainly due to frontal lobe degeneration and other forms of dementia [7,8].

Majorly dementias can be further classified into:

- Primary (diseases and conditions in which dementia is the main illness).
- Secondary (dementia due to another disease or condition).

1. Primary dementia includes:
   - Alzheimer's disease (AD)
   - Lewy body dementia (LBD)
   - Vascular dementia (VaD)
   - Frontotemporal dementia (FTD)
   - Mixed dementia
2. Dementia due to other diseases or conditions includes:
   - Parkinson's disease dementia (PDD)
   - Huntington's disease
   - Creutzfeldt–Jakob disease
   - Wernicke's–Korsakoff syndrome
   - Traumatic brain injury-induced dementia

TABLE 2.1 Types of dementia with their symptoms and prevalence rate.

S. no.	Type of dementia	Sign and symptoms	Prevalence rate
1.	Alzheimer's disease (AD)	Cognitive impairment, forgetfulness, confusion, and impaired thinking skills	60–80%
2.	Lewy body dementia (LBD)	Rapid eye movement sleep behavior disorder	5–10%
3.	Vascular dementia (VaD)	Memory impairment, difficulty in performing simple tasks, misplacing items, hallucinations, difficulty in reading and writing	5–10%
4.	Frontotemporal dementia (FTD)	Lack of judgment, apathy, loss of empathy, inappropriate social behavior	5–10%
5.	Mixed dementia • Parkinson's disease dementia (PDD) • Creutzfeldt–Jakob disease • Huntington's disease • Wernicke's–Korsakoff syndrome • Traumatic brain injury-induced dementia	• Hallucination, blanking out • Jerky muscles, mood swings • Judgment, planning, and organizing related problem • Memory altered • Amnesia, thinking capacity altered	5%

For more information, the dementias and their symptoms are elaborated in Table 2.1. The major focus of this chapter is to detail about the major forms as detailed in primary dementia.

2.3 Alzheimer's disease

AD is the most common form of dementia comprising up to 80% of total cases [9]. Mainly AD is an age-related progressive neurodegenerative disorder. According to "The Silver Book" from the alliance of aging research, Alzheimer is the seventh leading cause of death worldwide among all ages while fifth leading cause of death among people of age group 65 and above. AD can be caused due to many reasons, there could be genetic reasons behind it or it could be sporadic. Extracellular amyloid-β (Aβ) plaque deposits and intracellular neurofibrillary tangles (NFTs) of tau protein majorly in the hippocampus are the main clinical hallmarks of AD [10]. So let's understand these pathways and associated pathologies responsible for initiation and progression of disease in this chapter.

AD is classified into two types, that is, familial AD (early onset AD) and sporadic AD (late onset AD). Familial AD is common in younger people before the age of 65. The familial AD occurs mainly due to mutations in genes, that is, presenilins (PSEN) or amyloid precursor protein (APP) genes and accounts for about 5% of total AD cases. Whereas sporadic AD is the most common form occurs above the age of 65. Sporadic AD accounts for about 95% of total AD cases [11]. Alzheimer initiates with mild loss of memory and cognitive disabilities so a person might forget the places and things, but eventually situation may get more worsen, such as impaired judgment or reasoning, difficulty in initiating/continuing a conversation and decline in cognition and also motor functions. AD is further divided into different stages based on the appearance of symptoms [12], such as preclinical AD, mild cognitive impairment/MCI, mild AD, moderate AD, and severe AD the detailed symptoms are discussed in Table 2.2 [13]. Initially, the damages appear to take place in hippocampus and entorhinal cortex which are actually important for learning and memory. Eventually the problem spreads all over the brain and causes the atrophy of brain [14]. Furthermore, the accumulation of Aβ deposits and tau tangles aggravates other pathologies such as release of proinflammatory markers, increased reactive oxygen/nitrogen species, neurotransmitter imbalance, and other cellular and molecular dysfunctions. These pathologies are further explained in the etiopathogenesis for making a better understanding toward AD.

2.4 Etiopathogenesis

Although pathogenic mechanisms are wide but there in we have tried to discuss in brief. As discussed earlier extracellular deposits of Aβ and intracellular accumulations of NFTs of tau proteins are the major hallmarks of AD pathology [15]. Aβ is formed by the cleavage of APP, a transmembrane protein (neuronal cells). The cleavage of APP is carried out by three enzymes, that is, α, β, and ɣ secretases. Cleavage of APP by α and ɣ secretase produce soluble protein, which is being digested easily, whereas cleavage by β/ɣ secretases leading to Aβ formation [16].

Earlier, it was thought that Aβ is a "junk protein" and not useful for brain but it is now clear that Aβ is not a "junk protein," playing important role in neuronal trafficking of nutrients and give strength to the neuronal cells [17]. However, accumulation of Aβ due to increased synthesis through cleavage by β-secretases and the impaired clearance mechanisms disturb neuronal functioning and trigger activation of various deleterious pathways leading to neuronal death.

Indeed increased β-secretase activity and impaired clearance leading to increased production and deposits of Aβ have been reported to occur in AD brain. On the other hand, tau is a microtubule-associated protein and helps in holding the neuronal membrane microtubules together. The solid gripping

TABLE 2.2 Stages of Alzheimer's diseases.

S. no.	Alzheimer's stage	Symptoms	Brain changes	Brain regions affected
1.	Preclinical AD	Appears normal but biological changes in brain	Hippocampus	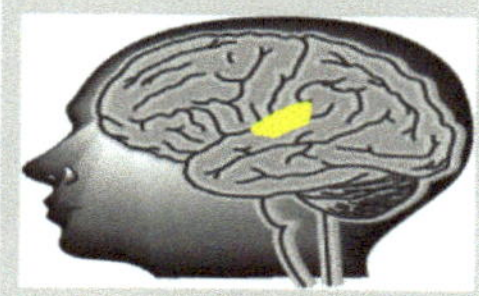
2.	MCI	Will begin to experience forgetfulness but do not interfere with everyday activities	Hippocampus and entorhinal cortex (medial temporal lobe)	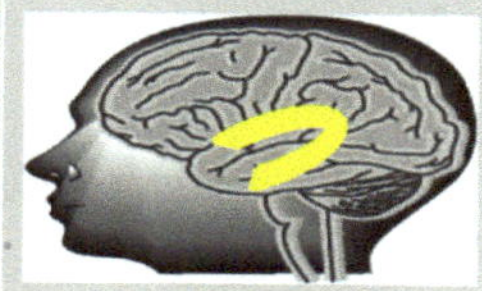
3.	Mild AD	Forgetfulness, reading problems, poor object recognition, forgetting familiar places, can be diagnosed	Lateral temporal and parietal lobes	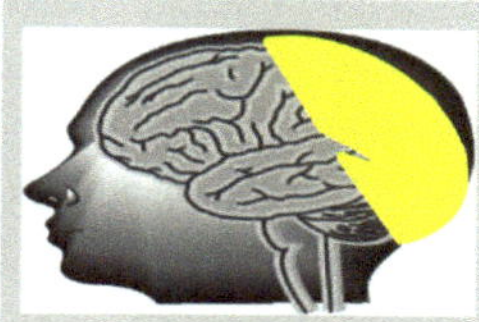
4.	Moderate AD	Clear signs and symptoms, poor judgment, impulsivity, difficulty in communication, confusion, behavior changes	Spreads to frontal lobe	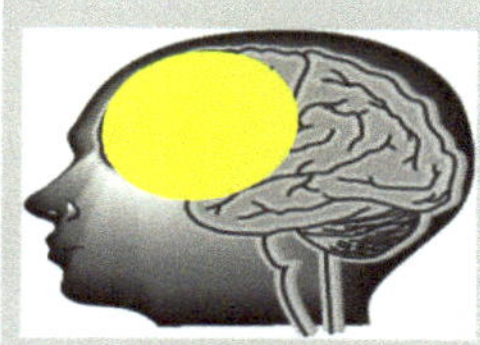
5.	Severe AD	Loss of motor functions, difficulty in performing daily activities, unaware of time and place, increased assistance and care, may result in death	Spreads to occipital lobe and widespread brain atrophy	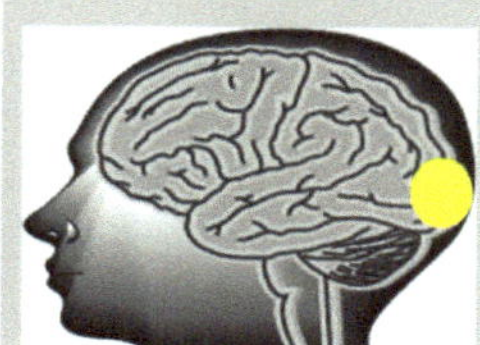

ability of tau protein is based on the controlled phosphorylation events. The tau phosphorylation is being regulated by Pi3K/AKT/GSK-3β signaling [18]. GSK-3β remains active and continuously phosphorylate tau protein and is inhibited by Pi3K/AKT signaling. Impaired Pi3K/AKT signals allow GSK-3β to over phosphorylate tau protein which makes them to lose the grip over microtubules and starts accumulating with the neurons, which are said to be NFTs. Overphosphorylation of tau protein due to increased GSK-3β activity have been reported in AD brains [19].

Increased deposits of Aβ and NFT formation have been reported to impair functional ability of neurons through various mechanisms. Aβ deposits attract more of glial cells around the periphery and trigger neuroinflammatory events, elevation in oxidative stress, mitochondrial dysfunction, and many more which ultimately results into neuronal death [20]. While tau made NFTs impair neuronal trafficking and do not allow transfer of nutrients, neurotransmitters within the cellular system. Both of these events impair the neuronal communication at first and slowly progress toward neuronal degeneration.

2.5 Lewy body dementia

LBD is the one of most common cause of dementia with 7.5% of all dementia cases in clinical population [21]. In general LBD is more prominent in males than in females and is observed above the age of 50 years. LBD is often called as an α-synucleinopathy characterized by abnormal deposits of α-synuclein [6]. In normal physiology α-synuclein helps in cell membrane remodeling at neuronal terminal. Accumulation of α-synuclein in neurons or surrounding glial cells forms the Lewy bodies resulting in neuronal cell death [22].

LBD is a broader term that includes both dementia with Lewy bodies and Parkinson's disease dementia. Lewy bodies are found in brain stem, subcortical, and cortical regions. LBD is a progressive disease, symptoms starts slowly and worsen over time with the progression of age. Lewy body deposits affect neurochemicals whose changes, in turn, can lead to problems with thinking, mood, movement, and behavior. LBD shows early symptoms like rapid eye movement sleep behavior disorder that remains undiagnosed. The stages 1 and 2 show autonomic and olfactory dysfunction, stages 3 and 4 show sleep and motor disturbances, while stages 5 and 6 show emotional and cognitive dysfunctioning. In later stages, people suffering with LBD are completely dependent on others for assistance and care [21,23]. The pathology of LBD is not yet clear and needs extensive research for early diagnosis and prevention of this form of dementia. Thus, further understanding of its etiopathogenesis may help in its early diagnosis and prevention.

2.6 Etiopathogenesis

The α-synuclein neuronal deposits are the major hallmarks of LBD. The misfolded and overexpressed α-synuclein starts accumulating in the dorsal IX and X motor nucleus/adjoining intermediate reticular zone [24]. These inclusions then spreads to brain stem (substantia nigra and basal ganglia) also activate surrounded glial cells leading to gliosis, and further extends to limbic system and neocortex. The increased Lewy body neurites lead to neuronal loss, gliosis in different parts of brain such as substantia nigra pars-compacta, locus coeruleus, and nucleus basalis of Meynert. These alterations cause loss of dopaminergic neurons in basal ganglia and acetyl choline transferase in cerebral cortex. The studies also showed the presence of NFTs in the LBD brain. While the density of NFTs in LBD brain is lesser than AD brain [25,26].

Genetic mutations in certain genes, that is, synuclein alpha (SNCA), leucine-rich repeat kinase-2 (LRRK-2) responsible for alteration in motor functioning while mutations in glucocerebrosidase gene and association of SNCA and SCARB-2 gene and increased expression of APOE4 gene produces AD like memory and cognitive deficits [27]. Other genetic alterations are observed in microtubule-associated protein tau (MAPT), scavenger receptor class B member 2, and apolipoproteins [21,28] (Fig. 2.1).

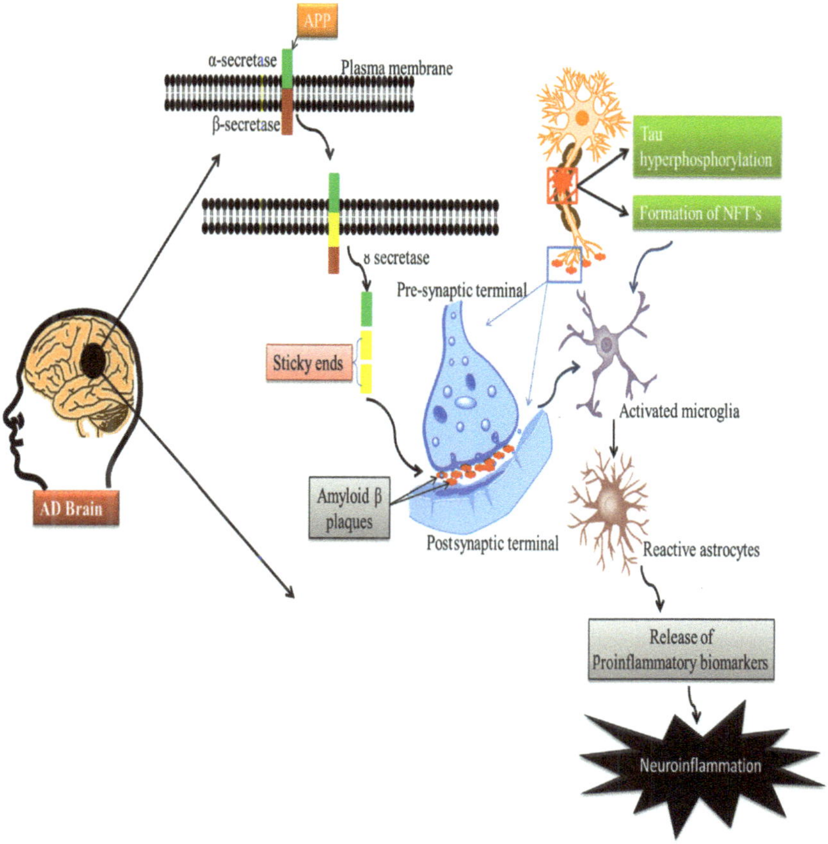

FIG. 2.1 Etiopathogenesis of AD. APP a transmembrane protein when cleaved with alpha secretase and beta secretase produces soluble fragments and are further degraded and cleared by various enzymes. Under pathological conditions such as in AD brain, APP when cleaved with the beta secretase and gamma secretase produces sticky ends which are more prone to the plaque formation. These plaques when gets deposited in the synapse interferes with the signal transmission and synaptic plasticity. Simultaneously tau a microtubular protein when gets aggregated intracellularly. These events further activates microglia and astrocytes becomes reactive which further releases proinflammatory cytokines and causes neuroinflammation.

Apart from this, LBD is also associated with the loss of certain neurons and neurotransmitters such as acetylcholine and dopamine [29]. Acetylcholine plays an important role in learning and memory, while dopamine plays an important role in movement, sleep, and behavior functions. Thus LBD affects brain regions controlling both cognitive and motor functions. LBD is characterized by bradykinesia, tremors, rigidity, progressive dementia with often extrapyramidal signs, hallucinations, and sometimes loss of visual and auditory functions as depicted in Fig. 2.2 [30,31]. LBD is linked to cognitive deficit associated with motor disabilities.

The current available treatments only provide symptomatic relief but no complete cure [29,9]. Here we have enlisted the current treatments available enlisted with their mechanisms in Table 2.3 and those under clinical investigations in Fig. 2.5 that could help the readers or researchers for deeper and easy understanding of the LBD.

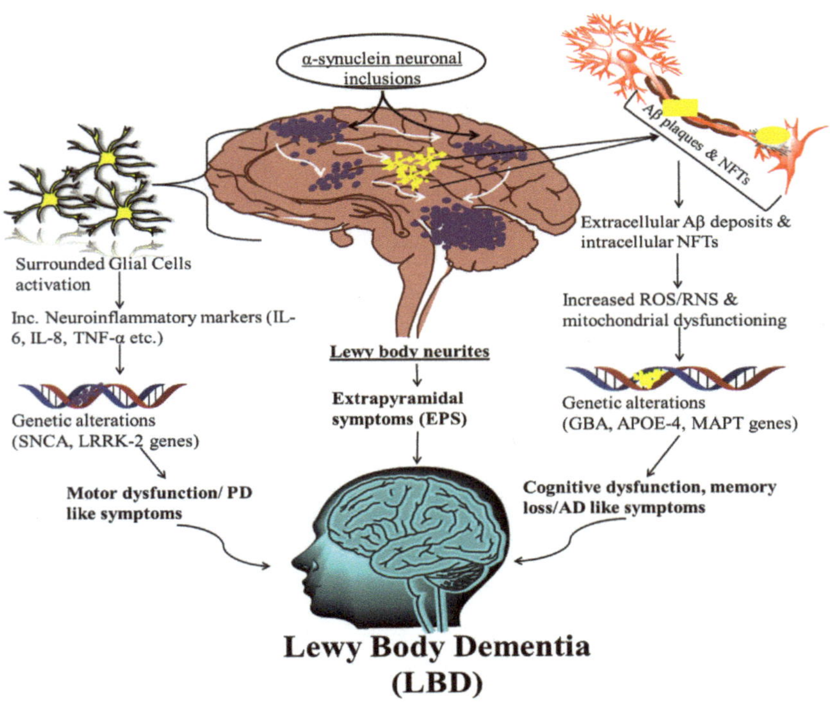

FIG. 2.2 Etiopathogenesis of Lewy body dementia. The alpha synuclein neuronal inclusions, Lewy body neurites, extracellular amyloid beta, and intracellular neurofibrillary tangle deposition causes glial cell activation, increases levels of neuroinflammatory markers, causes genetic alterations in synuclein alpha (SNCA), leucine-rich repeat kinase-2 (LRRK-2), glucosylceramidase beta (GBA), apolipoprotein E (APOE-4), and microtubule-associated protein tau (MAPT) genes responsible for extrapyramidal symptoms (EPS), motor and cognitive deficits.

TABLE 2.3 Types of FTD with their symptoms.

S. no.	Types of FTD	Symptoms
1.	Behavioral-variant frontotemporal dementia (BV-FTD)	• Inappropriate behavioral • Apathy • Loss of empathy • Stereotypical, compulsive behavior • Dietary changes • Executive deficits with relative sparing of visuospatial skills and memory
2.	Primary progressive aphasia (PPA)	• Prominent language impairment • Language deficits impair daily functioning
2a	Semantic-variant primary progressive aphasia (SVPPA)	• Aphasia is the most prominent • Impaired confrontation naming • Impaired single-word comprehension At least *three:*
2b	Nonfluent variant primary progressive aphasia (NFPPA)	• Impaired object knowledge • Surface dyslexia or dysgraphia • Spared repetition • Spared speech production *At least one:* • Agrammatism in production • Apraxia of speech *At least two:* • Impaired comprehension of complex sentences • Spared single-word comprehension • Spared object knowledge

2.7 Vascular dementia

VaD is the second most common type of dementia after AD plaguing geriatric population with 20% suffers [32] also with higher mortality rate and slow rate of progression when compared to AD [4,33]. VaD is the consequence of mainly cardiovascular disorders that abolish the blood supply of brain, depriving the neurons with nutrients which ultimately results to neuronal cell death or shrinking of neurons [34,35]. The major sign and symptoms of VaD comprised of memory impairment, difficulty in performing simple tasks, misplacing items, hallucinations, difficulty in reading and writing, changes in personality, behavior, mood, agitation, etc. [36]. There are numerous risk factors or etiological factors which contribute to the progression of VaD, some of them are age, coronary artery disease, high dietary saturated fat intake and cholesterol intake, head trauma, midlife diabetes mellitus, midlife hypertension, obesity, arteriosclerosis, smoking, etc. [37,38]. According to the Canadian Study of Health, age-standardized prevalence estimates for VaD ranged from 0.6% in 65–74 year olds to 4.8% in those over the age of 85 years. The annual incidence of VaD was estimated to be 2.5–3.8 cases per thousand. It is estimated that VaD accounts for 15–20% of dementia cases in Europe and North America, with the number closer to 30% in Asia and emerging countries [37] (Fig. 2.3).

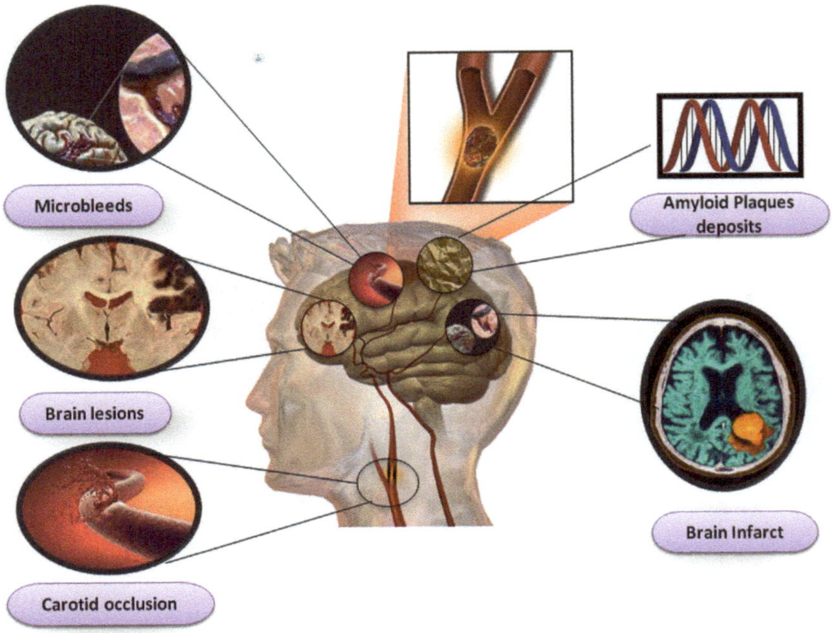

FIG. 2.3 Etiopathogenesis of vascular dementia. Various pathological alterations of VaD. Microbleeds, brain leisons, carotid occlusion, Aβ plaque deposits, and brain infarcts are the major hallmarks of AD.

2.8 Etiopathogenesis

There are pathological alterations in the brain that got triggered by various etiological factors. The idea of Tomlinson and colleagues [39] was re proposed by Hachinski and colleagues [40] who proposed that the VaD is caused in those patients who experience vascular risk factors such as cardiac disorders like hypertension, stroke, diabetes mellitus, obesity, etc. Till now there is no specific pathological criteria for the development of VaD but it is a lifestyle-based consequence which develop cerebral lesions, infraction, white matter lesions and collectively these contribute to the cognitive decline and other associated major symptoms.

Cerebral blood supply is important for the functioning and working of brain, and it is not at all surprising that blockade in the cerebral blood supply can lead to brain dysfunctioning. Any type of vascular alterations such as reduced cerebral perfusion due to cardiac arrest, cardiac failure, hypotension, arrhythmia, and atherosclerosis impair the cognition may be temporary or permanently depending on the extent and duration. Any occlusion of carotid arteries can lead to ischemic condition [41] which further cause the shortage of blood supply causing the neuronal cells to shrink and ultimately contributes to the symptoms of VaD [42].

There are some other linked alteration in vessels like leukoaraiosis and lacunar infarcts. Leukoaraiosis is a condition of white matter infarcts caused by perfusion disturbances while lacunar infarcts are small infarcts (2–20 mm in diameter) in the deep cerebral white matter, basal ganglia, or pons, results from the occlusion of small perforating artery supplying the subcortical areas of the brain. Both of these lesions of brain are strongly associated with cardiovascular risk factors, especially hypertension, diabetes, hyperlipidemia, and smoking. The white matter lesions or infarcts lead to vacuolation, demyelination, axonal loss leading to VaD [43].

Oxidative stress due to lifestyle or environmental factors cause an imbalance between ROS and endogenous antioxidants which further activated microglia and cause hypoperfusion via hypoxia, inflammatory reactions further aggravates the blood–brain barrier breakdown contributing to microvascular occlusion [44].

Amyloid plaques are well-known hallmark of AD but to lesser extent cerebral amyloid deposits are observed in elder age that are more prone to smoking or cardiovascular disorders [45]. Cerebral amyloid deposits are the main cause of microbleeds and large hemorrhages which both are responsible for the vascular type of dementia. White matter and gray matter infarcts, lesions, microbleeds, hemorrhage, blood–brain barrier permeability, oxidative stress, inflammation, etc. all cumulatively affect the neuronal plasticity, decline the glucose utilization, cerebral atrophy, neuronal cell shrinking, myelin damage ultimately contributes to major symptoms that are associated with VaD discussed in Fig. 2.2.

2.9 Frontotemporal dementia

The first case of FTD was observed in 1892 by Arnold Pick [46]. FTD is a heterogeneous neurodegenerative disorder characterized by alterations mainly in behavior, language, and motor coordination by severe atrophy of the frontal and temporal lobes. FTD is a genetic disorder affecting approximately 25–50% of people who experience family history [47]. Below 60 years, FTD is most prevalent and common type of dementia but it is rare with an estimated lifetime risk of 1 in 742. FTD can develop as early as the second decade of life, with 13% of cases occurring before the age of 60. Instances with earlier onset are more likely to have behavioral variant FTD (bvFTD), while cases with late onset are more likely to have nonfluent variant primary progressive aphasia syndrome. FTD advances faster than AD in general [48]. Although the prevalence of FTD is generally thought to be highest in the age groups 45–64 years, other population-based studies have found a higher prevalence and incidence of bvFTD in the elderly than previously thought, implying that bvFTD is more prevalent, in the senior population, it is relatively undiagnosed [49]. The main sign and symptoms of FTD are lack of judgment, apathy, loss of empathy, inappropriate social behavior, etc., and the rest symptoms depends on the further classification of FTD discussed in Table 2.2.

2.10 Etiopathogenesis

The pathogenesis of FTD is further classified into transactivation response DNA-binding protein 43 kDa (TDP-43), fused in sarcoma (FUS) and tau. Tau is found in neurons and have a physiological function in dendrites, in FTD these tau proteins get hyperphosphorylated and forms insoluble filamentous misfolded protein aggregates [50]. There are six different isoforms of tau generated from single gene, that is, MAPT gene. Genetic mutation in MAPT causes the splicing and decrease the microtubules binding affinity of tau and thus hyperphosphorylation elevates the detachment of tau and ultimately potentiate the cytoplasmic insoluble aggregates of tau [51].

TDP-43 accumulates in 50% population of FTD was discovered in 2006 and believed to be the most frequent pathological alterations in development of FTD. TDP-43 creates a strong link between FTD and amyotrophic lateral sclerosis (ALS). TARDBP gene on chromosome 1 encodes for the TDP-43 which is a 414 amino acid chain. It is ubiquitous ribonucleoprotein which helps for the RNA maintenance and its processing while RNA splicing and maintain the level of intron which are crucial for neuronal activity [52]. In pathological condition, the normal localization of TDP-43 gets disturbed and the affected neurons and glial cells experience the cytoplasmic aggregates leads to nuclear clearance. In the cortex and hippocampus there is accumulation of the full length phosphorylated C-terminal fragments of TDP-43 predominates which is the main and ultimate cause of FTD [53].

As like of TDP-43 remain a genetic factor of FTD, FUS is also a DNA/RNA-binding protein present in 5–10% cases of FTD and 4% of ALS again creating a link between FTD and ALS [47]. FUS is a 526 amino acid, ubiquitously expressed ribonucleoprotein and belongs to the FET (FUS, EWS; Ewing sarcoma protein, TAF-15; TATA-binding protein-associated factor 15). Being similar to TDP-43 functionally, FUS is linked with transcriptional repression, splicing regulation, and micro-RNA processing. In the pathological state, the FUS depletion is linked with MAPT gene mutation leading to longer tau isoforms [54]. FUS is localized in nucleus of healthy brain while in pathological state the cytoplasmic aggregates of FUS predominate causing loss of nuclear protein [55]. The above discussed pathologies are the major hallmarks in the development of FTD in Fig. 2.4.

2.11 Current treatments and drugs under clinical investigations

Treatment of dementia depends on its cause. Early detection of symptoms of dementia is thus important, as some causes can be treated [24]. However, in many cases, the cause of dementia is unknown or remained untreated. Treatment of dementia is a matter of debate as the exact cause of dementia is unknown. Various scientist associations are working hard to develop some treatment by considering the pathogenesis and cause of same but till now there are few drugs

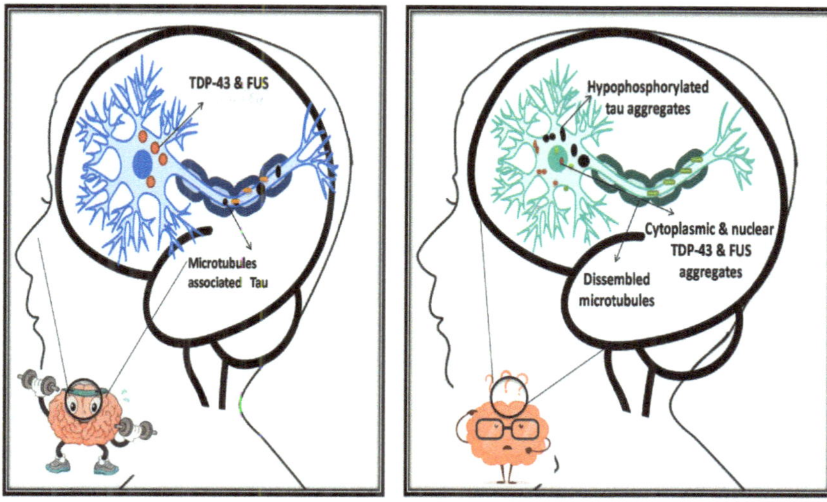

FIG. 2.4 Etiopathogenesis of frontotemporal dementia. The three main types of FTD pathology are characterized by the accumulation of distinct protein aggregates, TDP-43. (b) FUS are primarily found in the nucleus, where they are involved in several steps of RNA metabolism but on abnormal working form cytoplasmic accumulation and following aggregation and (c) tau hyperphosphorylation where the protein is dissociated from microtubules and accumulates into pathogenic tangles in the cytoplasm.

which provide symptomatic relief and are discussed below [56]. Based on the type of symptoms and diagnosis, different treatments are available in the market for each dementia discussed below.

1. *Alzheimer's disease*: There are few drugs available in the market which provides symptomatic relief for AD pathologies varying from mild to moderate or moderate to severe AD stages as enlisted in Table 2.4. Tacrine was the first approved drug for mild to moderate AD symptoms but now banned due to liver toxicity [57]. Recently, US FDA has approved Biogen's Aducanumab in 2021, a monoclonal antibody for the treatment of mild to moderate AD [58,59]. It acts by tagging and clearing the amyloid plaques. But still there is no complete cure for the disease thus searches for the newer therapeutics are still underway as given in Fig. 2.5.
2. *Lewy body dementia*: The available treatments for the LBD are mentioned in Table 2.4 and the drugs under clinical investigation are enlisted in Fig. 2.5.
3. *Vascular dementia*: Available symptomatic treatments for VaD are given in Table 2.4 and agents currently under clinical trials for VaD (Fig. 2.5).
4. *Frontotemporal dementia*: Agents currently under clinical trials for FTD are given in Fig. 2.5.

TABLE 2.4 Available treatments for major dementia types.

Dementia type	Drug	Brand name	Class	MOA
Alzheimer's disease (AD)	Donepezil	Aricept	Acetylcholinesterase inhibitors (AChEI)	Inhibits acetylcholinesterase-mediated breakdown of ACh.
	Galantamine	Razadyne ER	AChEI	Inhibits breakdown of ACh and also simulate nicotinic receptor for ACh release.
	Rivastigmine	Exelon	AChEI	Inhibits breakdown of both acetylcholine and butrylcholine.
	Tacrine	Cognex	AChEI	Reversible inhibition of AChE.
	Memantine	Mamenda	NMDA antagonist	Decreases the glutamate-mediated neurotoxicity by blocking NMDA receptors.
	Aducanumab	Aduhelm	Monoclonal antibody	Targets and remove the toxic Aβ plaques.
	Ibuprofen	Advil	NSAIDs	Decreases Aβ plaque-mediated neuroinflammation.
	Nitric oxide flurbiprofen (NFP)	Ocufen	NSAIDs	Decreases Aβ plaque-mediated neuroinflammation.
Lewy body dementia (LBD)	Donepezil	Aricept	Acetylcholinesterase inhibitors (AChEI)	Inhibits acetylcholinesterase-mediated breakdown of ACh.
	Galantamine	Razadyne ER	AChEI	Inhibits breakdown of ACh and also simulate nicotinic receptor for ACh release.
	Rivastigmine	Exelon	AChEI	Inhibits breakdown of both acetylcholine and butrylcholine.
	Memantine	Mamenda	NMDA antagonist	Decreases the glutamate-mediated neurotoxicity by blocking NMDA receptors.

Dementia type	Drug	Brand name	Class	MOA
	Aducanumab	Aduhelm	Monoclonal antibody	Targets and remove the toxic Aβ plaques.
	Carbidopa-levodopa	Sinemet, Rytary, Duopa	Decarboxylase inhibitors	Increases dopamine levels and improves PD like symptoms.
	Quetiapine	Seroquel	Antipsychotic	Improves both depressive and manic symptoms.
	Clozapine	Clozaril, Versacloz	Antipsychotic	Blocks D2 and D4 receptors and produces antipsychotic actions.
	Pimavanserin	Nuplazid	Antipsychotic	Improvement of PD like psychosis via inverse agonism of serotonin receptor.
	Clonazepam	Klonopin	Anticonvulsant	Modulation of GABA function and prevention of seizure attacks.
	Melatonin	Meloprax	Hyponotics	For insomnia.
Vascular dementia (VaD)	Memantine	Mamenda	NMDA antagonist	Decreases the glutamate-mediated neurotoxicity by blocking NMDA receptors.
	Donepezil	Aricept	Acetylcholinesterase inhibitors (AChEI)	Inhibits acetylcholinesterase-mediated breakdown of ACh.

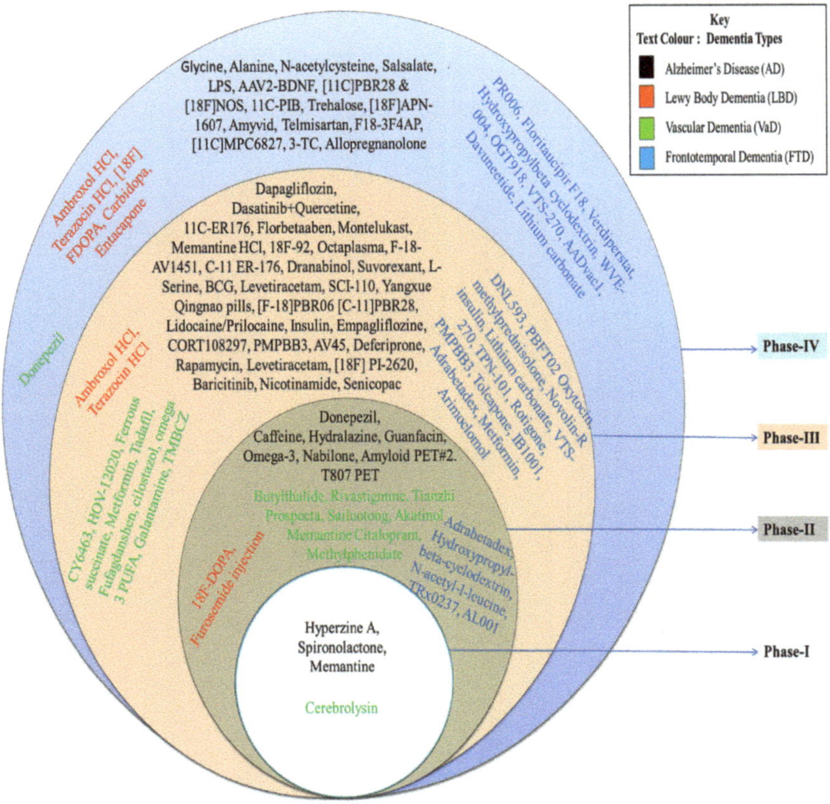

FIG. 2.5 Drugs under clinical investigation for different dementia types.

2.12 Conclusion

Dementia is the seventh leading cause of death without any specific known etiopathologies. The current chapter summarizes the types, prevalence, etiopathologies, and treatments for the varying types of dementia. The diagnosis and treatments vary with the cause and type of dementia. The current available treatments only provide symptomatic management of dementia; however, a wide number of therapeutics are still under clinical investigation for dementia. A few of them are enlisted here with their targets and treatment approaches. This book chapter will help the readers and researchers working in different fields to understand the etiopathologies and targets for treatments for further research.

References

[1] Ravindranath V, Sundarakumar JS. Changing demography and the challenge of dementia in India. Nat Rev Neurol 2021;17:747–58. https://doi.org/10.1038/s41582-021-00565-x.

[2] Nichols E, Steinmetz JD, Vollset SE, Fukutaki K, Chalek J, Abd-Allah F, Abdoli A, Abu-alhasan A, Abu-Gharbieh E, Akram TT, Al Hamad H, Alahdab F, Alanezi FM, Alipour V, Almustanyir S, Amu H, Ansari I, Arabloo J, Ashraf T, Astell-Burt T, Ayano G, Ayuso-Mateos JL, Baig AA, Barnett A, Barrow A, Baune BT, Béjot Y, Bezabhe WMM, Bezabih YM, Bhagavathula AS, Bhaskar S, Bhattacharyya K, Bijani A, Biswas A, Bolla SR, Boloor A, Brayne C, Brenner H, Burkart K, Burns RA, Cámera LA, Cao C, Carvalho F, Castro-de-Araujo LFS, Catalá-López F, Cerin E, Chavan PP, Cherbuin N, Chu DT, Costa VM, Couto RAS, Dadras O, Dai X, Dandona L, Dandona R, De la Cruz-Góngora V, Dhamnetiya D, Dias da Silva D, Diaz D, Douiri A, Edvardsson D, Ekholuenetale M, El Sayed I, El-Jaafary SI, Eskandari K, Eskandarieh S, Esmaeilnejad S, Fares J, Faro A, Farooque U, Feigin VL, Feng X, Fereshtehnejad SM, Fernandes E, Ferrara P, Filip I, Fillit H, Fischer F, Gaidhane S, Galluzzo L, Ghashghaee A, Ghith N, Gialluisi A, Gilani SA, Glavan IR, Gnedovskaya EV, Golechha M, Gupta R, Gupta VB, Gupta VK, Haider MR, Hall BJ, Hamidi S, Hanif A, Hankey GJ, Haque S, Hartono RK, Hasaballah AI, Hasan MT, Hassan A, Hay SI, Hayat K, Hegazy MI, Heidari G, Heidari-Soureshjani R, Herteliu C, Househ M, Hussain R, Hwang BF, Iacoviello L, Iavicoli I, Ilesanmi OS, Ilic IM, Ilic MD, Irvani SSN, Iso H, Iwagami M, Jabbarinejad R, Jacob L, Jain V, Jayapal SK, Jayawardena R, Jha RP, Jonas JB, Joseph N, Kalani R, Kandel A, Kandel H, Karch A, Kasa AS, Kassie GM, Keshavarz P, Khan MA, Khatib MN, Khoja TAM, Khubchandani J, Kim MS, Kim YJ, Kisa A, Kisa S, Kivimäki M, Koroshetz WJ, Koyanagi A, Kumar GA, Kumar M, Lak HM, Leonardi M, Li B, Lim SS, Liu X, Liu Y, Logroscino G, Lorkowski S, Lucchetti G, Lutzky Saute R, Magnani FG, Malik AA, Massano J, Mehndiratta MM, Menezes RG, Meretoja A, Mohajer B, Mohamed Ibrahim N, Mohammad Y, Mohammed A, Mokdad AH, Mondello S, Moni MAA, Moniruzzaman M, Mossie TB, Nagel G, Naveed M, Nayak VC, Neupane Kandel S, Nguyen TH, Oancea B, Otstavnov N, Otstavnov SS, Owolabi MO, Panda-Jonas S, Pashazadeh Kan F, Pasovic M, Patel UK, Pathak M, Peres MFP, Perianayagam A, Peterson CB, Phillips MR, Pinheiro M, Piradov MA, Pond CD, Potashman MH, Pottoo FH, Prada SI, Radfar A, Raggi A, Rahim F, Rahman M, Ram P, Ranasinghe P, Rawaf DL, Rawaf S, Rezaei N, Rezapour A, Robinson SR, Romoli M, Roshandel G, Sahathevan R, Sahebkar A, Sahraian MA, Sathian B, Sattin D, Sawhney M, Saylan M, Schiavolin S, Seylani A, Sha F, Shaikh MA, Shaji KS, Shannawaz M, Shetty JK, Shigematsu M, Shin JIl, Shiri R, Silva DAS, Silva JP, Silva R, Singh JA, Skryabin VY, Skryabina AA, Smith AE, Soshnikov S, Spurlock EE, Stein DJ, Sun J, Tabarés-Seisdedos R, Thakur B, Timalsina B, Tovani-Palone MR, Tran BX, Tsegaye GW, Valadan Tahbaz S, Valdez PR, Venketasubramanian N, Vlassov V, Vu GT, Vu LG, Wang YP, Wimo A, Winkler AS, Yadav L, Yahyazadeh Jabbari SH, Yamagishi K, Yang L, Yano Y, Yonemoto N, Yu C, Yunusa I, Zadey S, Zastrozhin MS, Zastrozhina A, Zhang ZJ, Murray CJL, Vos T. Estimation of the global prevalence of dementia in 2019 and forecasted prevalence in 2050: an analysis for the Global Burden of Disease Study 2019. Lancet Public Heal 2022;7:e105–25. https://doi.org/10.1016/S2468-2667(21)00249-8.

[3] Cao Q, Tan C-C, Xu W, Hu H, Cao X-P, Dong Q, Tan L, Yu J-T. The prevalence of dementia: a systematic review and meta-analysis. J Alzheimer's Dis 2020;73:1157–66.

[4] Inzitari M, Inzitari D. Vascular dementia. Pathy's Princ Pract Geriatr Med 2022;2:811–21.

[5] Ruano L, Araújo N, Branco M, Barreto R, Moreira S, Pais R, Cruz VT, Lunet N, Barros H. Prevalence and causes of cognitive impairment and dementia in a population-based cohort from Northern Portugal. Am J Alzheimers Dis Other Demen 2019;34:49–56. https://doi.org/10.1177/1533317518813550.

[6] Taylor JP, McKeith IG, Burn DJ, Boeve BF, Weintraub D, Bamford C, Allan LM, Thomas AJ, O'Brien JT. New evidence on the management of Lewy body dementia. Lancet Neurol 2020;19:157–69. https://doi.org/10.1016/S1474-4422(19)30153-X.

[7] Dementia PM. Dementia 2. Gerontologist 2016;56:536. https://doi.org/10.1093/geront/gnw162.2164.

[8] Gnanalingham KK, Byrne EJ, Thornton A, Sambrook MA, Bannister P. Motor and cognitive function in Lewy body dementia: comparison with Alzheimer's and Parkinson's diseases. J Neurol Neurosurg Psychiatry 1997;62:243–52. https://doi.org/10.1136/jnnp.62.3.243.

[9] Watts KE, Storr NJ, Barr PG, Rajkumar AP. Systematic review of pharmacological interventions for people with Lewy body dementia. Aging Ment Heal 2022;0:1–14. https://doi.org/10.1080/13607863.2022.2032601.

[10] Frozza RL, Lourenco MV, de Felice FG. Challenges for Alzheimer's disease therapy: insights from novel mechanisms beyond memory defects. Front Neurosci 2018;12:1–13. https://doi.org/10.3389/fnins.2018.00037.

[11] Kvartsberg H, Lashley T, Murray CE, Brinkmalm G, Cullen NC, Höglund K, Zetterberg H, Blennow K, Portelius E. The intact postsynaptic protein neurogranin is reduced in brain tissue from patients with familial and sporadic Alzheimer's disease. Acta Neuropathol 2019;137:89–102. https://doi.org/10.1007/s00401-018-1910-3.

[12] Assefa BT, Gebre AK, Altaye BM. Reactive astrocytes as drug target in Alzheimer's disease. Biomed Res Int 2018;2018:8–12.

[13] Wilson H, Pagano G, Politis M. Dementia spectrum disorders: lessons learnt from decades with PET research. J Neural Transm 2019;126:233–51. https://doi.org/10.1007/s00702-019-01975-4.

[14] Raskin J, Cummings J, Hardy J, Schuh K, Dean R. Neurobiology of Alzheimer's disease: integrated molecular, physiological, anatomical, biomarker, and cognitive dimensions. Curr Alzheimer Res 2015;12:712–22. https://doi.org/10.2174/1567205012666150701103107.

[15] Bjørklund G, Aaseth J, Dadar M, Chirumbolo S. Molecular targets in Alzheimer's disease. Mol Neurobiol 2019;56:7032–44.

[16] Baranello RJ, Bharani KL, Padmaraju V, Chopra N, Lahiri DK, Greig NH, Pappolla MA, Sambamurti K. Amyloid-beta protein clearance and degradation (ABCD) pathways and their role in Alzheimer's disease. Curr Alzheimer Res 2015;12:32–46. https://doi.org/10.2174/1567205012666141218140953.

[17] Koudinova NV, Koudinov AR, Berezov TT. Amyloid beta: functional protein or biological junk?. Biochem Suppl Ser B Biomed Chem 2007;1:185–91.

[18] Lloret A, Fuchsberger T, Giraldo E, Vina J. Molecular mechanisms linking amyloid β toxicity and Tau hyperphosphorylation in Alzheimer' s disease. Free Radic Biol Med 2015;83:186–91.

[19] Weller J, Budson A. Current understanding of Alzheimer's disease diagnosis and treatment. F1000Research 2018;7:1161. https://doi.org/10.12688/f1000research.14506.1.

[20] Sharma C, Kim S, Nam Y, Jung UJ, Kim SR. Mitochondrial dysfunction as a driver of cognitive impairment in Alzheimer's disease. Int J Mol Sci 2021;22:4850. https://doi.org/10.3390/ijms22094850.

[21] Menšíková K, Matěj R, Colosimo C, Rosales R, Tučková L, Ehrmann J, Hraboš D, Kolaříková K, Vodička R, Vrtěl R, Procházka M, Nevrlý M, Kaiserová M, Kurčová S, Otruba P, Kaňovský P. Lewy body disease or diseases with Lewy bodies? NPJ Park Dis 2022;8:1–11. https://doi.org/10.1038/s41531-021-00273-9.

[22] Walker Z, Possin KL, Boeve BF, Aarsland D. Lewy body dementias. Lancet 2015;386:1683–97. https://doi.org/10.1016/S0140-6736(15)00462-6.

[23] Sanford AM. Lewy body dementia. Clin Geriatr Med 2018;34:603–15. https://doi.org/10.1016/j.cger.2018.06.007.

[24] Kane JPM, Surendranathan A, Bentley A, Barker SAH, Taylor JP, Thomas AJ, Allan LM, McNally RJ, James PW, McKeith IG, Burn DJ, O'Brien JT. Clinical prevalence of Lewy body dementia. Alzheimer's Res Ther 2018.;10:1–8 https://doi.org/10.1186/s13195-018-0350-6.

[25] Chan KY, Wu JJ, Liu L, Theodoratou E, Car J, Middleton L, Russ TC, Deary IJ, Campbell H, Wang W, Rudan I. Epidemiology of Alzheimer's disease and other forms of dementia in China, 1990-2010: a systematic review and analysis. Lancet 2013;381:2016–23. https://doi.org/10.1016/S0140-6736(13)60221-4.

[26] Perry RH, Irving D, Blessed G, Fairbairn A, Perry EK. Senile dementia of Lewy body type. A clinically and neuropathologically distinct form of Lewy body dementia in the elderly. J Neurol Sci 1990;95:119–39. https://doi.org/10.1016/0022-510X(90)90236-G.

[27] Gibb WRG, Esiri MM, Lees AJ. Clinical and pathological features of diffuse cortical Lewy body disease (Lewy body dementia). Brain 1987;110:1131–53. https://doi.org/10.1093/brain/110.5.1131.

[28] Ballard C, Ziabreva I, Perry R, Larsen JP, O'Brien J, McKeith I, Perry E, Aarsland D. Differences in neuropathologic characteristics across the Lewy body dementia spectrum. Neurology 2006;67:1931–4. https://doi.org/10.1212/01.wnl.0000249130.63615.cc.

[29] Gan J, Liu S, Wang X, Shi Z, Shen L, Li X, Guo Q, Yuan J, Zhang N, You Y. Clinical characteristics of Lewy body dementia in Chinese memory clinics. BMC Neurol 2021;21:1–11.

[30] Howard E, Irwin DJ, Rascovsky K, Nevler N, Shellikeri S, Tropea TF, Spindler M, Deik A, Chen-Plotkin A, Siderowf A. Cognitive profile and markers of Alzheimer disease–type pathology in patients with Lewy body dementias. Neurology 2021;96:e1855–64.

[31] Milán-Tomás Á, Fernández-Matarrubia M, Rodríguez-Oroz MC. Lewy body dementias: a coin with two sides. Behav Sci (Basel) 2021;11:94.

[32] Akhter F, Persaud A, Zaokari Y, Zhao Z, Zhu D. Vascular dementia and underlying sex differences. Front Aging Neurosci 2021;583:08.

[33] Gallaway PJ, Miyake H, Buchowski MS, Shimada M, Yoshitake Y, Kim AS, Hongu N. Physical activity: a viable way to reduce the risks of mild cognitive impairment, Alzheimer's disease, and vascular dementia in older adults. Brain Sci 2017;7:22.

[34] Calabrese V, Giordano J, Signorile A, Laura Ontario M, Castorina S, De Pasquale C, Eckert G, Calabrese EJ. Major pathogenic mechanisms in vascular dementia: roles of cellular stress response and hormesis in neuroprotection. J Neurosci Res 2016;94:1588–603.

[35] Tian D, Gao Q, Chang Z, Lin J, Ma D, Han Z. Network pharmacology and in vitro studies reveal the pharmacological effects and molecular mechanisms of Shenzhi Jiannao prescription against vascular dementia. BMC Complement Med Ther 2022;22:1–18.

[36] Budson AE, Solomon PR. Memory loss, Alzheimer's disease, and dementia-E-book: a practical guide for clinicians. Philadelphia: Elsevier Health Sciences; 2021.

[37] Bir SC, Khan MW, Javalkar V, Toledo EG, Kelley RE. Emerging concepts in vascular dementia: a review. J Stroke Cerebrovasc Dis 2021;30:105864.

[38] Wichansawakun S, Chupisanyarote K, Wongpipathpong W, Kaur G, Buttar HS. Antioxidant diets and functional foods attenuate dementia and cognition in elderly subjects. Funct Foods Nutraceut Metab Non-Commun Dis 2022;1:533–49.

[39] Tomlinson BE, Blessed G, Roth M. Observations on the brains of demented old people. J Neurol Sci 1970;11:205–42.

[40] Hachinski VC, Lassen NA, Marshall J. Multi-infarct dementia: a cause of mental deterioration in the elderly. Lancet 1974;304:207–9.

[41] Parsi MM, Duval C, Ariëns RAS. Vascular dementia and crosstalk between the complement and coagulation systems. Front Cardiovasc Med 2021;8:803169.

[42] Tiwari N, Upadhyay J, Ansari MN, Raza SS, Ahmad W, Ansari MA. Experimental rodent models of vascular dementia: a systematic review. CNS Neurol Disord Targets (Formerly Curr Drug Targets-CNS Neurol Disord 2021;20:657–72.

[43] Lecordier S, Manrique-Castano D, El Moghrabi Y, ElAli A. Neurovascular alterations in vascular dementia: emphasis on risk factors. Front Aging Neurosci 2021;13:556.

[44] Rajeev V, Fann DY, Dinh QN, Kim HA, De Silva TM, Lai MKP, Chen CL-H, Drummond GR, Sobey CG, Arumugam TV. Pathophysiology of blood brain barrier dysfunction during chronic cerebral hypoperfusion in vascular cognitive impairment. Theranostics 2022;12:1639.

[45] Charidimou A, Gang Q, Werring DJ. Sporadic cerebral amyloid angiopathy revisited: recent insights into pathophysiology and clinical spectrum. J Neurol Neurosurg Psychiatry 2012;83:124–37.

[46] Pick A. Uber die Beziehungen der senilen Hirnatrophie zur Aphasie. Prag Med Wochenschr 1892;17:165–7.

[47] Hock E, Polymenidou M. Prion-like propagation as a pathogenic principle in frontotemporal dementia. J Neurochem 2016;138:163–83.

[48] Kramer AO, Alioto AG, Kramer JH. Neurodegenerative conditions. In: Wiley encyclopedia healing psychology. USA: Wiley Online Books; 2020. https://doi.org/10.1002/9781119057840.ch25.

[49] Balachandran S, Matlock EL, Conroy ML, Lane CE. Behavioral variant frontotemporal dementia: diagnosis and treatment interventions. Curr Geriatr Rep 2021;10:1–7.

[50] Riku Y, Seilhean D, Duyckaerts C, Boluda S, Iguchi Y, Ishigaki S, Iwasaki Y, Yoshida M, Sobue G, Katsuno M. Pathway from TDP-43-related pathology to neuronal dysfunction in amyotrophic lateral sclerosis and frontotemporal lobar degeneration. Int J Mol Sci 2021;22:3843.

[51] Rademakers R, Cruts M, Van Broeckhoven C. The role of tau (MAPT) in frontotemporal dementia and related tauopathies. Hum Mutat 2004;24:277–95.

[52] Berning BA, Walker AK. The pathobiology of TDP-43 C-terminal fragments in ALS and FTLD. Front Neurosci 2019;13:335.

[53] de Boer EMJ, Orie VK, Williams T, Baker MR, De Oliveira HM, Polvikoski T, Silsby M, Menon P, van den Bos M, Halliday GM. TDP-43 proteinopathies: a new wave of neurodegenerative diseases. J Neurol Neurosurg Psychiatry 2021;92:86–95.

[54] Hofmann JW, Seeley WW, Huang EJ. RNA binding proteins and the pathogenesis of frontotemporal lobar degeneration. Annu Rev Pathol Mech Dis 2019;14:469–95.

[55] Nicolas G, Sévigny M, Lecoquierre F, Marguet F, Deschênes A, Del Pelaez MC, Feuillette S, Audebrand A, Lecourtois M, Rousseau S. A postzygotic de novo NCDN mutation identified in a sporadic FTLD patient results in neurochondrin haploinsufficiency and altered FUS granule dynamics. Acta Neuropathol Commun 2022;10:1–18.

[56] Hendriks S, Peetoom K, Bakker C, Van Der Flier WM, Papma JM, Koopmans R, Verhey FRJ, De Vugt M, Köhler S, Withall A. Global prevalence of young-onset dementia: a systematic review and meta-analysis. JAMA Neurol 2021;78:1080–90.

[57] Patocka J, Jun D, Kuca K. Possible role of hydroxylated metabolites of tacrine in drug toxicity and therapy of Alzheimer's disease. Curr Drug Metab 2008;9:332–5.

[58] Association A. 2020 Alzheimer's disease facts and figures. Alzheimer's Dement 2020;16:391–460.

[59] Padda IS, Parmar M. Aducanumab. In: StatPearls [Internet]. Treasure Island (FL): StatPearls Publishing; 2021. p. 1–12.

Chapter 3

Receptor attacking ligands for active targeting to brain

Tushar Kanti Rajwar, Biswakanth Kar, Goutam Ghosh, Goutam Rath
Department of Pharmaceutics, School of Pharmaceutical Sciences, Siksha 'O' Anusandhan (Deemed to be University), Bhubaneswar, Odisha, India

3.1 Introduction

Brain-related disorders are recognized as one of society's most increasingly high-risk disorders under neurological diseases. According to the global estimations, neurological diseases were the main contributors to "Disability-adjusted life-years (DALYs are defined as the sum of years lived with impairment due to a neurological disorder and healthy years lost due to premature mortality and disability)" almost 276 million, and fatalities almost 9 million worldwide in 2016. About 42.2% stroke, 16.2% migraine, 10.4% Alzheimer's diseases and other dementias, and 7.9% meningitis were the largest contributors to neurological DALYs [1,2].

The problem is uncontrollable because of the complex drug permeation issue over the "blood–brain barrier (BBB) to the brain parenchyma." Though few drugs with low molecular weight can pass across BBB, still it is a major issue. Various brain disorders including tumors, Alzheimer's disease, Parkinson's disease, dementia, epilepsy, mental disorder, stroke, transient ischemic attack, etc. are hard to treat for this problem. The BBB's restriction on the chemicals that flow past it is assumed to evolve as a natural defensive mechanism against poisons or diseases. The permeability of the BBB is controlled by tight junctions between capillary endothelial cells. Two main roadblocks for drug transport over the BBB are P-glycoprotein (P-gp) and breast cancer resistance protein, as their efflux pumps play a major role in the efflux of chemotherapeutic and other central nervous system (CNS)-acting medicines. A two transporters system has been developed for drug administration to circumvent the activity of efflux pumps in the brain. P-gp is an ATP-driven membrane transporter produced at the luminal membranes of brain capillary endothelial cells (BCECs) that perform two roles. First, it extrudes a range of substrates from the brain parenchyma. Second, it stops particular molecules from being taken up by endothelial cells on the luminal side. To control the entry and departure of tiny molecules,

Nanomedicine-Based Approaches for the Treatment of Dementia. https://doi.org/10.1016/B978-0-12-824331-2.00009-1
Copyright © 2023 Elsevier Inc. All rights reserved.

the BBB has distinct transcellular transport pathways/systems. Drugs can be transported to the brain by conjugating them with enzymatic components that assure the drug's functionality after it has passed through the digestive system. For example, glucose transporter 1 (GLUT1) transports 2-deoxyglucose, "large amino acid transporter 1 (LAT1)" transports L-DOPA, and monocarboxylate transporter 1 (MCT1) transports probenecid, among other things. Receptors play a major role and are commonly used to transport essential chemicals such as hormones over the BBB and can also transport therapeutic molecules across it. Therapeutic molecules like hormones and drugs can pass through it by various brain receptors, including, insulin receptors, transferrin receptors, folate receptors, lipoprotein receptors, interleukin receptors, etc. as they are overexpressed in various brain diseases. Furthermore, the BBB's unique trait of allowing the transcytosis of huge macromolecules for nutrition transfer is occasionally used to avoid the lysosomal pathway. The advantage of a receptor-mediated method is that it allows for a significant increase in the amount of drug or substance delivered across the BBB. Another benefit of this approach is its adaptability, it can be used to conjugate liposomes, polymer systems, or nanoparticles (NPs). Many receptors on the BBB are overexpressed, including "folate receptors, transferrin receptors (Tf), low-density receptors, growth receptors, choline receptors, insulin receptors, scavenger receptors, and diphtheria toxin receptors." These receptors can help ligand-conjugated nanocarriers pass through the BBB. Major reports have been found on brain cancer, moreover, other diseases like Alzheimer's disease, dementia, epilepsy, Parkinson's disease, etc. are also included. For example, folate receptor alpha (FRα, a subtype of folate receptor) has been reported as an overexpressed brain receptor, mainly in the case of brain glioma, which helps in folic acid transportation into the cells. Folic acid plays a role in developing and spreading cancer through its function in nucleotide production, giving methyl groups for DNA methylation in cell division, proliferation, and tumor suppression in malignant cells. Overexpression of FRα is associated with increased signaling of signal transducer and activator of transcription 3, a human transcription factor, implying that FRα may play a role in cancer cell malignancy transcriptional regulation is involved in cell cycle control. When activated in gliomas, FRα has a comparable effect—albeit on a scale 500 times that of noncancerous tissue receptors [3]. Similarly, transferrin (Tf) and transferrin receptors (TfR) have been extensively studied in terms of gliomas and their treatment because TfR overexpressed upon BCECs and tumor cells, by facilitating more Tf to cross BBB, and also could be used to target therapy. TfR1 (a subtype of transferrin receptor) promotes tumor growth and increases iron buildup in gliomas by increasing proliferation and glutamate synthesis. TfR1 is the most common iron-binding mechanism in most cells, but various investigations have shown that iron intake varies by cell type. If TfRs cannot bind to Tf and carry iron into cells, iron transport throughout the body is impaired if they are defective. This will lead to anemia and iron shortage in the body, etc. [4].

To overcome these transportation challenges across BBB, several physical, physiological, and pharmacological approaches have been evolved. The physiological approaches of transport across BBB are the most applicable and widely accepted. Different types of approaches are used to bypass the BBB to supply therapeutics inside it, including invasive (intracerebral injection or implants, intracerebroventricular infusion, convection-enhanced delivery, BBB disruption, etc.), noninvasive (chemical and colloidal techniques, etc.), and miscellaneous (intranasal delivery) techniques. Invasive methods are expensive, necessitate anesthesia and hospitalization, and are not patient friendly. These methods may aid tumor dispersion by successfully disrupting the BBB. Neurons in the brain may be permanently destroyed if undesired blood components enter the brain. Logical design of polymer-based drug delivery system has lately improved the drug delivery directly to the brain interstitium. Nanocarriers are the ideal alternative for patient compliance, administration of a drug without anesthesia, no need for hospitalization, nanosize range, NPs can penetrate the brain's small capillaries and be absorbed into cells for noninvasive active targeting, protecting drugs from chemical and enzymatic breakdown. The nanocarriers are proving themselves as active targeting weapon for noninvasive brain-targeting strategies.

Prabhu et al. developed a highly magnetic iron oxide NP of temozolomide to target glioblastoma for drug influx for selective tumor targeting, by tagging antibodies against nestin and transferrin to penetrate BBB. The functionalized nanocarriers showed sustained release and resulted from a significant reduction in tumor cells than the free drug [5].

Functionalization of nanocarriers with suitable components can make them specifically targeted and suitable to pass across BBB. Muro and colleagues developed a dual-targeting DDS by fusing peptide-functionalized novel polyester-based NPs loaded with paclitaxel, which can overcome the limitations of current chemotherapeutics. Paclitaxel has a strong affinity for the low-density lipoprotein receptor (LDLR), getting over the gaps in current anticancer drugs, to transfer the drug from bloodstream to the brain, and subsequently to glioma cells [6].

Different receptor-mediated transport systems utilizing insulin, folate, transferrin, lipoprotein, and other receptors to treat brain illnesses; like Kuo et al. prepared carmustine (BCNU) filled "solid lipid nanoparticles (SLNs)" grafted with 85-14 monoclonal antibodies (MAbs) for brain-targeting delivery by targeting insulin receptor, as an antitumor drug delivery approach to treat brain cancer. Dixit and colleagues designed gold nanoparticles (Au NPs) charged with the photodynamic pro10 medication for photosensitizer delivery to the glioma cancer cell by targeting transferrin peptide (Tfpep) receptor. Sonali et al. prepared temozolomide (TMZ) loaded, lactoferrin protein (Lf) nanoparticles (TMZ-LfNPs) to treat devastating cancerous gliomas, etc. The drug administration site is generally located far away from the target location. As a result, the delivered medicine must reach the desired site in sufficient concentration.

NPs attached with ligands or groups can bind to specific receptors, causing NPs to be internalized by the cells. The most effective technique of delivering drugs is in nanocarrier forms to the brain via the BBB has been found as a receptor-mediated DDS as a result of receptor–ligand interaction mechanisms. The overexpressed receptors on BBB can help ligand-conjugated nanocarriers pass through the BBB. NPs carrying conjugated ligands or moieties can bind to specific receptors, causing the NPs to be internalized by the cells.

3.2 Receptor-mediated nanocarrier platforms for brain drug delivery

A variety of drug delivery studies are underway for active brain-targeted drug delivery. Nanocarrier-based techniques for active brain targeting of brain receptors have gained traction and are being used in a variety of ways. Different therapeutic ways to target medications to reach the brain via crossing the BBB have been investigated to treat neurological illnesses. Drug targeting by NPs may be able to overcome unmet challenges in drug transport through BBB. To increase drug transport to the brain, nanocarriers, particularly lipid nanocarriers such as polymeric NPs, liposomes, micelles, gold NPs, magnetic NPs, and others with sizes ranging from 1 to 100 nm, are commonly used. Transferrin receptors, folate receptors, lipoprotein receptors, insulin receptors, choline receptors, scavenger receptors are some of the overexpressed brain receptors on the BBB that can allow ligand-conjugated nanocarriers to pass through. Conjugated ligands or moieties containing NPs can specifically bind to the appropriate receptor, and stimulate cellular manifestation of the carriers. Table 3.1 represents the recently researched active targeting strategies for brain drug delivery.

3.2.1 Insulin receptor

Insulin is recognized to play a role in brain function regulation. Glial cells and brain cells have been shown to have regulatory effects on circulating insulin's activity. This shows that insulin interacts with insulin receptors on BBB's luminal side, causing transcytosis uptake. The plasma membrane is made up of coated pits, a specific region of insulin receptors where insulin binds. Followed by ligand–receptor binding, the pits invaginate into the cell and eventually detach from the plasma membrane, creating coated vesicles. Acidification of the cell's endosomes causes ligand–receptor dissociation, allowing insulin to pass through the membrane to the opposite side. Two alpha and beta transmembrane subunits make up the heterotetrameric receptor. When the receptor is targeted, endogenous insulin metabolism is interrupted, hence MAbs with affinity for an insulin receptor epitope must be utilized. Drugs, which cannot penetrate the BBB, have been conjugated to insulin receptor-specific MAbs, resulting in a breakthrough. Ulbrich and colleagues prepared "insulin or anti-insulin receptor MAb (29B4) coupled loperamide-loaded human serum albumin nanoparticles

TABLE 3.1 The recently researched active targeting strategies for brain drug delivery.

Brain receptors	Nanocarrier	Drug	Disease condition	Outcome	References
Insulin receptor	Human serum albumin nanoparticles	Loperamide		Pretreatment with the antibody might completely block loperamide transport over the BBB utilizing NP with covalently linked insulin	[7]
Insulin receptor	Solid lipid nanoparticles	Carmustine	Brain malignancies	The formulation was able to cross BBB and able to treat malignant cells	[8]
Transferrin receptor	Micelles	Docetaxel	Brain cancer	Drug release from the prepared particles was sustained for more than 24 hours with 50% release and proved its efficacy as an anticancer delivery	[9]
Transferrin receptor	Gold nanoparticles	Photodynamic prodrug	Brain cancer	In vitro study showed increased cellular uptake of the prepared nanocarriers. Drug accumulation continued for more than 4 hours	[10]
Folate receptor	Pegylated nanoparticles	Poly-(ethylene glycol)-b-poly (ε-caprolactone) (PEG-b-PCL)	BBB impermeability	The prepared nanoparticles showed greater transport and uptake into human choroid plexus epithelial cells as compared to unmodified ones	[11]
Folate receptor	Pegylated gold nanoparticles	Doxorubicin	Folate receptor cancer	Drug release was in controlled way from the prepared nanoparticles. They showed a higher cytotoxic effect on the folate cancer cells than the noncancer cells	[12]
Lipoprotein receptor	Lactoferrin nanoparticles	Temozolomide	Glioma	The prepared nanoparticles were able to cross BBB and their release was pH dependent which signified enhanced therapeutic efficacy	[13]

Brain receptors	Nanocarrier	Drug	Disease condition	Outcome	References
Lipoprotein receptor	Lipoprotein nanocarrier	Apolipoprotein E	Alzheimer's disease	The prepared nanocarriers showed efficient efficacy in lowering amyloid deposition	[15]
Leptin receptor	Pegylated dendrigraft	Leptin30	Brain targeting gene delivery	The prepared nanoparticles proved to transport across BBB in vitro model effectively and accumulate more in brain cells	[17]
Leptin receptor	Pegylated liposome	Doxorubicin	Brain tumor	In vitro study of the prepared liposomes showed increased cytotoxicity, cellular uptake, and tumor cell growth suppression as compared to the drug	[18]
Nicotinic-acetyl-choline receptors	PLGA nanoparticle	Doxorubicin		This study paved the path for development of nanocarriers as a noninvasive approach for various brain diseases in future	[19]
Scavenger receptor	PF32-DNA nano complex	Perfect 32, peptide-based vector		The study showed that scavenger receptor was also involved in the uptake of peptide–DNA nano complex	[21]
Scavenger receptor	Iron oxide nanoparticles	Aβ oligomer-specific scfv antibody	Alzheimer's disease	The prepared nanoparticles showed the highest efficiency for antibody oligomer targeting with increased antibody oligomer uptake by microglia	[22]
Interleukin receptors	Liposome	Doxorubicin	Brain cancer	In cell culture models, the prepared liposomes specifically target and deliver the drug to the cancer cells	[23]

(HAS-NP)" using "NHS-PEG-MAL-5000 crosslinker." In the tail-flick test of mice, the produced loperamide-laden HAS-NPs with covalently bound insulin or 29B4 incited a considerable antinociception effect, concluding drug penetration across BBB with insulin coupled HAS-NPs, as compared to control loperamide-loaded HAS-NPs [7]. In another study, Kuo and coresearchers developed carmustine (BCNU)-loaded nanoparticles (SLNs) (83-14 Mab/BCNU-SLNs), and grafted with 85-14 MAb and applied them for brain-targeting delivery, as an antitumor drug delivery system in the treatment of brain cancer. Human brain microvascular endothelial cells were stained after incubation with "83-14 MAb/BCNU-SLNs" to show the interaction of nanocarriers with expressed insulin receptors. As per the in vitro study findings, increasing the weight percentage of tween 80 improved the transportability of "83-14 MAb/BCNU-SLNs" across BBB [8]. Although the insulin receptor has been proved as a potential medication delivery target, the receptor's necessary involvement in glucose homeostasis makes it difficult to regard it as a feasible choice.

3.2.2 Transferrin receptor

It is one of the most widely utilized drug delivery techniques. In cells like erythrocytes and monocytes, the transferrin receptor is functional. It helps transferrin-bound iron to be absorbed. It is found on the BBB's endothelial cells as a glycoprotein with two 90-kDa subunits connected by a disulfide bridge. There are two approaches to use transferrin receptors for medication delivery: (1) with a targeted ligand, and (2) with an antibody that recognizes the receptor. The receptor is responsible for coordinating the uptake of transferrin-bound iron. Iron is considered to be transferred across the BBB as iron-transferrin complexes by capillary endothelial cells, via receptor-mediated endocytosis. As a result, this technology has the potential to be used to distribute drugs effectively. The presence of high concentrations of transferrin receptors on BBB endothelial cells and their ability to transport across the BBB is very preferable for effective drug administration across the BBB. For targeted brain cancer treatment, Sonali and her colleagues developed "transferrin-conjugated docetaxel-loaded D-alpha-tocopheryl polyethylene glycol 1000 succinate (vitamin E TPGS or TPGS) micelles." The drug release profile showed sustained release for more than 24 hours with 50% release of drug from transferrin-conjugated micelles. In comparison to nontargeted micelles and commercialized formulations, produced TPGS micelles were found to be a suitable carrier for brain delivery due to their nanosize, solubility improvement, and better permeability, which enabled better and sustained brain targeting of docetaxel [9].

Metal NPs were also tested as brain delivery weapons for active targeting. For example, in another work, Dixit and colleagues created gold nanoparticles (Tfpep-Au NPs) loaded with "Pc 4 (photodynamic pro drug)," which can target transferrin peptide (Tfpep). They compared them with untargeted AuNPs for delivering the photosensitizer to glioma cells. According to in vitro studies of

LN229 and U87 (human glioma cancer cell lines) overexpression of transferrin receptor, targeted conjugates showed much higher cellular uptake than untargeted particles. Internalized in Tf-containing endosomes, Tfpep-Au NPs-Pc 4 accumulate in glioma cells' mitochondria. Over 4 hours, Pc 4 continues to accrue [10]. After all, transferrin receptors have been highly researched concerning various brain disorders, which resulted in improved and prolonged targeting. Recent research has focused on employing immunoliposomes to transport neuroactive medication molecules to the brain as encapsulated cargo via the transferrin receptor.

3.2.3 Folate receptor

Folates are pterin compounds that are required for de novo nucleotide synthesis and function as vitamins. Folic acid is the most common form of folate that is added to the diet as a supplement. A glycoprotein receptor is the folate receptor, which controls folic acid and various types of folate endocytosis. According to study, the folate receptor is overexpressed on both the BBB and glioma cells, in contrast to normal settings. Due to the high affinity toward folate receptor of folic acid is an ideal and appealing excipient for coating a drug delivery vehicle by enhancing drug uptake via folate receptor-facilated endocytosis. Kuplennik and colleagues used a simple nanoprecipitation method to make a highly hydrophobic block copolymer, "poly- (ethylene glycol)-b-poly(-caprolactone) (PEG-b-PCL)," in which the PEG block edge was functionalized with an amine moiety. They investigate a new mechanism of folate receptor alpha (FR)-mediated folate uptake for nanomedicine delivery to the CNS. The uptake of FR-conjugated NPs by "human choroid plexus epithelial cells" was investigated. Human choroid plexus epithelial cells absorbed FR-modified NPs more than their nonmodified counterparts. The result showed the conjugation of the "folic receptor alpha-folic acid (FRα-FA) complex" to the NP surface increases accumulation in the brain, indicating the potential of "FRα-FA NPs" as a weapon for delivering active chemicals from the systemic circulation to the CNS [11]. To deliver doxorubicin to cancer cells with positive folate receptors, Asadishad and colleagues developed folate-modified PEGylated gold NPs. Activated-folate and activated-PEG were used to conjugate doxorubicin and folate, respectively. The doxorubicin nanocarriers exhibited a stronger fatal effect on KB cells (FR positive cells) as compared to A549 cells (negative cells). Drug-loaded NPs increased cell viability in healthy cells (HFF cells), than free drug [12].

3.2.4 Lipoprotein receptor

The BBB and the surface of BCECs contain LDLRs. They serve a variety of functions as signaling receptors and play a variety of roles. Lactoferrin, melanotransferrin, TAT protein, ApoE, and other molecules have been shown to interact with them. Sonali et al. prepared temozolomide (TMZ) loaded, lactoferrin protein (Lf) nanoparticles (TMZ-LfNPs) to treat devastating cancerous gliomas. The findings imply that using "lactoferrin nanoparticles (LfNPs)" for their potential of crossing BBB, pH-dependent drug release, and tumor targeting could improve TMZ therapeutic efficacy while reducing adverse effects. In an orthotopic glioma model, On GL261 cells, LfR specific uptake and toxicity (glioma model) resulted in significant tumor reduction, proving the formulation's efficacy in glioma treatment [13].

The LRP1 and LRP2 lipoprotein receptor-related proteins are frequently employed for targeted delivery across the BBB [14]. To achieve the aforesaid goals, Song and colleagues created a biomimetic apolipoprotein E (ApoE) nanocarrier (ANC) for BBB penetration and amyloid-beta (Aβ)-targeted delivery using recombinant ApoE and synthetic lipids. "α-mangostin (α-M)" is a polyphenolic compound which blocks the development of Aβ oligomers and fibrils by accelerating cellular breakdown, which is a primary target for Alzheimer's disease treatment. In vitro, ANC had a 54-fold higher cellular absorption than the control liposome, and in vivo, it had a much higher brain transport efficiency. Addition of α-M increases Aβ binding affinity of the nanoformulation (ANC-α-M) rather than diminishing it. When compared to the nontreated control and ANC, "ANC-α-M" enhanced microglia-mediated absorption and breakdown of Aβ by 336% and 29-fold, respectively. Low-density lipoprotein and ApoE-modified albumin NPs have also been found in receptor-mediated transcytosis to penetrate the BBB [15].

3.2.5 Leptin receptor

Leptin is an appetite and energy-regulating hormone. It is 16 kDa in size. An immunoglobulin-like domain and a transmembrane anchoring region make up the leptin receptor family, with a cytoplasmic tail. They are thought to be comparable to cytokine receptors because of their orientation. The short and long forms of leptin receptors have been identified as a result of differences in splicing patterns. Through endocytosis, leptin can get to parts of brain which regulates energy balance. It passes through the endothelium that lines the brain's capillaries. Peptides derived from a parent leptin molecule are employed as targets for drugs that target the leptin receptor [16]. Liu and coworkers derived "leptin-derived 30-amino-acid peptide-modified pegylated poly-l-lysine dendrigraft for brain targeted gene delivery." Leptin30 is a 30-amino-acid peptide derived from leptin that is utilized as a brain-targeting ligand by intravenous injection. This study used the nonviral gene vector dendrigraft poly-l-lysine. NPs were created by combining "dendrigraft poly-l-lysine–PEG–Leptin30 with plasmid DNA (pDNA)." The characteristics and methods of cellular absorption were studied in leptin-expressing "BCECs." The targeted NPs were shown to penetrate the BBB successfully in vitro and accumulate more in brains following i.v. administration resulted. In vitro and in vivo, gene transfection efficiency is comparatively high. Furthermore, during in vitro transfection, the

NPs showed reduced cytotoxicity [17]. In another work, Darban et al. investigated the antitumor activity of Doxil in "C26 (colon carcinoma) tumor model" using a leptin-derived peptide (LP16, Leptin 91-110) as PEGylated liposomal doxorubicin (PLD, Doxil) targeted ligand for surface decoration. As a result, Doxil was synthesized and described successfully with different LP16 peptide densities (25, 50, 100, and 200 peptides on the surface of each liposome). In vitro study resulted improved cytotoxicity, cellular binding, and uptake in C26 cells of LP16-targeted doxilformulations (LP16-Doxil) in comparison to free Doxil [18].

3.2.6 Nicotinic-acetylcholine receptors

The nicotinic-acetylcholine receptor is another CNS receptor with a significant expression. Its main function is to transfer acetylcholine. The receptor's molecular weight is 290 kDa. This is made up of five subunits, each having transmembrane and cytoplasmic regions. These subunits are organized in a circular pattern around a central channel. Nicotine and acetylcholine are both ligands for these receptors.

Huey et al. formulated a NP-based targeted DDS utilizing a ligand that targets specific brain cells and nicotinic acetylcholine receptors (nAChRs) to treat "rabies virus-derived peptide (RDP)." It was discovered that the RDP facilitated effects of this drug delivery method are dependent on the activity of the nAChR, implying a cellular absorption mechanism. RDP's ability to target specific neuronal cells via the nAChR provides a nontoxic, noninvasive, and promising strategy for brain drug delivery. These receptors have been shown "RVG (rabies virus glycoprotein)" transport into target cells in studies. This led to the development of RVG29, a 29-mer peptide that was the prime reason behind using receptor-mediated transcytosis to deliver therapeutic compounds to brain parenchyma [19].

Hawkins and colleagues used endothelial nAChRs to control cerebral microvascular permeability. Nicotine enhances the permeability of the BBB in vivo. This shows that nAChRs are involved in brain microvascular permeability modulation. Immunofluorescence microscopy studied the expression of AChRs subunits in cerebral microvessels. The findings revealed that in the cerebral microvasculature, nAChRs are expressed, they increase BBB permeability in response to nicotine administration, and that peripheral nAChR antagonism is sufficient to block nicotine's effect on the BBB [20].

3.2.7 Scavenger receptor

Scavenger receptors are predominantly located on endothelial cells of the BBB surfaces, glycoproteins in nature. Based on their structures they generate several classes and subclasses. Scavenger receptors from both classes A and B are expressed in BBB. Because they do not have any specific binding ligand, so, these receptors have a lot of potential as drug delivery mechanisms. They can recognize and bind to a variety of chemicals, ranging from LDL-based compounds to apoptotic residues. Transcytosis, which can be caveolae or clathrin-mediated depending on the ligand, is how they internalize ligands and carrier molecules.

Srimanee et al. used a peptide-based vector PepFect 32 (PF32), modified with a targeting ligand (Angiopep-2) binding to LDLR-related protein-1 to examine the role of scavenger receptors in pDNA delivery across the BBB (LRP-1). PF32-pDNA complexes speculated the internalization via lipoprotein LRP-1 receptor. "Scavenger receptor class A and B (SCARA3, SCARA5, and SR-BI) and LRP-1 receptor" mediated endocytosis transport PF32-pDNA nanocomplexes into brain endothelial cells, according to the researchers. SCARA3, SCARA5, and SR-BI are all found in endothelial cells of the brain. The transfection rate is reduced when these receptors are inhibited [21].

Other disorders can benefit from active brain targeting, in addition to cancer. Liu et al. created multifunctional magnetic iron oxide NPs (W20/XD4-SPIONs) by conjugating a "oligomer-specific scFv antibody W20 and class A scavenger receptor (SR-A) activator XD4 onto superparamagnetic iron oxide nanoparticles (SPIONs)" for their early diagnostic potentials for Alzheimer's disease. When compared to "W20-SPIONs" or "XD4-SPIONs," "W20/XD4-SPIONs" had the best AOS-targeting efficiency and significantly boosted AOs uptake by microglia. "W20/XD4-SPIONs" selectively and sensitively bind to AOs in AD brains, generating an MRI signal, indicating that "W20/XD4-SPIONs" could be used as early-stage AD diagnostic agents [22].

3.2.8 Interleukin receptors

The cytokine interleukin is linked to the upregulation of carcinogenic molecules. In brain tumor samples and glioma cell lines, "interleukins (such as IL-1b, IL-4, IL-6, and IL-8)" have been reported to be overexpressed. Activated T cells release interleukin-13 (IL-13), which plays an important role in the immune response. IL-13R1 and IL-13R2 are the receptors that combine with IL-4a and IL-4Rb to form the receptor. The binding of IL-13 causes endocytosis to happen. Normal cells express IL-13/4R, while glioblastoma cells express IL-13R2. IL-13 binds to IL-13R2 with a high affinity. It has a large molecular weight and is easy to denature. A substitute ligand for IL-13, the Il-13 peptide, has been produced. NPs are conjugated with this interleukin peptide and charged with doxorubicin, as a result, glioma cells showed enhanced absorption via the IL-13 receptor.

Madhankumar et al. described the overexpression of the IL-13 receptor $\alpha 2$ protein by liposomes, conjugated with human IL-13 that binds to brain cancer cells. Glioblastoma multiforme tissue specimens adhere to the conjugated liposomes, but the normal cortex does not. The liposomes are conjugated with human IL-13, which enables selective binding to glioma cells and endocytosis uptake. When doxorubicin is delivered to glioma cells using IL-13–conjugated liposomes, cytotoxicity and drug accumulation and retention are increased compared to when the drug is delivered free. Glioma tumor mouse model was used to investigate the therapeutic potential and targeted efficacy of IL-13–conjugated liposomes delivering doxorubicin in vivo [23].

3.3 Conclusion

Various brain disorders need active targeted drug delivery strategies for treatment, but BBB is a major restriction over brain drug delivery. Receptors play a major role and are commonly used to transport essential chemicals such as hormones over the BBB and can also transport therapeutic molecules across it. Therapeutic molecules like hormones and drugs can pass through it by various brain receptors, including, insulin receptors, transferrin receptors, folate receptors, lipoprotein receptors, interleukin receptors, etc. as they are overexpressed in various brain diseases. To overcome these transportation challenges across BBB, several physical, physiological, and pharmacological approaches have been evolved. The physiological approaches of transport across BBB are the most applicable and widely accepted. For active targeting strategies, lipidic nanocarriers have proven themselves as an effective weapon. For the nanosize range, NPs can penetrate the brain's small capillaries and be absorbed into cells for noninvasive active targeting, protecting drugs from chemical and enzymatic breakdown. Different metallic nanocarriers also have been studied, and they have shown good results, including greater cellular uptake, prolonged drug accumulation, controlled release, higher cytotoxic effect on cancer cells, better efficacy, etc. So, nanocarriers can be further studied as an alternative to active brain-targeting strategies, in the treatment of different brain disorders.

References

[1] Feigin VL, Vos T. Global burden of neurological disorders: from global burden of disease estimates to actions. Neuroepidemiology 2019;52:1–2. https://doi.org/10.1159/000495197.

[2] Feigin VL, Vos T, Nichols E, Owolabi MO, Carroll WM, Dichgans M, Deuschl G, Parmar P, Brainin M, Murray C. The global burden of neurological disorders: translating evidence into policy. Lancet Neurol 2020;19:255–65. https://doi.org/10.1016/S1474-4422(19)30411-9.

[3] McCord E, Pawar S, Koneru T, Tatiparti K, Sau S, Iyer AK. Folate receptors' expression in gliomas may possess potential nanoparticle-based drug delivery opportunities. ACS Omega 2021;6:4111–8 https://doi.org/10.1021/acsomega.0c05500.

[4] Koneru T, McCord E, Pawar S, Tatiparti K, Sau S, Iyer AK. Transferrin: biology and use in receptor-targeted nanotherapy of gliomas. ACS Omega 2021;6:8727–33. https://doi.org/10.1021/acsomega.0c05848.

[5] Prabhu S, Goda JS, Mutalik S, Mohanty BS, Chaudhari P, Rai S, Udupa N, Rao BSS. A polymeric temozolomide nanocomposite against orthotopic glioblastoma xenograft: tumor-specific homing directed by nestin. Nanoscale 2017;9:10919–32. https://doi.org/10.1039/C7NR00305F.

[6] Di Mauro PP, Cascante A, Brugada Vilà P, Gómez-Vallejo V, Llop J, Borrós S. Peptide-functionalized and high drug loaded novel nanoparticles as dual-targeting drug delivery system for modulated and controlled release of paclitaxel to brain glioma. Int J Pharm 2018;553:169–85. https://doi.org/10.1016/j.ijpharm.2018.10.022.

[7] Ulbrich K, Knobloch T, Kreuter J. Targeting the insulin receptor: nanoparticles for drug delivery across the blood–brain barrier (BBB). J Drug Targeting 2011;19:125–32. https://doi.org/10.3109/10611861003734001.

[8] Kuo Y-C, Shih-Huang C-Y. Solid lipid nanoparticles carrying chemotherapeutic drug across the blood–brain barrier through insulin receptor-mediated pathway. J Drug Targeting 2013;21:730–8. https://doi.org/10.3109/1061186X.2013.812094.

[9] Sonali, Agrawal P, Singh RP, Rajesh CV, Singh S, Vijayakumar MR, Pandey BL, Muthu MS. Transferrin receptor-targeted vitamin E TPGS micelles for brain cancer therapy: preparation, characterization and brain distribution in rats. Drug Deliv 2016;23:1788–98. https://doi.org/10.3109/10717544.2015.1094681.

[10] Dixit S, Novak T, Miller K, Zhu Y, Kenney ME, Broome A-M. Transferrin receptor-targeted theranostic gold nanoparticles for photosensitizer delivery in brain tumors. Nanoscale 2015;7:1782–90. https://doi.org/10.1039/C4NR04853A.

[11] Kuplennik N, Lang K, Steinfeld R, Sosnik A. Folate receptor α-modified nanoparticles for targeting of the central nervous system. ACS Appl Mater Interfaces 2019;11:39633–47. https://doi.org/10.1021/acsami.9b14659.

[12] Asadishad B, Vossoughi M, Alemzadeh I. Folate-receptor-targeted delivery of doxorubicin using polyethylene glycol-functionalized gold nanoparticles. Ind Eng Chem Res 2010;49:1958–63. https://doi.org/10.1021/ie9011479.

[13] Kumari S, Ahsan SM, Kumar JM, Kondapi AK, Rao NM. Overcoming blood brain barrier with a dual purpose temozolomide loaded lactoferrin nanoparticles for combating glioma (SERP-17-12433). Sci Rep 2017;7:6602. https://doi.org/10.1038/s41598-017-06888-4.

[14] Hu K, Li J, Shen Y, Lu W, Gao X, Zhang Q, Jiang X. Lactoferrin-conjugated PEG–PLA nanoparticles with improved brain delivery: in vitro and in vivo evaluations. J Controlled Release 2009;134:55–61. https://doi.org/10.1016/j.jconrel.2008.10.016.

[15] Song Q, Song H, Xu J, Huang J, Hu M, Gu X, Chen J, Zheng G, Chen H, Gao X. Biomimetic ApoE-reconstituted high density lipoprotein nanocarrier for blood–brain barrier penetration and amyloid beta-targeting drug delivery. Mol Pharm 2016;13:3976–87. https://doi.org/10.1021/acs.molpharmaceut.6b00781.

[16] Tosi G, Badiali L, Ruozi B, Vergoni AV, Bondioli L, Ferrari A, Rivasi F, Forni F, Vandelli MA. Can leptin-derived sequence-modified nanoparticles be suitable tools for brain delivery. Nanomedicine 2012;7:365–82. https://doi.org/10.2217/nnm.11.98.

[17] Liu Y, Li J, Shao K, Huang R, Ye L, Lou J, Jiang C. A leptin derived 30-amino-acid peptide modified pegylated poly-l-lysine dendrigraft for brain targeted gene delivery. Biomaterials 2010;31:5246–57. https://doi.org/10.1016/j.biomaterials.2010.03.011.

[18] Amiri Darban S, Nikoofal-Sahlabadi S, Amiri N, Kiamanesh N, Mehrabian A, Zendehbad B, Gholizadeh Z, Jaafari MR. Targeting the leptin receptor: to evaluate therapeutic efficacy and anti-tumor effects of Doxil, in vitro and in vivo in mice bearing C26 colon carcinoma tumor. Colloids Surf B 2018;164:107–15. https://doi.org/10.1016/j.colsurfb.2018.01.035.

[19] Huey R, O'Hagan B, McCarron P, Hawthorne S. Targeted drug delivery system to neural cells utilizes the nicotinic acetylcholine receptor. Int J Pharm 2017;525:12–20. https://doi.org/10.1016/j.ijpharm.2017.04.023.

[20] Hawkins BT, Egleton RD, Davis TP. Modulation of cerebral microvascular permeability by endothelial nicotinic acetylcholine receptors. Am J Physiol-Heart Circ Physiol 2005;289:H212–9. https://doi.org/10.1152/ajpheart.01210.2004.

[21] Srimanee A, Regberg J, Hällbrink M, Vajragupta O, Langel Ü. Role of scavenger receptors in peptide-based delivery of plasmid DNA across a blood–brain barrier model. Int J Pharm 2016;500:128–35. https://doi.org/10.1016/j.ijpharm.2016.01.014.

[22] Liu X-G, Zhang L, Lu S, Liu D-Q, Zhang L-X, Yu X-L, Liu R-T. Multifunctional superparamagnetic iron oxide nanoparticles conjugated with Aβ oligomer-specific scFv antibody and class A scavenger receptor activator show early diagnostic potentials for Alzheimer's disease. IJN 2020;15:4919–32. https://doi.org/10.2147/IJN.S240953.

[23] Madhankumar AB, Slagle-Webb B, Mintz A, Sheehan JM, Connor JR. Interleukin-13 receptor–targeted nanovesicles are a potential therapy for glioblastoma multiforme. Mol Cancer Ther 2006;5:3162–9. https://doi.org/10.1158/1535-7163.MCT-06-0480.

Chapter 4

Dendrimers in the effective management of Alzheimer's and dementia

Rakesh Kumar Sahoo, Vinay Kumar, Sanya Batheja, Umesh Gupta
Department of Pharmacy, School of Chemical Sciences and Pharmacy, Central University of Rajasthan, Bandarsindri, Ajmer, Rajasthan, India

4.1 Introduction

Neurodegenerative disorders involve a wide range of conditions that result from progressive damage to cells and nervous system connections that play an integral function in mobility, coordination, strength, sensation, and cognition. Alzheimer's disease and Parkinson's disease are the most common neurodegenerative diseases. According to the Alzheimer's Association [2], it is observed that approximately 6.2 million US population (age ≥65 years) are suffering from dementia which is majorly caused by "Alzheimer's disease" (AD) and other neurodegenerative disorders [2]. AD is the most common type of dementia. It is noticeable by severe memory loss and cognitive impairment; and currently, it has limited effective therapeutic options for managing the patient's condition. It is accountable for approximately 60–80% of all dementia cases [3]. Dementia is a particular term used for the impaired functionalities of the brain. The characteristic symptom of dementia indulges difficulty in thinking, recalling, and decision making; it may vary person to person. The mortality rates of AD patients causing dementia have amplified to 16% more than the average mortality rate in the current COVID-19 pandemic situation 2020. As per official records, 271,872 US individuals were died due to dementia among which 121,499 individuals faced AD as the cause of death. Hence, AD has become a prominent cause of dementia involving various risk factors such as age-related, family history, genetic, social and cognitive environment, traumatic brain injury, and other modifiable factors [2].

Currently, there are no FDA-approved pharmacologic therapies for the cure or prevention of dementia or AD. While, many marketed interventions are available either for the delay of onset of dementia or reducing the

Nanomedicine-Based Approaches for the Treatment of Dementia. https://doi.org/10.1016/B978-0-12-824331-2.00003-0
Copyright © 2023 Elsevier Inc. All rights reserved.

symptoms. Several USFDA-approved cholinesterase inhibitor drugs such as donepezil, rivastigmine, tacrine, and galantamine are utilized for reducing the symptoms of mild to severe type of AD [4]. Till date, oral route has been exploited by the formulations commercialized which have been shifting to nasal route for bypassing the side effects. Recently, many nanoformulations are considered for bypassing the adverse effects which incorporates nanoemulsions, dendrimers, nanostructured lipid carriers, in situ hydrogels, etc. [5].

4.2 History and definition of dendrimers

In the field of nanotechnology, dendrimers are one of the most promising innovations for biomedical applications especially drug delivery [9]. The term dendrimers evolved from the Greek word "dendron" meaning "tree-like" and "meros" meaning "part" which eventually means architecture with numerous branching units [13]. The framework of dendrimers encompasses highly branched, nanosized, and monodispersed structures with a diameter of 2–10 nm. Originally, it was first discovered by Fritz Vogtle in 1978, and later in the early 1980s, it was independently discovered by Donald A. Tomalia and George R. Newkome. Dendrimers were also named star-like polymer and cascade molecules as it follows a cascade reaction for the formation of a star-like structure. PAMAM dendrimers also called starburst dendrimers was the first discovered and patented dendritic molecule by Tomalia and coworkers. The synthesis of dendrimers can be consummated either by convergent method or by divergent method [1,12]. A unique architectural motif of dendritic molecule incorporates three main parts which are the innermost core, peripheral units, and functional groups. The peripheral units are repetitive branching units that act as a backbone of the structure by protecting the core moiety from exogenous elements and connecting the core moiety with the functional group. On the basis of these repetitive branching units, the dendrimers were classified in different generations such as G0.5, G1, G2, etc. While the functional groups at the terminals are the recognition sites that tend to initiate pharmacological activity by binding or any other process. Also, the functional group at the terminals grants the inclusion of additional moieties for active targeting and improvising the drug delivery system [10]. The escalation of technology along with the presence of unique properties of dendrimer labels it as an ideal carrier for the targeted delivery of therapeutic and diagnostic agents.

4.3 Properties of dendrimers

Dendrimers have some attributed properties owing to their nanometric size and highly organized monodispersed architecture (Fig. 4.1). The most important

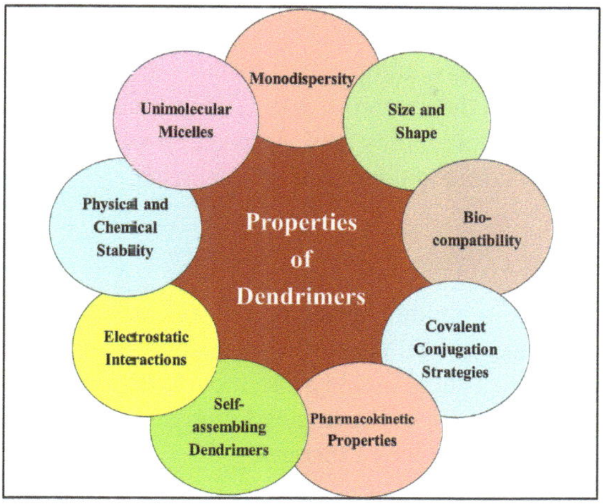

FIG. 4.1 Properties of dendrimers.

distinctive properties of dendrimers that are particularly relevant to their drug delivery applications are listed below:

Monodispersity

The construction of a well-defined molecular structure of the dendritic assembly exhibits monodispersity of dendrimers. It can be confirmed using analytical techniques such as mass spectroscopy (MALDI-TOF), gel electrophoresis, transmission electron microscopy, and size exclusion chromatography.

Size and shape

The unique architecture of dendritic assembly is an ideal nanocarrier due to its uniform size and compact shape. The size of dendrimers varies systematically from 1 to 100 nm in diameters depending upon their generation number. The predefined size and shape help to cross cell membranes and prevent premature clearance from the human body [15,16].

Biocompatibility

A dendritic assembly is said to be biocompatible with the cellular system as it exhibits a therapeutic effect at the site of action with reduced side effects. Dendrimers are widely used as nanocarriers in the diagnosis and treatment of cancer. Also, many research groups have established that the biocompatibility of dendrimers is compromised with an extended stay in the human body [7].

Covalent conjugation strategies

These are utilized for encapsulation of therapeutics in dendrimers which can be covalently conjugated to the receptors at the site of tumor exhibiting acidic pH. The conjugated dendritic assembly acts as a prodrug which gets activated in the body, and that delivers drug at the site of action [1,14].

Pharmacokinetic properties

It is considered to be a promising factor for the fabrication of dendrimers. Generally, the pharmacokinetic properties of dendrimers depend on the physicochemical properties of the assembly and their biological interaction. It also helps in reducing adverse effects by targeted drug delivery, photodynamic therapy, diagnosis, and neutron capture therapy.

Self-assembling dendrimers

Dendrimers have an advantage of self-assembly that has gained interest to circumvent the obstacles of phased synthesis. The well-defined layers of dendrimers are developed using different strategies that may differ the stability of dendrimers based on generation number.

Electrostatic interactions

Dendrimers are composed of distinct layers among which the periphery contains functional group moieties providing surface charge to the molecule. The surface charge allows molecular recognition and formation of dendritic assembly or dendriplexes using electrostatic interactions [8].

Chemical and physical stability

The stability of dendrimers varies with the type of dendrimers and their generation number. Lower the generation number, better stability is observed. In contrast, the unique architecture of dendrimers possesses excellent stability against external stimuli. It is also observed to produce stable conjugates of therapeutic agents, imaging agents, or targeting agents with dendrimers [11].

Unimolecular micelles

Formation of a molecule using a single moiety is called unimolecular. The micellar structure of dendrimers is formed of a single moiety, hence referred to as unimolecular micelles, for example, PAMAM dendrimers are composed of repetitive units of ethylenediamine. It aids in cellular accumulation and encompasses as a potential carrier for the drug delivery system [6].

4.4 Types of dendrimers

4.4.1 PAMAM dendrimers

Polyamidoamine dendrimers, well-known as PAMAM dendrimers, are one of the most explored dendrimer category in the field of drug delivery. The hyper branched structure of PAMAM dendrimers is comprised of ethylene diamine core, amide group branching, and surface functional groups like amine group ($-NH_2$), hydroxyl group (–OH), and carboxylic group (–COOH). PAMAM dendrimers possess multiple surface functional groups depending on the generation number, which can be modified with different ligands to achieve targeted delivery of therapeutic agents. The hydrophobic core is capable of encapsulating the poorly aqueous soluble drugs. The cationic nature of these dendrimers imparts inherent cytotoxicity, but can be overcome by fabrication of biocompatible molecules like polyethylene glycol [13,17].

4.4.2 PPI dendrimers

Polypropyleneimine dendrimers, well-known as PPI dendrimers, are the oldest commercially available dendrimers for drug delivery. The core of these dendrimers consists of di-amino butane (hence, also called as DAB dendrimers) and the repeating units are of propyleneimine. The $-NH_2$ groups present at the surface of PPI dendrimers enhance their aqueous solubility. Like PAMAM dendrimers, these are also capable of encapsulating the hydrophobic drugs. However, the stability of PPI dendrimers limits their use in drug delivery. PEGylation and acetylation strategies are used to overcome the stability and low encapsulation challenges [18,19].

4.4.3 PLL dendrimers

Dendrimers consisting of lysine residues are referred as poly-l-lysine or PLL dendrimers. In comparison to PAMAM and PPI dendrimers, these dendrimers possess enhanced biocompatibility and reduced cytotoxicity. Modification of specific amino acid sequences in PLL dendrimers provides the additional advantage of stimuli responsiveness. These dendrimers are basically used in gene delivery. Gene transfection efficiency of PLL dendrimers increases with the increase in generation number [20,21].

4.4.4 PPH dendrimers

Dendrimers which are synthesized keeping phosphorus atoms at each branching point are known as phosphorous or PPH dendrimers. These especially designed dendrimers are unique in terms of straightforward fabrication and the rich chemistry diversity with peripheral reactive groups like aldehydes and $P(S)Cl_2$ groups. Hydrophobic interior and hydrophilic surface of these dendrimers promote their cellular internalization [22]. Studies revealed that PPH dendrimers affect the aggregation of amyloid peptide and tau protein in neurodegenerative disorders [23].

4.4.5 Carbosilane dendrimers

Carbosilane dendrimers are the synthesized dendrimers based on silicon chemistry. The idea of this specialized category is based on the principle that the electrophilic silicon (Si^+) can be readily accessible by nucleophilic moieties. Carbosilane dendrimers have exhibited remarkable thermal stability. The hydrophobic skeleton of these dendrimers can be changed to hydrophilic through surface functionalization [24].

4.4.6 Other types of dendrimers

Along with the above-mentioned major categories of dendrimers, there are other dendrimers which are also being used for their diagnostic and therapeutic applicability. It includes Janus dendrimers, linear-dendritic block copolymers, peptide dendrimers, glycol dendrimers, and PAMAMOS dendrimers [25].

4.5 Dendrimer-mediated brain delivery approaches

Brain delivery of therapeutic moieties is very challenging due to the presence of blood–brain barrier (BBB). BBB is composed of complex tight junctions formed by cerebral endothelial cells between blood and the brain. Among all USFDA-approved small molecule drugs, only 2% is permitted to cross the BBB [26]. Nanocarriers have exhibited remarkable results in developing drug delivery systems to deliver drugs for the treatment of brain diseases. Dendrimers are of nanometric size with monodispersity and possess a number of peripheral functional groups which can be engineered as per the need of drug delivery [25]. For the effective brain delivery, drug molecules can either be physically encapsulated in the internal cavities of dendrimers or chemically conjugated to the peripheral functional groups [27]. Additionally, surface engineering of dendrimers can impart specific features to the nanocarrier, which thereby enhances their biocompatibility, drug-release kinetics, and targeting efficiency in brain delivery. This section will enlighten different approaches for the effective brain delivery of active pharmaceutical ingredients.

4.5.1 Bypassing the BBB with invasive approaches

Brain delivery of drugs through invasive approaches can be an answer for bypassing BBB. There are certain invasive routes of administration like intracerebroventricular route (ICV) [27], intracerebral/intraparenchymal route [28], convection-enhanced delivery (CED) [29], and intrathecal route [30], and intratympanic route [31], which can directly deliver the drugs into targeted region of the brain. In case of ICV route, drug can be delivered to the brain from an implantable reservoir or through a pump monitored catheter. Thereby it allows the drug to follow an extended release pattern through diffusion. Administration of drugs via ICV route has shown reduced systemic toxicity. It also provided additional protection to the drug from getting metabolized in the blood serum [32]. In comparison to diffusion-based drug delivery strategies, CED possesses certain advantages such as reduced dose-related toxicity and increased intratumoral distribution. The molecular weight or diffusivity of the drugs does not affect the drug penetration to the brain region, when administered via CED [29]. To explore the diagnostic efficacy of dendrimers administered via CED, Yang et al. grafted epidermal growth factor to boronated hyperbranched PAMAM dendrimer for boron neutron capture therapy. The intratumoral uptake of the synthesized diagnostic moiety was evidenced to be significantly higher in glioma-bearing rats [33]. Risk of infection and undesired fluid flow to more sensitive regions of brain are some major challenges associated with CED. Furthermore, drugs can also be delivered directly to the brain parenchyma via intracerebral or intraparenchymal implant or injectable [28]. Regino et al. investigated the in vitro and in vivo efficacy of gadolinium (Gd)-based PAMAM dendrimers of generation 8 via CED. Gd-based agents were observed to have almost 1.6 times higher in vitro CT attenuation values in comparison to iodine-based agents. Use of Gd-based dendrimers exhibited elevated visibility through both CT and MR in less than 100 mM range. Determination of volume of distribution was found to have greater sensitivity in case of MR than CT [34]. Dendrimer-based nanoparticle formulations have shown effective results in drug delivery via non-invasive approaches [35].

4.5.2 Bypassing the BBB with non-invasive approaches

Along with the invasive approaches, non-invasive approaches like intranasal delivery may have potential to bypass BBB. Drugs which are administered through nasal route possess several advantages. Unlike drugs administered through oral route, drugs can avoid enzymatic degradation and fast pass metabolism through nasal delivery and can get directly absorbed into the systemic circulation. This may also lead to earlier onset of therapeutic effect and increased bioavailability of the drug [36,37]. There is a direct and unique anatomical connection between the nasal cavity and the brain, which can be utilized to deliver certain drugs directly into the central nervous system without crossing the BBB [38,39]. The olfactory neurons and trigeminal nerves come into play when the drugs basically get deposited at the nasal mucosa [40]. After intranasal administration, the major pathways followed for brain delivery of therapeutic is represented in Fig. 4.2. Exploring the nose-to-brain delivery route, there are several formulations which are presently at preclinical and clinical stages, and available in different dosage forms like nasal spray, gels, powders, etc. [41,42]. Implementation of nanotechnology can potentiate nose-to-brain delivery of therapeutic agents. Nanoparticulate carriers are capable of shielding the active

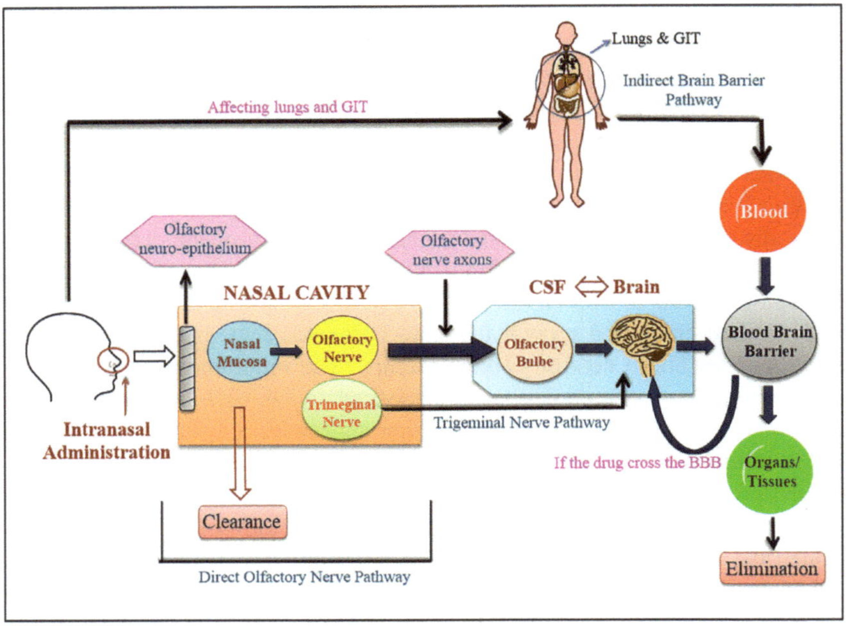

FIG. 4.2 Graphical representation of major pathways to target the brain regions after intranasal administration.

moiety from degradation along with increment in its nasal cavity retention. Additionally, the efflux of drug into the nasal cavity can also be prevented through nanotechnology-based approaches. The nanometric size and surface functionalities of dendrimers make these nanocarriers a potential candidate for nose-to-brain delivery of drugs. Dong and coworkers explore the in vivo efficacy of PAMAM dendrimers (of different generations) in the intranasal delivery of poorly aqueous soluble drug, that is, insulin. The pharmacokinetic behavior observed after administration were found to be concentration- and generation-dependent. However, PAMAM dendrimers of generation 3 exhibited significant nasal absorption of macromolecules [43]. Another research group, Katare et al. performed comparative investigation between intranasal and intraperitoneal administration of a poorly soluble antipsychotic drug haloperidol through PAMAM dendrimers. Problem associated with the aqueous solubility of the drug was resolved as it enhanced the solubility by more than 100 times. The developed formulation administered via intranasal route exhibited remarkable behavioral responses in comparison to the drug-loaded formulation administered via intraperitoneal route [44]. Researchers also investigated the intranasal brain delivery of siRNA complexed with PAMAM dendrimers considering high mobility group box-1 as the target. After 1 hour of nasal administration, the fluorescent-tagged formulation was markedly observed in the cytoplasm of glial cells in many brain regions, incorporating the amygdala, cerebral cortex, and striatum. The outcomes of in vivo experiments performed on rats with cerebral ischemia revealed that the cerebral infract volume was noticeably reduced and behavioral deficits were also recovered on administration of siRNA complexed dendrimers [45]. In situ gel based on dendrimers has also exhibited interesting outcomes in drug delivery via nose-to-brain route. PEGylated PAMAM dendrimers of generation 5 were utilized to deliver a poorly water soluble natural neuroprotective agent, paeonol to the brain via intranasal route. A stable 3D network space structure was observed on rheological characterization of the in situ gel formulation with cytotoxic effects upon in vitro analysis [46].

4.5.3 Traversing the BBB with non-invasive approaches

Dendrimer-mediated invasive and non-invasive approaches have shown their capabilities to bypass BBB for diagnostic and therapeutic efficacy. However, there are several non-invasive approaches like carrier-mediated transport (CMT), adsorptive-mediated transcytosis (AMT), receptor-mediated transcytosis (RMT), cell-mediated transport, para-cellular transport, and passive transcellular diffusion, which are capable of traversing the BBB through dendrimer-mediated drug delivery systems [47,48].

In case of CMT, an endogenous solute binds to a protein carrier or transporter present on the luminal side of BBB, which thereby permits the passage of ingredients, such as glucose, vitamins, and amino acids [35]. Dendrimer-mediated brain uptake was explored by Sharma and coworkers using CMT approach. Mannose-conjugated PAMAM dendrimers (–OH terminated) exhibited excellent in vitro uptake, possibly due to carrier-mediated mannose endocytosis [49]. In case of AMT, positively charged nanoformulations get internalized through endocytosis and traversed through the BBB. To achieve AMT mechanism, therapeutic moiety or nanocarrier can be modified to impart cationic charge on the surface. However, the nonselectivity of the adsorption process increases the chances of toxic effects, thereby limits the efficacy of AMT [50]. In case of RMT, vesicles containing receptor ligand conjugates are formed through endocytosis followed by membrane invagination and subsequently the ligand enters into the brain traversing the BBB. There are several receptors present on the BBB, which are involved in the process of brain drug delivery through RMT. Some of the receptors are insulin receptor, transferrin receptor neonatal Fc receptor, apolipoprotein E receptor 2, and melanotransferrin receptor [25, 51–53]. Researchers investigated the comparative brain targeting potency of concanavalin A, glucosamine, and sialic acid-conjugated PPI dendrimers in the delivery of paclitaxel. Sialic acid functionalization demonstrated maximum brain targeting with enhanced therapeutic effect [54]. Gothwal et al. explored the brain targeting efficiency of lactoferrin-conjugated PAMAM dendrimers in the delivery of memantine. The outcomes of in vivo biodistribution studies revealed that maximum brain uptake was observed in lactoferrin-modified dendrimers. Additionally, significant improvement in behavioral changes was observed in $AlCl_3$-induced Alzheimer's mice model [55]. Similar results were obtained in case of lactoferrin anchored PPI dendrimers, which exhibited excellent in vitro brain uptake of pDNA [56]. Researchers also explored the brain delivery efficiency of transferrin-modified PPI dendrimers and found that the gene delivery and gene expression in cancer cells were enhanced significantly through transferrin receptors [57].

4.6 Dendrimers in Alzheimer's disease

4.6.1 Use of PAMAM dendrimers

Dendrimers are considered as a remarkable tool for a wide range of pharmaceutical applications [58]. Dendrimers have showcased an immense potential for the treatment of neurological disorders especially AD. PAMAM dendrimers have gained much attention due to their limitless benefits [59]. Researchers developed sialic acid-conjugated PAMAM dendrimers to assess the attenuation of sialic acid-derived amyloid-β (Aβ) toxicity [61]. It is noticed that Aβ deficit SH-SY-5Y neuroblastoma cells to show the higher attenuation against Aβ-dependent neuronal toxicity. The toxicity prevention properties of the sialic acid-modified dendrimers were a function of dendrimer size. Another similar investigation performed by the research group revealed that the sialic acid-grafted PAMAM dendrimer showed a greater efficacy for Aβ-induced neurotoxicity [62]. The author showed that sialic acid-functionalized dendrimeric polymers could mimic the cell surface sialic acid clusters and attenuate Aβ-induced neurotoxicity. This emphasizes the understanding of Aβ-cell surface binding and is subjected to newer opportunities in the prevention of Aβ toxicity in AD. Wang et al. developed phenyl surface-modified carboxyl terminated PAMAM dendrimers that showed the alteration in the $A\beta_{42}$ protein via conformation hydrophobic-binding electrostatic repulsion [63]. The well-balanced interactions indicated the dendrimer-mediated inhibition of β-sheet structure peptide, which was recognized by alterations at the level of the fibrillary framework. In another similar protocol, the author studied the phenyl derived generation-dependent dendrimer significant interference on the accumulation of Aβ peptide [40]. The phenyl-functionalized dendrimers of lower to higher generation dendrimers comprised of negative charges and hydrophobic groups available on their surface based on the HyBER mechanism. It was observed that higher generation dendrimers exhibited greater inhibition because high-generation dendrimers have compact surface functionalities. In contrast, low-generation dendrimers are comprised of sparse distributions of terminal functional moieties. Gothwal and coworkers developed lactoferrin engineered PAMAM dendrimers with an enhanced pharmacokinetic behavior and better bioavailability in Alzheimer's rat model [64]. The developed nanoscaffolds presented enhanced brain uptake and boosted memory in the management of AD. In another similar protocol, the author prepared the lactoferrin-conjugated PAMAM dendrimer for sustained administration of rivastigmine against the Alzheimer's induced mice model [65]. In another study, Gothwal et al. developed a smart multifunctional PAMAM dendrimer and evaluated their efficacy

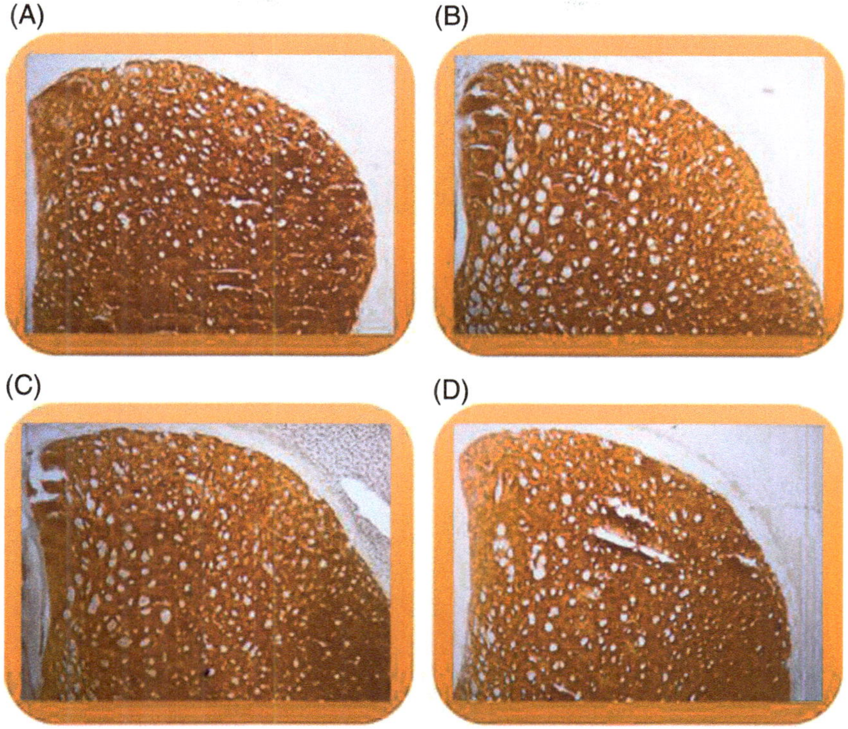

FIG. 4.3 Different forms of MEM on the AL-induced increase for AChE activity. Representative sections of striatum from (A) AL, (B) AL+MEM, (C) AL+PAMAM-MEM, and (D) AL+MEM-PAMAM-Lf groups. Densitometric analysis of the photographs of AChE staining is at the bottom as reprinted with permission reference no. (Reprinted with permission from [55].)

against aluminum chloride-derived Alzheimer's mice model (Fig. 4.3) [55]. The lactoferrin-functionalized dendrimers were evaluated for controlled drug release in mimicking the biological environment.

4.6.2 Use of PPI dendrimer

PPI dendrimers are amine-functionalized unimicellar macromolecules exploited for potential drug transport applications. It is synthesized mainly by a divergent approach. PPI dendrimers comprise two types of nitrogen atoms; sufficient primary amine is available at surface functionalities, and the tertiary amine is present in interior cavities. Importantly, tertiary nitrogen atoms are more acidic at pKa around 6–9, while primary nitrogen atoms are more basic at pKa around 10. In their synthesis, repeated reactions result in an exponential increase in the number of primary amines, which comprised 1,4-diaminobutane as the multifunctional core. In an interesting investigation, Klajnert et al. explored the effect of polypropylene imine dendrimers on the formation of amyloid fibrils as a function of pH to gain further insight into the aggregation mechanism of its

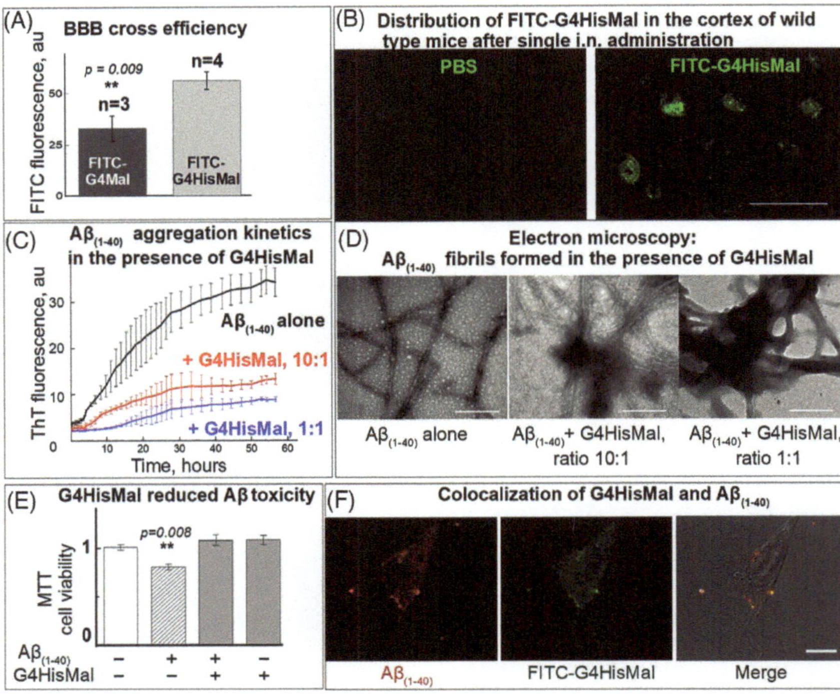

Fig. 4.4 G4HisMal dendrimers cross the BBB and inhibit Aβ(1–40) induced cell toxicity. (A) FITC fluorescence of brain tissue homogenates after i.n. administration of FITC-G4HisMal and FITC-G4Mal. Statistics: Student's *t* test, data are expressed as a mean ± SD; $n = 3$ per group. (B) Fluorescence microscopy images show the presence of FITC-G4HisMal in the cortex after i.n. administration of FITC-G4HisMal. The bar is 10 μm. (C) Aggregation of 20 μm $A\beta_{(1-40)}$ in the presence of G4HisMal. (D) Transmission electron microscopy (TEM): samples were collected at the end of ThT kinetics as shown in (C). Bar =1 00 nm. (E) MTT assay of $A\beta_{(1-40)}$ toxicity in the absence (dashed bar) and the presence of G4HisMal (gray bars). White columns correspond to control SH–SY5Y cells; these values are taken as one of cell viability. The experiment was repeated twice in triplicate. Statistics: one-way ANOVA followed by Tukey's post hoc test, data are expressed as a mean ± SD. (F) Colocalization of FITC-G4HisMal dendrimers with $A\beta_{(1-40)}$ in SH–SY5Y cells. SH–SY5Y cells were treated with 10 μmol $A\beta_{(1-40)}$ and 1 μmol G4HisMal after 24 hours of incubation, then cells were fixed and labeled with specific antibodies against $A\beta_{(1-40)}$ (red) 1 μmol and FITC against FITC-labeled dendrimers (green). Merge shows colocalization of $A\beta_{(1-40)}$ and FITC-G4HisMal. (Reprinted with permission from [66].)

inhibition [60]. At the in vitro level, PrP 185-208 and $A\beta_{1-28}$-derived amyloid fibrils formation evaluated utilizing thioflavin T assay. The researcher found concentration-dependent dendrimer effect against the fibril formations for both Alzheimer's peptides and prion. Also, the results concluded that the level of protonation of His, Glu, and Asp residues played a vital role in the desired inhibition effect. Aso et al. investigated dual functionalized poly (propylene imine) dendrimers for the ability to transverse the BBB for superior therapeutic potential in memory deficient transgenic mice-derived AD (Fig. 4.4) [66]. In one of the experiments, Wrobel et al. studied histidine and maltose dual functionalized PPI dendrimer significantly assured biocompatibility and capability to transverse the BBB in vivo to prevent the progression of AD [67]. It was noticed that developed multifaceted dendrimers demonstrated important features for synapse and memory protection in in vivo transgenic mice. Researchers further examined the formulation, as mentioned earlier for in situ examination, to reduce early-stage amyloid aggregates in transgenic mice-derived AD [74]. It was observed that nanoformulations studied for significant attenuation in vitro $A\beta_{1-40}$ and showed better antiamyloidal activity in both APP/PS1 transgenic and wild-type mice.

4.6.3 Use of other dendrimers

There are other kind of cationic dendrimers, which are also explored for their efficacy against AD. For instance, one interesting investigation, synthesized cationic phosphorous dendrimer were studied for better anti-amyloidal action, which prevent the AD. The biophysical and biochemical analysis including circular dichroism, fluorescence measurement inferred that better anti-amyloidal action were observed against amyloid peptide ($A\beta_{1-28}$) and MAP-tau protein. In another experiment, Neelov et al. investigated PLL dendrimers of different generation for significant restriction of aggregation of amyloid peptide [68]. The in vitro studies emphasized both dendrimer effects on cell viability and their preventive role against Aβ-insult SH-SY-5Y human neuroblastoma cells. For instance, Al-Azzawi et al. studied the poly(epsilon-lysine) dendrimer-based nanoscaffolds to augment the administering of the flurbiprofen across the BBB and selective targeting at diseased tissue [69]. The researchers synthesized the dendrimer architecture utilizing the solid-phase peptide protocol, which was characterized by fourier-transform infrared spectroscopy and mass spectroscopy. The in vitro experiment concluded that drug-bearing dendrimeric nanoformulations showed the higher γ-secretase enzyme activity at targeted cells and evidently supported by precise drug release. Another investigation, the Wasiak et al. studied the cationic dendrimer macromolecules have been proven to attenuates the amyloidogenesis and prevent the aggregation of tau protein [70]. The in vitro examination illustrated the foregoing properties of dendrimer that restricted the acetylcholinesterase activity, restricted the secretion of TNF-α, and also exhibited minimal antioxidant properties.

4.7 Dendrimers in dementia

Dementia is a type of neurological disorder, in which the patient shows impaired ability to remember, think, or loses his/her decision-making ability in performing the daily activities. Use of dendrimer-based nanocarriers against the most common type of dementia, that is, Alzheimer's is explained in detail in the above-mentioned section [71]. HIV infection of central nervous system leads to the incidence of HIV-associated dementia in adults. Researchers explored the utilization of therapeutic siRNA-based gene therapy to inhibit the HIV infection. Carbosilane dendrimers of generation-2 were successfully utilized as non-viral vector to deliver siRNA and transfect to HIV-infected human astrocytes through the BBB [72]. The efficiency of newly designed moieties to counter neurodegeneration can be estimated on the basis of their inhibition capability against acetylcholinesterase and butyrylcholinesterase. Viologen–phosphorus dendrimers exhibited generation and size dependent inhibitory effect on cholinesterase activities, which thereby opened way for their future exploration [73]. Although dendrimers have been used against different neurological disorders, their efficacy against dementia has not been explored till date.

4.8 Conclusion

BBB is crucial in regulating pivotal functions of the brain, and its disruption leads to a progression of severe brain disorders. Considering the benefits of the current facts and knowledge, BBB impairment is crucial in regulating the expression of specific abundant receptors in the epithelial cells from brain capillaries. The prominent research goal in designing and developing nanoformulations should consider the safety profile that will make a major impact in the preclinical research and clinical arena. In the current decade, surface-modified dendrimers are gaining huge attention in the pharmaceutical field by improving the bioavailability and brain uptake of therapeutic agent. Dendrimers have exhibited a capacity to overcome the shortcomings, considering the restricted delivery of nanotherapeutic agents in the AD conditions. The in vivo studies reported that dendrimers have ability to significantly transport both chemotherapeutic and neuroprotective molecules to combat the neurodegenerative diseases. Also, further investigation in the development of nanoparticles like dendrimers that can target specific brain cells, especially microglia, neural stem, cholinergic neurons, might enhance its therapeutic value. Moreover, utilization of dendrimers in the treatment of dementia can be explored by researchers. Overall, there is a need to focus on developing nanoplatforms by developing more efficient non-invasive and brain-directed therapies for clinical neurodegenerative benefits.

References

[1] Abbasi E, Aval SF, Akbarzadeh A, Milani M, Nasrabadi HT, Joo SW, Hanifehpour Y, Nejati-Koshki K, Pashaei-Asl R. Dendrimers: synthesis, applications, and properties. Nanoscale Res Lett 2014;9(1):1–10.

[2] Alzheimer's Association. Alzheimer's disease facts and figures. Alzheimer's Dement 2021; 17(3):327–406.

[3] Breijyeh Z, Karaman R. Comprehensive review on Alzheimer's disease: causes and treatment. Molecules 2020;25(24):5789.

[4] Camps P, Formosa X, Galdeano C, Gómez T, Muñoz-Torrero D, Scarpellini M, Viayna E, Badia A, Clos MV, Camins A, Pallàs M, Bartolini M, Mancini F, Andrisano V, Estelrich J,

Lizondo M, Bidon-Chanal A, Luque FJ. Novel donepezil-based inhibitors of acetyl- and butyrylcholinesterase and acetylcholinesterase-induced beta-amyloid aggregation. J Med Chem 2008;51(12):3588–98.
[5] Cunha S, Ben Forbes B, Lobo JMS, Silva AC. Improving drug delivery for Alzheimer's disease through nose-to-brain delivery using nanoemulsions, nanostructured lipid carriers (NLC) and in situ hydrogels. Int J Nanomed 2021;16:4373–90.
[6] Fan X, Li Z, Loh XJ. Recent development of unimolecular micelles as functional materials and applications. Polym Chem 2016;38:5898–919.
[7] Gothwal A, Malik S, Gupta U, Jain NK. Toxicity and biocompatibility aspects of dendrimers. In: Chauhan A, Kulhari H, editors. Pharmaceutical applications of dendrimers. USA: Elsevier Inc.; 2019:251–74.
[8] Jain K. Dendrimers smart nanoengineered polymers for bioinspired applications in drug delivery. In: Jana S, Maithi S, Jana S, editors. Biopolymer-based composites, 1st ed. UK: Woodhead Publishing Ltd.; 2017:169–220.
[9] Kesharwani P, Jain K, Jain NK. Dendrimer as nanocarrier for drug delivery. Prog Polym Sci 2014;39:268–307.
[10] Palmerston Mendes L, Pan J, Torchilin VP. Dendrimers as nano carriers for nucleic acid and drug delivery in cancer therapy. Molecules 2017;22:1409.
[11] Sharma A, Liaw K, Sharma R, Spriggs T, Appiani La Rosa S, Kannan S, Kannan RM. Dendrimer-mediated targeted delivery of rapamycin to tumor-associated macrophages improves systemic treatment of glioblastoma. Biomacromolecules 2020;21:5148–61.
[12] Tomalia DA, Baker H, Dewald J, Hall M, Kallos G, Martin S, Smith P. Dendritic macromolecules: synthesis of starburst dendrimers. Macromolecule 1986;19(9):2466–8. doi:10.1021/ma00163a029.
[13] Tomalia DA, Fréchet JMJ. Discovery of dendrimers and dendritic polymers: a brief historical perspective. J Polym Sci Part A: Polym Chem 2002;40:2719–28.
[14] Yang WJ, Cheng YY, Xu TW, Wang XY, Wen LP. Targeting cancer cells with biotin-dendrimers conjugates. Eur J Med Chem 2008;44:862.
[15] Zahin N, Anwar R, Tewari D, Kabir T, Sajid A, Mathew B, Uddin S, Aleya L, Abdel-Daim M. Nanoparticles and its biomedical applications in health and diseases: special focus on drug delivery. Environ Sci Pollut Res 2020;27:19151–68.
[16] Tomalia DA, Fréchet JM. Discovery of dendrimers and dendritic polymers: a brief historical perspective. J Polym Sci Part A Polym Chem 2002;40(16):2719–28.
[17] Maiti PK, Çağın T, Wang G, Goddard WA. Structure of pamam dendrimers: generations 1 through 11. Macromolecules 2004;37(16):6236–54.
[18] Ziemba B, Janaszewska A, Ciepluch K, Krotewicz M, Fogel WA, Appelhans D, Voit B, Bryszewska M, Klajnert B. In vivo toxicity of poly (propyleneimine) dendrimers. J Biomed Mater Res Part A 2011;99(2):261–8.
[19] Kaur D, Jain K, Mehra NK, Kesharwani P, Jain NK. A review on comparative study of PPI and PAMAM dendrimers. J Nanopart Res 2016;18(6):1–14.
[20] Ryan GM, Kaminskas LM, Bulitta JB, McIntosh MP, Owen DJ, Porter CJ. PEGylated polylysine dendrimers increase lymphatic exposure to doxorubicin when compared to PEGylated liposomal and solution formulations of doxorubicin. J Controlled Release 2013;172(1):128–36.
[21] Byrne M, Victory D, Hibbitts A, Lanigan M, Heise A, Cryan SA. Molecular weight and architectural dependence of well-defined star-shaped poly (lysine) as a gene delivery vector. Biomater Sci 2013;1(12):1223–34.
[22] Caminade AM, Majoral JP. Nanomaterials based on phosphorus dendrimers. Acc Chem Res 2004;37(6):341–8.

[23] Wasiak T, Ionov M, Nieznanski K, Nieznanska H, Klementieva O, Granell M, Cladera J, Majoral JP, Caminade AM, Klajnert B. Phosphorus dendrimers affect Alzheimer's (Aβ1–28) peptide and MAP-Tau protein aggregation. Mol Pharm 2012;9(3):458–69.

[24] Zhou LL, Roovers J. Synthesis of novel carbosilane dendritic macromolecules. Macromolecules 1993;26(5):963–8.

[25] Zhu Y, Liu C, Pang Z. Dendrimer-based drug delivery systems for brain targeting. Biomolecules 2019;9(12):790.

[26] Sharma G, Sharma AR, Lee SS, Bhattacharya M, Nam JS, Chakraborty C. Advances in nanocarriers enabled brain targeted drug delivery across blood brain barrier. Int J Pharm 2019;559:360–72.

[27] Siegal T, Rubinstein R, Bokstein F, Schwartz A, Lossos A, Shalom E, Chisin R, Gomori JM. In vivo assessment of the window of barrier opening after osmotic blood–brain barrier disruption in humans. J Neurosurg 2000;92(4):599–605.

[28] Bennewitz MF, Saltzman WM. Nanotechnology for delivery of drugs to the brain for epilepsy. Neurotherapeutics 2009;6(2):323–36.

[29] Bobo RH, Laske DW, Akbasak A, Morrison PF, Dedrick RL, Oldfield EH. Convection-enhanced delivery of macromolecules in the brain. Proc Natl Acad Sci 1994;91(6):2076–80.

[30] Yi X, Manickam DS, Brynskikh A, Kabanov AV. Agile delivery of protein therapeutics to CNS. J Controlled Release 2014;190:637–63.

[31] Zhang X, Chen G, Wen L, Yang F, Shao AL, Li X, Long W, Mu L. Novel multiple agents loaded PLGA nanoparticles for brain delivery via inner ear administration: in vitro and in vivo evaluation. Eur J Pharm Sci 2013;48(4-5):595–603.

[32] Furtado D, Björnmalm M, Ayton S, Bush AI, Kempe K, Caruso F. Overcoming the blood–brain barrier: the role of nanomaterials in treating neurological diseases. Adv Mater 2018;30(46):1801362.

[33] Yang W, Barth RF, Adams DM, Ciesielski MJ, Fenstermaker RA, Shukla S, Tjarks W, Caligiuri MA. Convection-enhanced delivery of boronated epidermal growth factor for molecular targeting of EGF receptor-positive gliomas. Cancer Res 2002;62(22):6552–8.

[34] Regino CAS, Walbridge S, Bernardo M, Wong KJ, Johnson D, Lonser R, Oldfield EH, Choyke PL, Brechbiel MW. A dual CT-MR dendrimer contrast agent as a surrogate marker for convection-enhanced delivery of intracerebral macromolecular therapeutic agents. Contrast Media Mol Imaging 2008;3(1):2–8.

[35] Fang F, Zou D, Wang W, Yin Y, Yin T, Hao S, Wang B, Wang G, Wang Y. Non-invasive approaches for drug delivery to the brain based on the receptor mediated transport. Mater Sci Eng: C 2017;76:1316–27.

[36] Grassin-Delyle S, Buenestado A, Naline E, Faisy C, Blouquit-Laye S, Couderc LJ, Le Guen M, Fischler M, Devillier P. Intranasal drug delivery: an efficient and non-invasive route for systemic administration: focus on opioids. Pharmacol Ther 2012;134(3):366–79.

[37] Bitter C, Suter-Zimmermann K, Surber C. Nasal drug delivery in humans. Top Applic Mucosa 2011;40:20–35.

[38] Kim YS, Sung DK, Kim H, Kong WH, Kim YE, Hahn SK. Nose-to-brain delivery of hyaluronate–FG loop peptide conjugate for non-invasive hypoxic-ischemic encephalopathy therapy. J Controlled Release 2019;307:76–89.

[39] Sukumar UK, Bose RJ, Malhotra M, Babikir HA, Afjei R, Robinson E, Zeng Y, Chang E, Habte F, Sinclair R, Gambhir SS. Intranasal delivery of targeted polyfunctional gold–iron oxide nanoparticles loaded with therapeutic microRNAs for combined theranostic multimodality imaging and presensitization of glioblastoma to temozolomide. Biomaterials 2019;218:119342.

[40] Wang Z, Xiong G, Tsang WC, Schätzlein AG, Uchegbu IF. Nose-to-brain delivery. J Pharmacol Exp Ther 2019;370(3):593–601.

[41] Patel A, Surti N, Mahajan A. Intranasal drug delivery: novel delivery route for effective management of neurological disorders. J Drug Deliv Sci Technol 2019;52:130–7.

[42] Mignani S, Shi X, Karpus A, Majoral JP. Non-invasive intranasal administration route directly to the brain using dendrimer nanoplatforms: an opportunity to develop new CNS drugs. Eur J Med Chem 2021;209:112905.

[43] Dong Z, Katsumi H, Sakane T, Yamamoto A. Effects of polyamidoamine (PAMAM) dendrimers on the nasal absorption of poorly absorbable drugs in rats. Int J Pharm 2010;393(1-2):245–53.

[44] Katare YK, Daya RP, Sookram Gray C, Luckham RE, Bhandari J, Chauhan AS, Mishra RK. Brain targeting of a water insoluble antipsychotic drug haloperidol via the intranasal route using pamam dendrimer. Mol Pharm 2015;12(9):3380–8.

[45] Kim ID, Shin JH, Kim SW, Choi S, Ahn J, Han PL, Park JS, Lee JK. Intranasal delivery of HMGB1 siRNA confers target gene knockdown and robust neuroprotection in the postischemic brain. Mol Ther 2012;20(4):829–39.

[46] Xie H, Li L, Sun Y, Wang Y, Gao S, Tian Y, Ma X, Guo C, Bo F, Zhang L. An available strategy for nasal brain transport of nanocomposite based on PAMAM dendrimers via in situ gel. Nanomaterials 2019;9(2):147.

[47] Gao H. Progress and perspectives on targeting nanoparticles for brain drug delivery. Acta Pharm Sin B 2016;6(4):268–86.

[48] Fang F, Zou D, Wang W, Yin Y, Yin T, Hao S, Wang B, Wang G, Wang Y. Non-invasive approaches for drug delivery to the brain based on the receptor mediated transport. Mater Sci Eng: C 2017;76:1316–27.

[49] Sharma A, Porterfield JE, Smith E, Sharma R, Kannan S, Kannan RM. Effect of mannose targeting of hydroxyl pamam dendrimers on cellular and organ biodistribution in a neonatal brain injury model. J Controlled Release 2018;283:175–89.

[50] Wang ZH, Wang ZY, Sun CS, Wang CY, Jiang TY, Wang SL. Trimethylated chitosan-conjugated PLGA nanoparticles for the delivery of drugs to the brain. Biomaterials 2010; 31(5):908–15.

[51] Pardridge WM. Blood–brain barrier delivery. Drug Discov Today 2007;12(1-2):54–61.

[52] Qian ZM, Li H, Sun H, Ho K. Targeted drug delivery via the transferrin receptor-mediated endocytosis pathway. Pharmacol Rev 2002;54(4):561–87.

[53] Yu Y, Jiang X, Gong S, Feng L, Zhong Y, Pang Z. The proton permeability of self-assembled polymersomes and their neuroprotection by enhancing a neuroprotective peptide across the blood–brain barrier after modification with lactoferrin. Nanoscale 2014;6(6):3250–8.

[54] Patel HK, Gajbhiye V, Kesharwani P, Jain NK. Ligand anchored poly (propyleneimine) dendrimers for brain targeting: comparative in vitro and in vivo assessment. J Colloid Interface Sci 2016;482:142–50.

[55] Gothwal A, Kumar H, Nakhate KT, Ajazuddin, Dutta A, Borah A, Gupta U. Lactoferrin coupled lower generation pamam dendrimers for brain targeted delivery of memantine in aluminum-chloride-induced Alzheimer's disease in mice. Bioconjug Chem 2019;30(10):2573–83.

[56] Somani S, Robb G, Pickard BS, Dufès C. Enhanced gene expression in the brain following intravenous administration of lactoferrin-bearing polypropylenimine dendriplex. J Controlled Release 2015;217:235–42.

[57] Somani S, Blatchford DR, Millington O, Stevenson ML, Dufès C. Transferrin-bearing polypropylenimine dendrimer for targeted gene delivery to the brain. J Controlled Release 2014;188:78–86.

[58] Fana M, Gallien J, Srinageshwar B, Dunbar GL, Rossignol J. PAMAM dendrimer nanomolecules utilized as drug delivery systems for potential treatment of glioblastoma: a systematic review. Int J Nanomed 2020;15:2789.

[59] Mignani S, El Kazzouli S, Bousmina M, Majoral JP. Expand classical drug administration ways by emerging routes using dendrimer drug delivery systems: a concise overview. Adv Drug Deliv Rev 2013;65:1316–30.

[60] Klajnert B, Cladera J, Bryszewska M. Molecular interactions of dendrimers with amyloid peptides: pH dependence. Biomacromolecules 2006;7:2186–91.

[61] Patel D, Henry J, Good T. Attenuation of β-amyloid induced toxicity by sialic acid-conjugated dendrimeric polymers. Biochim Biophys Acta (BBA)-General Subjects 2006;1760:1802–9.

[62] Patel DA, Henry JE, Good TA. Attenuation of β-amyloid-induced toxicity by sialic-acid-conjugated dendrimers: role of sialic acid attachment. Brain Res 2007;1161:95–105.

[63] Wang Z, Dong X, Sun Y. Hydrophobic modification of carboxyl-terminated polyamidoamine dendrimer surface creates a potent inhibitor of amyloid-β fibrillation. Langmuir 2018;34:14419–27.

[64] Gothwal A, Nakhate KT, Alexander A, Ajazuddin, Gupta U. Boosted memory and improved brain bioavailability of rivastigmine: targeting effort to the brain using covalently tethered lower generation pamam dendrimers with lactoferrin. Mol Pharm 2018;15:4538–49.

[65] Gothwal A, Singh H, Jain SK, Dutta A, Borah A, Gupta U. Behavioral and biochemical implications of dendrimeric rivastigmine in memory-deficit and Alzheimer's induced rodents. ACS Chem Neurosci 2019;10(2019):3789–95.

[66] Aso E, Martinsson I, Appelhans D, Effenberg C, Benseny-Cases N, Cladera J, Gouras G, Ferrer I, Klementieva O. Poly (propylene imine) dendrimers with histidine-maltose shell as novel type of nanoparticles for synapse and memory protection. Nanomed: Nanotechnol Biol Med 2019;17:198–209.

[67] Wrobel D, Appelhans D, Signorelli M, Wiesner B, Fessas D, Scheler U, Voit B, Maly J. Interaction study between maltose-modified PPI dendrimers and lipidic model membranes. Biochim Biophys Acta (BBA)-Biomembr 2021;1848:1490–501.

[68] Neelov I, Janaszewska A, Klajnert B, Bryszewska M, Makova NZ, Hicks D, Pearson HA, Vlasov GP, Ilyash MY, Vasilev DS, Dubrovskaya NM. Molecular properties of lysine dendrimers and their interactions with aβ-peptides and neuronal cells. Curr Med Chem 2013;20:134–43.

[69] Al-Azzawi S, Masheta D, Guildford AL, Phillips G, Santin M. Dendrimeric poly (epsilon-lysine) delivery systems for the enhanced permeability of flurbiprofen across the blood-brain barrier in Alzheimer's disease. Int J Mol Sci 2018;19:3224.

[70] Wasiak T, Marcinkowska M, Pieszynski I, Zablocka M, Caminade AM, Majoral JP, Klajnert-Maculewicz B. Cationic phosphorus dendrimers and therapy for Alzheimer's disease. New J Chem 2015;39:4852–9.

[71] Chen JH, Lin KP, Chen YC. Risk factors for dementia. J Formos Med Assoc 2009;108(10):754–64.

[72] Jiménez JL, Clemente MI, Weber ND, Sanchez J, Ortega P, de la Mata FJ, Gómez R, García D, López-Fernández LA, Muñoz-Fernández MÁ. Carbosilane dendrimers to transfect human astrocytes with small interfering RNA targeting human immunodeficiency virus. BioDrugs 2010;24(5):331–43.

[73] Ciepluch K, Weber M, Katir N, Caminade AM, El Kadib A, Klajnert B, Majoral JP, Bryszewska M. Effect of viologen–phosphorus dendrimers on acetylcholinesterase and butyrylcholinesterase activities. Int J Biol Macromol 2013;54:119–24.

[74] Benseny-Cases N, Álvarez-Marimon E, Aso E, Carmona M, Klementieva O, Appelhans D, et al. In situ identification and G4-PPI-His-Mal-dendrimer-induced reduction of early-stage amyloid aggregates in Alzheimer's disease transgenic mice using synchrotron-based infrared imaging. Sci Rep 2021;11(1):1–9.

Chapter 5

Polymeric nanoparticles as drug delivery systems for dementia

Gerard Esteruelas[a,b], Eliana B. Souto[c,d], Amanda Cano[a,b,e,f], Miren Ettcheto[e,g], Marta Espina[a,b], Antonio Camins[e,g], Maria Luisa García[a,b,e], Elena Sánchez-López[a,b,e,h]

[a]Department of Pharmacy, Pharmaceutical Technology & Physical Chemistry, Faculty of Pharmacy & Food Sciences, University of Barcelona, Barcelona, Spain, [b]Institute of Nanoscience & Nanotechnology (IN2UB), Barcelona, Spain, [c]Department of Pharmaceutical Technology, Faculty of Pharmacy, University of Porto, Porto, Portugal, [d]REQUIMTE/UCIBIO, Faculty of Pharmacy, University of Porto, Porto, Portugal, [e]Biomedical Research Networking Centre in Neurodegenerative Diseases (CIBERNED), Madrid, Spain, [f]Ace Alzheimer Center Barcelona – International University of Catalunya (UIC), Barcelona, Spain, [g]Department of Pharmacology, Toxicology & Therapeutic Chemistry, Faculty of Pharmacy & Food Sciences, University of Barcelona, Barcelona, Spain, [h]Unit of Synthesis and Biomedical Applications of Peptides, IQAC-CSIC, Barcelona, Spain

5.1 Introduction

Nanomaterials and nanomedicine have gradually gained importance as a pharmacotherapeutic tool for treatment, diagnosis, and prevention of different types of diseases [1,2]. Proof of which is the enormous increase of the demand that has occurred in nanomaterials at a commercial and industrial level [3]. This phenomenon can be explained due to the imperative need for novel therapeutic strategies for the treatment of different diseases, such as those that affect the central nervous system (CNS). For this type of pathologies or syndromes, such as dementia, in average the pharmacological activities of the drugs currently used are reduced by more than 98% as a consequence of the blood–brain barrier (BBB) [4,5]. This entails not only a decrease in the desired therapeutic efficacy, but can also lead to a safety problem for the patient, since this active molecule, by not being able to fully access its therapeutic target, can interact with other tissues or molecules and cause unwanted effects ([2,6]).

Moreover, in the recent decades life expectancy has alarmingly increased, which has led to an increase in the incidence of neurodegenerative pathologies [7]. According to data from the World Health Organization (WHO), dementia is one of the 10 main causes of death worldwide, being the second in developed countries with high economic levels [8]. This fact makes dementia an important public health problem for which there is currently no therapeutic strategy or

Nanomedicine-Based Approaches for the Treatment of Dementia. https://doi.org/10.1016/B978-0-12-824331-2.00006-6
Copyright © 2023 Elsevier Inc. All rights reserved.

completely effective treatment, and there are no tools available that allow an effective early diagnosis [9–11].

For all the above, nanomedicine is essential for the crucial development of effective therapies and specially controlled drug delivery systems such as polymeric nanoparticles (NPs) [6,12]. Using this tool, we can improve the efficacy and bioavailability of current and future treatments, due to the fact that it allows to control the drug pharmacokinetic profile and, at the same time, to guide the active molecule to its therapeutic target. Thus facilitating the passage through the most restrictive physiological barriers of the body such as the BBB, achieving a potential increase in efficiency and reducing toxicity [13].

5.2 Dementia

Dementia is a syndrome where there is a deterioration or loss of cognitive function, beyond what is predictable by aging. It interferes with the day-to-day life of the patient, affecting memory, comprehension, visual perception, language, learning capacity, ability to solve problems, and judgment. In addition to this deterioration, dementia can affect emotional control as well as social skills [10,14].

Dementia is currently one of the most frequent chronic diseases. According to WHO data, it is estimated that there are approximately 50 million people who suffer from it, and each year there are almost 10 million new cases worldwide [8,15].

In addition to the data presented, it should be noted that due to the general aging of society, it is estimated that in countries like the United States by 2050 the cases of people suffering from dementia could double. Reaching 152 million case worldwide [15].

This syndrome produces a huge impact, not only on the person who suffers from it, but also on their environment, because it is one of the main causes of dependency and disability within the older population. The demands of dementia can be devastating at the physical, psychological, and economic level of the environment closest to the patient [16,17].

The symptomatology will depend on the region of the brain that is affected, the type of dementia, the magnitude, the time elapsed, and even the personality of the person who suffers it. In the initial stages of dementia, symptoms may be disregarded, such as occasional forgetfulness or loss of notion of time, but as time passes the symptoms worsens, producing difficulty in communication, forgetting names of people or even family members, changes in behavior among others. Finally, in more advanced stages, in addition to the memory and physical deterioration, the patient can become completely dependent [18–20].

In general, the long-term prognosis of a patient diagnosed with dementia is not very promising. In this area, with the current therapies, the decline of these patients can be delayed, and symptoms can be ameliorated but they do not offer a cure to this disease [21,22].

Dementia is the result of a wide variety of diseases and injuries that primarily or secondarily affect the brain, such as Alzheimer's disease (AD) or dementia resulting from a stroke.

Therefore, we find a very heterogeneous scenario between the different types of dementia. AD is the most widely known thus being attributed to the highest percent of total cases [23]. Other major types of dementia are vascular dementia, Lewy body dementia (LBD) (abnormal aggregates of proteins that develop within nerve cells), and frontotemporal dementia (FTD) (degeneration of the frontal lobe of the brain). However, the boundaries between the different forms of dementia are unclear and mixed forms often coexist [24–27].

As can be seen in Fig. 5.1, AD is the most common type of dementia affecting around 60–80% of the people who suffer from dementia [29]. Briefly, AD occurs with a loss of cognitive function as well as memory loss due to a neurodegenerative process involving death of neuronal cells. In this disease, the formation of neurofibrillary tangles of aggregates of the hyperphosphorylated tau protein and aggregates of oligomers of the Aβ-amyloid protein occurs, resulting in the formation of senile plaques [30–32]. At the macroscopic level,

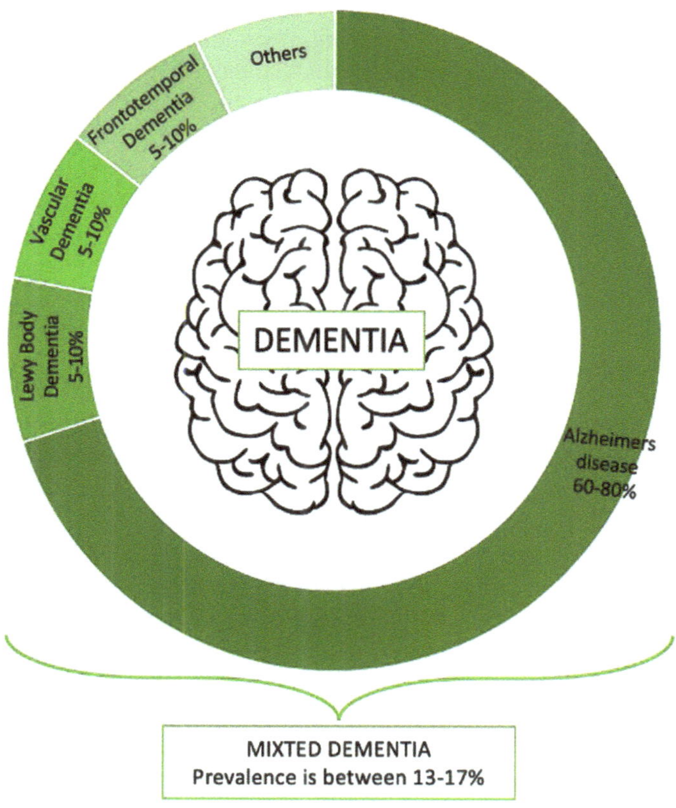

FIG. 5.1 Main types of dementia, adapted from [23,28].

a progressive bilateral atrophy, a thinning of the cortical lamina, and the weight of the brain are observed [33–35].

LBD is produced by the accumulation of Lewy bodies. These are formed by a protein called α-synuclein which, when accumulated in certain brain regions, inhibits the formation of neurotransmitters such as dopamine, thus affecting movement, mood, and sleep. It also inhibits the formation of acetylcholine causing memory impairment. LBD, usually concurs with hallucinations during the initial stages and, in general, there is no short-term memory loss [9,36–38].

Like LBD, vascular dementia is another one of the most frequent types of dementia, affecting between 5% and 10% of patients. This type of dementia is produced by the temporary blockage of oxygen and nutrients supply to the brain due to a decrease in blood flow. The symptoms will depend on the magnitude of the vascular injury produced and the affected region. Memory loss can be similar to AD [25,39,40].

Another relevant type of dementia is FTD that encompasses a group of diseases involving progressive neurodegeneration of neuronal cells in the frontal lobe, causing problems in speech, movement, planning ability, or control of emotions [9,41,42].

Other types of dementia with great relevance but a lower incidence are, on the one hand, the one known as Parkinson's disease (PD) with dementia where Lewys bodies appear, which means that movement problems and mental deterioration start earlier. On the other hand, dementia associated with Down syndrome, a prevalence what affects specially to young population. Moreover, other types of dementia such as the one caused by Huntington's disease, Creutzfeldt–Jakob disease, normal pressure hydrocephalus, Wernicke–Korsakoff syndrome [36,43], and posterior cortical atrophy are also worth mentioning. Among mixed dementias, the most frequent is AD and vascular dementia concomitantly [23].

5.3 Polymeric nanoparticles

Polymeric NPs generally are colloidal systems with a size ranged between 1 and 500 nm. These NPs can be formulated using different methods depending on the physicochemical characteristics of both the polymer, the drug and administration route [44–47].

In general, polymeric NPs are classified into two large subfamilies: nanocapsules and nanospheres, which differ in their morphology. The first is composed of a reservoir-type system, composed of a core, where the drug is generally dissolved, covered by a polymeric matrix that allows controlling the kinetic release profile of the drug. On the other hand, nanospheres are based on matrix systems where the drug is dispersed inside. The drug is released either by a diffusion process or degradation mechanism. Moreover, a combination of the two mechanisms can also occur. It is important to highlight that both NPs can have drug adsorbed on their surface, thus promoting a rapid initial release [48–51].

There is a great variety of biopolymers that could form the matrix core of the NPs. The most widely used polymers according to whether they are of natural or synthetic origin are classified below.

5.3.1 Natural polymers

This group of polymers are made from proteins, oligosaccharides, and polysaccharides from natural origin such as plants, bacteria, animals, and fungi. This type of polymers has shown high biocompatibility and biodegradability, the latter mediated by enzymatic degradation reactions. This phenomenon allows scientists to adjust polymer degradation rate modifying the kinetics of drug release. These characteristics make natural polymers an excellent option for food, cosmetic, and medical applications. Nevertheless this kind of polymers presents a great problem derived from the variability that may exist between the different batches, which can be harmful for the application in nanomedicine due to the variations of the physicochemical properties that this may present. Moreover, often these polymers require chemical modifications to improve their properties and decrease their immunogenicity [51–53]. The most widely used naturals polymers are listed below (Fig. 5.2):

- *Chitosan* is produced from a controlled deacetylation process in a basic medium of chitin, which is a polymer that is found very abundantly in the exoskeletons of crustaceans and insects, as well as in the cell wall of fungi. Chitosan is a copolymer formed by a linear chain of polysaccharides through the bond between D-glucosamine and N-acetylglucosamine (Fig. 5.2) [1–4]. This polymer can be modified by changing the degree of acetylation and molecular weight to obtain the desired properties. In general, chitosan is soluble in the majority of organic solvents as well as in acid solutions at pH <6.5 [54].

  This biopolymer of natural origin is one of the most widely used in both the textile and pharmaceutical industries. Especially in the latter, it has aroused great interest due to its potential for biomedical applications, since it is a polymer that is considered to have practically no toxicity. It allows protease-mediated biodegradation producing oligosaccharides that can be reused as glycoprotein components or excreted. Finally, due to the deacetylation reaction used during its synthesis, this polymer acquires a positive charge, which allows it to improve cell absorption, adhesion, and subsequent permeability in the mucosa. These offer a great potential to administer medications orally and increase its intestinal permeability [55].
- *Dextran* is a complex glucan of microbial origin, formed by glycosidic bonds of branched α-D-glucose units. It is a polymer with a large number of hydroxyl groups, offering hydrophilic proprieties. The high number of hydroxyl chains allows a large number of possible chemical modifications to vary its properties. Some of the most prominent are acetylation in order to change its affinity for water and transform it into a hydrophobic polymer, or

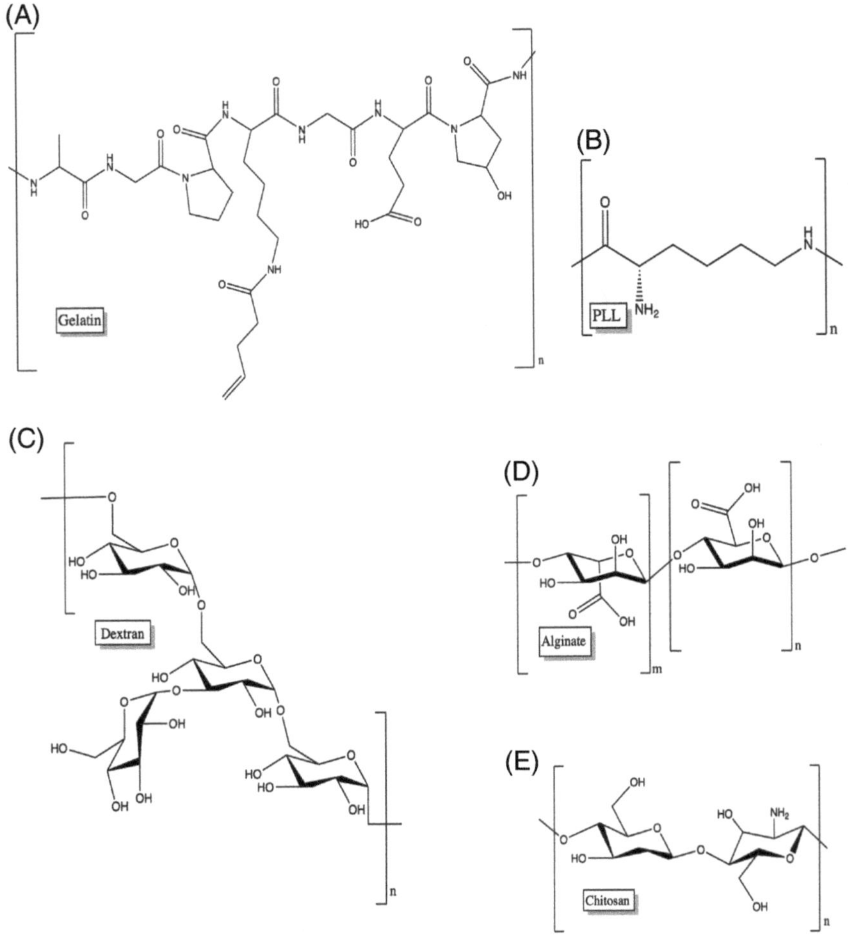

FIG. 5.2 Chemical structure of the different most widely used natural polymers. A: Gelatin, B: PLL, C: dextran, D: alginate, and E: chitosan.

the introduction of a sulfate group. Dextran has excellent biological properties of biocompatibility and degradation to be used in the transport of drugs [50,56,57].

- *Alginate* is obtained by an economic process of purifying brown seaweed. It is a linear hydrophobic polysaccharide formed by bonds between monomers of β-D-mannuronic acid and α-L-glucuronic acid [1–4]. The physicochemical properties of this polymer are conditioned by the sequence and ratio of these monomers. The molecular weight can also vary from 200 to 500 kDa. It is considered a very versatile polymer that allows its large number of modifications thanks to the large number of hydroxyl and carboxylic groups. These allow the modification of its physicochemical and biological properties. It is a polymer of interest in the biomedical industry due to its high biocompatibility, nonimmunogenicity nor toxicity, which also has good biodegradation and high mucoadhesiveness that allows high cell bonding [58,59].

- Other natural polymers used are *poly-L-lysine*, this polymer is a homopolymer of lysines, it is used mainly for the formation of nanocapsules to increase the absorption of negatively charged molecules, such as nucleic acids. Finally, another polymer that can be used is *gelatin* derived from collagen, which is a protein found in greater quantity in animals, especially in epithelial and bone tissue, it is a very biocompatible polymer that is easily degraded by physiological enzymes, present in numerous clinical applications, currently in the field of nanomedicine its use is limited by the lack of homogeneity in the sizes of the NPs obtained [50,51,60].

5.3.2 Synthetic polymers

This group of polymers is highly heterogeneous. They are designed with specific physicochemical properties to meet the desired objective, they can be optimized depending on the pathology to be targeted, the molecules to be encapsulated or the route of administration. They have numerous advantages, including their high stability, their ease of production scaling at an industrial level, high purity and little variability between different batches, the latter being one of the main problems of natural polymers. Currently, the synthetic polymers used have to meet a series of requirements, both the polymer itself and the different metabolites produced during their degradation. This constitutes the limiting point when using this type of polymers because in some cases the degradation metabolites do not meet the characteristics described. These polymers must be biocompatible with the recipient tissues, and, in addition, they must be stable in a physiological environment, and also biodegradable [48,51,61].

Among the different families of synthetic polymers that exist, the most promising in the field of nanomedicine are aliphatic polyesters. The synthetic polymers most widely used are described below (Fig. 5.3).

- *Polylactic acid (PLA)*, this polymer is produced by the polymerization reaction of the two chiral forms deriving in L-PLA and D-PLA. For drug delivery systems the most widely involved candidate is the one formed by the amorphous form L,D-PLA because the degradation reaction is faster and more adequate. This polymer is widely used in biomedical applications thanks to its practically absence of toxicity, biocompatibility and biodegradability, resulting in lactic acid that will later be metabolized and excreted from the body in the form of CO_2. Moreover, this polymer can be positively charged by introducing new functional groups in the backbone of the polymer such as amines. It is used for the transport of drugs and proteins and for genetic sequences of interest. Some limitations regarding the low encapsulation efficiency have been described in this polymer. As it has been shown that small NPs of this polymer could present a slight immunogenicity [61,62].

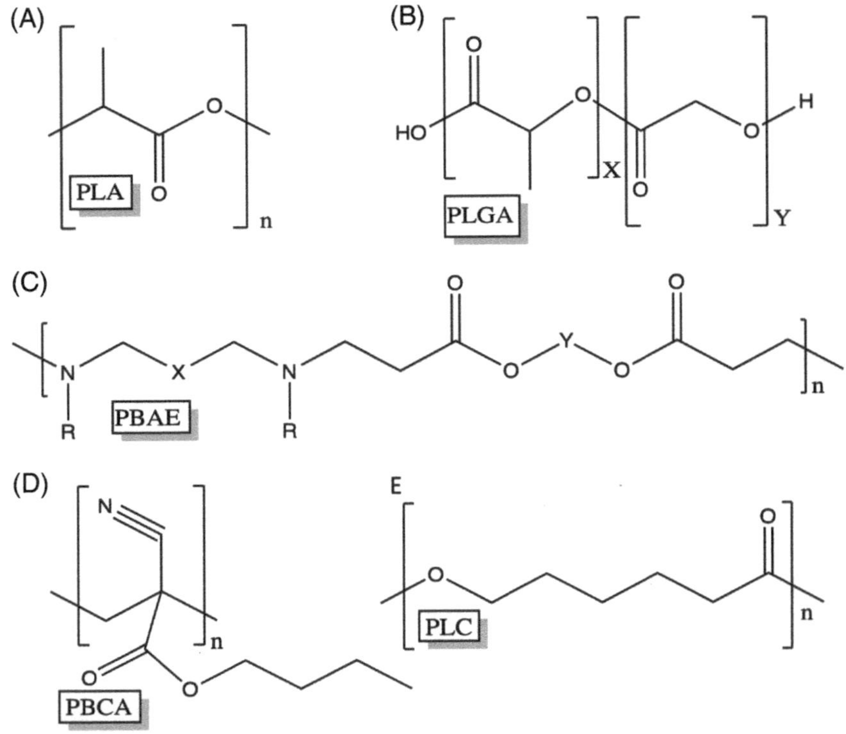

FIG. 5.3 Chemical structure of the most widely used synthetic polymers. A: PLA, B: PLGA, C: PBAE, D: PBCA, and E: PCL.

- *Poly-D,L-(lactic-co-glycolic acid) or PLGA* is one of the biodegradable synthetic polymers that is currently best characterized. It comes from the polymerization reaction of the heterocyclic dimers of lactic acid and glycolic acid, therefore combining PLA and polyglycolic acid PGA. There are different types of PLGA depending on the PLA/PGA ratio. This allows its molecular weight and polymer degradation rate to be modulated in order to be able to adjust the subsequent release kinetics of the encapsulated substance. This polymer has high stability and low toxicity. When metabolized it degrades into lactic acid and glycolic acid to later be transformed into CO_2 and water. PLGA allows the modification of its surface with the addition of cationic groups to improve the encapsulation efficiency of certain molecules. Despite this, PLGA may not be able to control the release of certain drugs or bioactive molecules. This polymer is approved by the different drug agencies for the administration of drugs with prolonged effect [51,63,64].
- *Polycaprolactone (PCL)* is a hydrophobic biopolymer synthesized from the polymerization of ε-caprolactone. It is considered a semicrystalline polymer that at room temperature has good solubility in organic solvents. This polymer, due to its good stability in biological fluids, its low toxicity and

high permeability, constitutes a great candidate for applications in the field of nanomedicine. It possesses ester bonds that are easily hydrolyzed under physiological conditions, and does not produce acid metabolites. However, at the end of its metabolization it is excreted in the form of CO_2, a fact that makes it an ideal polymer long-lasting for implants. PCL is a polymer is usually employed along with other polymers to modulate degradation processes [65].

- *Poly (β-amino ester)* is a synthetic polymer obtained through a conjugated addition of amine to acrylamide, which allows the modification of the polymer skeleton by adding different terminations, in order to modify its properties, such as charge, hydrophobicity, or molecular weight. This biopolymer, apart from its low toxicity, stands out for its insolubility at physiological pH but its high solubility at more acidic pH (below 6.5). This factor confers a high specificity for intracellular release, due to the fact that until the NPs are not phagocytosed or within an endosome where the pH is acidified, the polymer will not begin to solubilize and release the content [66,67].
- Finally, another synthetic polymer is poly (butylcyanoacrylate) (PBCA), this is a biodegradable biopolymer approved by the Food and Drug Administration for the closure of surgical wounds. This polymer also has suitable characteristics for the field of biomedical nanotechnology. It is a low molecular weight polymer formed mainly by chains of approximately 4 kDa. It is one of the synthetic biopolymers that degrades faster by enzyme-mediated hydrolysis of the ester groups, resulting in water-soluble compounds [68,69].

5.4 Polymeric nanoparticles for treatment and diagnosis of dementia

In the last decade, important advances have been made in order to improve the treatment and diagnosis of dementia, especially for AD, as this syndrome constitutes the majority of cases of dementia. In these advances, as can be observed in Table 5.1 the use of nanotechnology in particular of polymeric NPs stands out [70].

5.4.1 PLGA

A wide variety of studies have been carried out exploring the development of brain-target PLGA NPs. Especially, AD is one of the most widely studied pathologies for novel pharmacological therapies involving this type of NPs. In this area Aalinkeel et al. have developed and characterized PLGA NPs in order to be able to treat and diagnose AD. They encapsulated Ginsenoside Rg3 and Thioflavin T, being the former a powerful anti-inflammatory of natural origin with the potential to reduce AD plaques. On the other hand, Thioflavin T is a fluorescent marker for protein aggregation, as could be the case for protein Aβ-amyloid aggregations. These NPs were functionalized by incorporating cell

TABLE 5.1 Summary of polymeric NPs for the treatment of different types of dementia.

Polymer	Drug or active molecule	Characteristics	Type of dementia	Functionalization	In vitro assay	In vivo Assay	References
PLGA	Ginsenoside Rg3	Size: 115 nm, PDI: 0.081, EE: 65–70%, PZ: negative	AD	Angiopep2	Cellular uptake and viability. Model of crossing the BBB	-	[71]
	Quercetin	Size: 100–150 nm, PDI: not specified, EE: not specified, PZ: not specified	AD	-	Studying inhibition and dissolution efficiency by ThT. Disaggregation of αβ aggregates. Cytotoxicity studies	Model APP/PS1 mice	[90]
	Curcumin	Size: 204 nm, PDI: 0.07, EE: 60%, PZ: −13 mV	AD	G7	Uptake into neurons. Cellular toxicity. Disaggregation of αβ aggregates	-	[72]
	iAβ5	Size: 166 ± 2 nm, PDI: 0.10 ± 0.04, EE: 63 ± 9%, PZ: −13 ± 1 mV	AD	Antibodies (OX26) and anti-αβ (DE2B4)	Cellular uptake. Toxicity	-	[76]
	PHA-767491	Size: 145–155 nm, PDI: <0.15, EE: 18%, PZ: not specified	FTD	-	Permeability to the CNS and Neuroprotective efficacy in cell model	-	[42]

Polymer	Drug or active molecule	Characteristics	Type of dementia	Function-alization	In vitro assay	In vivo Assay	Refer-ences
	Peptides: QBP1, NT17, and PGQ9P2	Size: <200 nm, PDI: <0.1, EE: 60%, PZ: (−24.3) to (−27.5) mV	HD	ApoE	HD models cell. Model of crossing the BBB	Biodistribution in mice. *Drosophila* HD model	[77]
	-	Size: ≈ 100 nm, PDI: not specified, EE: not specified, PZ: −30.2, to −31.4 mV	PD	-	Cellular uptake. Flow cytometry. Lysosomal pH analysis.	-	[78]
	Vitamin D-binding protein (DBP)	Size 226.6 ± 44.4 nm, PDI: 0.039 ± 0.013, EE: 89.3 ± 3.3%, PZ: −0.144 mV	AD	-	MTT assay. ThT assay. Histological analysis	Effectivity with male transgenic mice (5XFAD)	[91]
PLGA-PEG	Memantine	Size: 152.6 ± 0.5 nm, PDI: 0.043 ± 0.009, EE: not specified, PZ: −22.4 mV	AD severe	-	Cytotoxicity studies. Transport across the BBB. Immunohisto-chemistry	Biodistribution in brain. Immu-nohistochemistry studies Morris water maze	[74]
	Curcumin	Size: 150 nm, PDI: not specified, EE: 15.6%, PZ: 3.83 ± 0.89 mV	AD	B6	Red blood cell (RBC) lysis. Cytotoxicity studies. Cellular uptake studies	Morris water maze	[73]
Chitosan	Tacrine	Size: 41 ± 7 nm, PDI: not specified, Drug-loading capacity: 10.86%, PZ: +34.7 ± 1.5 mV	AD	-	Release kinetics. Stability studies	Biodistribution	[80]

(Continued)

Table 5.1 Cont'd

Polymer	Drug or active molecule	Characteristics	Type of dementia	Functionalization	In vitro assay	In vivo Assay	References
	Memantine	Size: 43.65 nm, PDI: not specified, EE: not specified, PZ: not specified	AD	-	-	Biodistribution Morris water maze	[92]
	Donepezil	Size: ranging from 116.8 to 227.5 nm, PDI: not specified, EE: approx. 70%, PZ: not specified	AD	-	-	-	[93]
	Anti-HTT small interfering RNA	Size: 100–160 nm, PDI: not specified, EE: not specified, PZ: not specified	HD	-	-	Gen silencing experiments	[94]
	Rivastigmine	Size: <200 nm, EE: 96.36 ± 1.09%, PZ: 26.6,±,0.9 mV, PDI: <0.3	AD	-	-	Pharmacodynamic study. Drugs and treatment schedule. Elevated plus maze. Morris water maze. Measurement of locomotor activity	[95]
Chitosan (PEG-PLA)	Nerve growth factor (NGF), acteoside (ACT), and plasmid DNA (pDNA)	Size: 160 nm, PDI: not specified, EE: not specified, PZ: −20.33 mV	PD LBD	-	Activities and toxicities studies. MPP^+ + PC12 cells were used as the PD cell model to investigate the neuro-protective.	PD mouse model. The pole test. Tests for anxiety-like behaviors. Biodistribution	[82]

Polymer	Drug or active molecule	Characteristics	Type of dementia	Functionalization	In vitro assay	In vivo Assay	References
Chitosan-PLGA	-	Size: 203.45 ± 5.75 nm, PDI: not specified, EE: not specified, PZ: 8.0 ± 1.45 mV	AD cerebral amyloid angiopathy	Antibody anti-Aβ	Uptake of immuno-nanovesicles by polarized MDCK. Cell monolayer	-	[81]
PBCA	Coumarin	Size: 197 ± 2.3 nm, PDI: 0.18, PZ: −22.44 ± 2.3 mV, EE: 77.99 ± 0.91%	AD	ApoE3	MTT assay, with SH-SY5Y human neuroblastoma cells. Flow cytometry. Antiapoptotic activity	-	[85]
	Rivastigmine	Size: 146.8 ± 2.6 nm, PDI: not specified, PZ: −13.9 ± 0.58 mV, EE 43.59 ± 3.80%	AD	-	Drug release	Morris water maze (scopolamine mouse model)	[86]
	^{125}I clioquinol	Size: 45 nm, PDI: not specified, EE: not specified, PZ: not specified	AD	-	-	Efficient test	[87,88]
	Tioflavina T and Tioflavina S	Size: 90–100 nm, PDI: not specified, EE: not specified, PZ: not specified	AD	-	Enzymatic degradation. Histochemical analysis	Binding of αβ	[89]
PCL	Memantine	Size <200 nm, PDI: <0.2, EE: 80%, PZ: −26 mv	AD	-	-	-	[83]

(Continued)

Table 5.1 Cont'd

Polymer	Drug or active molecule	Characteristics	Type of dementia	Function-alization	In vitro assay	In vivo Assay	Refer-ences
PCL-PEG	NAP or Coumarin-6	Size: Nap: 88.4 ± 7.8 nm and Coumarin: 89.0 ± 5.7 nm, PDI: Nap: 0.22 ± 0.033, cumarin 0.20 ± 0.039, EE Nap: 47.61 ± 2.36%, PZ: approx. 23 mV	AD	Lactoferrin	Cellular uptake. Histology studies	Brain delivery of NPs after intranasal administration in rat model. Neuroprotective effect. Morris water maze	[84]
PCL -mPEG	Donepezil	Size: 123.45 ± 3.98, PDI: 0.20 ± 0.04, EE: 87.21 ± 4.37%, PZ: −3.31 ± 1.49 mV	AD	ApoE3	Cytotoxicity and cellular uptake studies. Proteolysis assay neuronal toxicity in cell lines SH-SY5Y cells	Morris water maze. Behavioral assessment for cognitive function. Passive avoidance task	[96]

EE, encapsulation efficiency, PDI, polydispersion index; PZ, zeta potential.

penetrating peptides (CPPs), specifically Angiopep2. The in vitro characterization studies showed a great potential of the NPs for the treatment of AD. The authors demonstrated that the NPs were able to cross the BBB and significantly reduce both plaque formation and the expression of genes that produce them. However, in vivo studies will be needed to confirm these results [71].

In the treatment of AD, one of the drugs that has been subject of study is curcumin due to its antiamylogenic capacity. Curcumin inhibits the formation of new plaques of β-amyloid and also, disaggregate existing ones. However, this molecule has a low ability to cross through the BBB. Therefore, Barbara et al. developed functionalized curcumin NPs using the g7 peptide attached to their surface. In in vitro studies they demonstrated NPs safety in hypothalamic cell cultures and also a high capacity to disaggregate amyloid aggregates, thus reducing the inflammation and oxidative stress. In this line of research [72], Fan et al. also encapsulated curcumin in PLGA NPs functionalized with polyethylene glycol (PEG) and with the CPP B6. In this work, they carried out in vitro studies where the compatibility of NPs with blood was demonstrated as well as the increase in cellular absorption of curcumin. They also carried out in vivo studies such as the Morris water maze test with double transgenic mice, where these presented a great improvement in memory and spatial capacity. Moreover the authors also carried out ex vivo studies demonstrating the potential of NPs to decrease the formation of β-amyloid plaques and aggregates of the hyperphosphorylated tau protein [73].

Using a similar approach, Sánchez-López et al. also developed PLGA-PEG NPs for AD. In this case they encapsulated memantine, a drug focused on the treatment of severe and moderated AD but with solubility and toxicity problems. In this case they optimized the formulation which did not show any toxicity in brain cell lines. They also demonstrated both in vitro and in vivo the ability of these NPs to cross the BBB. Finally, they carried out in vivo studies that revealed the improvement in memory with respect to the free memantine in the double transgenic mouse model. In addition, NPs were able to a decrease inflammation and the β-amyloid plaques characteristic of AD [74]. Although not mentioned in the article, these NPs may also have potential for the treatment of vascular dementia due memantine potential for this disease [75].

It is worth highlighting the work carried out by Loureiro et al. as an example where the PLGA NPs were functionalized by the binding of two antibodies (OX26) and anti-A2 (DE2B4) for the release of iAβ5 encapsulated in the NPs. These were aimed to block the formation of the fibrils, through the inhibition of the formation of oligomers [76].

PLGA NPs have also been developed for other types of dementia, such as FTD. Rojas-Prats et al. had recently published and excellent study based on the encapsulation of potent CDC7 kinase inhibitor called PHA-767491. This molecule has problems to be able to permeate through the BBB but is capable of reducing the transcription of the DNA of one of the main proteins that is accumulated in the cytoplasm of neuronal cells in FTD. In vitro studies demonstrated the ability of NPs to penetrate the BBB and their efficacy using a cellular model of TDP-43 phosphorylation [42].

Other study developed PLGA NPs loaded with the QBP1 or, NT17 or, PGQ9P2 peptides for the treatment of Huntington's disease. These peptides with inhibitory capacity for polyglutamine aggregation possess low penetration capacity to cross the BBB. These biocompatible formulations did not show cellular toxicity but demonstrated the ability to cross the BBB [77].

Finally, Zeng et al. propose a novel treatment approach for the treatment PD with the presence of Lewys bodies. They develop PLGA NPs by varying the PLA/PGA ratio without encapsulating any substance. In order to take advantage of the acidification that occurs when these NPs degrade in autophagic lysosome and to modulate the pH, it is common in these pathologies that their acidification is altered [78].

5.4.2 Chitosan

Chitosan is a widely interesting polymer for the development of controlled release systems for dementia. In this area, chitosan NPs were developed by Chowdhury et al. coupling chitosan with polyfluorene. The resulting NPs, in addition to being able to efficiently cross the BBB, also allowed neurotoxic amyloid oligomers to be modulated selectively through a nonpathological route, thus offering potential applications in both treatment and diagnosis of dementia such as of AD [79].

Focusing more specifically on this polymer, Radwan et al. carried out a highly interesting research for AD. They improved the therapeutic efficacy of memantine for the treatment of AD, developing of chitosan NPs through gamma radiation. After conducting the in vivo tests, the authors concluded that chitosan NPs loaded with memantine, transported this drug more effectively to the brain, thus constituting a therapeutic improvement both at behavioral and molecular level [80].

Also for the treatment of AD, NPs that combine PLGA with chitosan have been proven to be useful. Chitosan was used as a coating but showed an essential function improving the aqueous dispersibility and the stability in the lyophilization of the systems. About these NPs, Jaruszewski et al. conjugated an anti-Aβ antibody, an obtained a suitable vehicle for the transport of a therapeutic or diagnostic agent for both AD and cerebral amyloid angiopathy that can lead to dementia of vascular origin [81].

Moreover, chitosan NPs has been developed for the treatment of other types of dementia. Xue et al. obtained chitosan NPs that were combined with PEG-PLA that allowed the administration of nerve growth factor NGF, acteoside ACT, and plasmid DNA pDNA for the treatment of PD. These researchers, after conducting the different in vitro and in vivo studies, demonstrated the neuroprotective effect of these NPs that allowed the significant inhibition of T-Syn in vitro, which shows the potential of these chitosan NPs for the inhibition of the Lewys bodies in both PD and LBD [82].

5.4.3 PCL

PCL is a versatile polymer that stands out in the area of nanostructured systems for dementia. For the treatment of AD, for the first time, memantine NPs have only been developed used PCL as polymer by Mahmoudi et al. [83].

Moreover Liu et al. developed PCL-PEG NPs functionalized by binding of lactoferrin, a protein whose receptor is expressed mainly in respiratory epithelial cells and neuronal. These NPs allowed the intranasal administration of peptides or proteins with potential neuroprotectant agents such as the NAP peptide, presenting a greater accumulation in the CNS compared to nonfunctionalized NPs. In addition, the efficacy of these NPs is confirmed in vivo in preclinical behavior studies Morris water maze test [84].

5.4.4 PBCA

In general, at present, PBCA is a polymer which use has been discontinued for the preparation of NPs. However some studies have yet shown utility for dementia. In this area Mulik et al. developed NPs for the encapsulation of coumarin. This molecule is an antioxidant that inhibits the oxidative stress that occurs in AD. In this work they functionalized the NPs with the CPP ApoE3 that presents antiamyloid and antioxidant intrinsic activity. Moreover in vitro studies demonstrated that, when combining the effect of this peptide together with coumarin, an inhibition of cell cytotoxicity mediated by amyloid plaques is obtained. Additionally, NPs could also improve the bioavailability of the drug in the CNS offering it photoprotection, and improving its stability [85]. Also, for the treatment of AD, rivastigmine-loaded PBCA NPs have been optimized. The efficacy of these NPs was evaluated using behavioral in vivo test with an scopolamine-induced mouse model. Moreover, in this study they also obtained the NPs replaced PBCA by to PLGA, generally presenting similar characteristics. According to their results, both NPs constitute potential tools for the administration of rivastigmine in CNS for treatment of dementia [86].

PBCA-optimized NPs could also be used as a tool for the diagnosis of dementia. As is the case with the investigations carried out by Roney et al. and Kulkarni et al. who developed PBCA NPs that encapsulated ^{125}Iclioquinol (5-chloro-7-iodo-8-hydroxyquinoline), radiolabeled quinoline much showed affinity for Aβ-plaques, to be used as biomarkers. They were assessed in vivo and showed a greater accumulation in double transgenic mice, and in mice that were directly injected with the Aβ42 peptide than in control mice [87,88].

Another examples are the NPs developed by Siegemund et al. the authors produced a nanocapsules with a polystyrene and a PBCA shell. These allow the encapsulation of Thioflavin T and Thioflavin S. These compounds can bind to amyloid fibrillar peptides, therefore these nanos can be used for diagnosis and identification of amyloid plaques [89].

As has been shown, many possible combinations of polymeric NPs with or without drug are currently being studied, mainly for the treatment of AD but also different types of dementia. However, it is very important to continue investigating in this area of nanotechnology and nanomedicine, by both optimizing and adapting the properties of these NPs to the diagnosis and treatment objectives aimed to treat and prevent dementia.

5.5 Functionalization or modification strategies of polymeric nanoparticles for dementia

Polymeric NPs have the peculiarity of presenting a large surface area where the polymer is exposed against the tissues. As explained in Section 5.3, polymers present a great variety of functional groups that confer them some of their properties. At the same time these modification allow the modification and the union of multiple ligands on their surface, in order to design and confer the desired characteristics. Regarding this fact, different functional strategies are described.

The first one consists on modifying of the polymeric matrix or the surface of the NPs by introducing of PEG. As can be seen in Table 5.1, this is one of the most recurrent strategies. PEG is a polyether which gives NPs a hydrophilic coating to the hydrophobic core of the polymer used. This strategy allows an increase in the average half-life of NPs in plasma, by acting as a steric barrier preventing interactions with other molecules [97,98]. PEG, in addition to its low immunogenicity and antigenicity, can confer a greater interaction of NPs with the target tissue [99].

Another useful strategy is the attachment of CPP. These were discovered in 1988 [100]. In general, they are peptides of only about 6–30 aminoacids. These were aimed to increase the bioavailability and uptake of NPs. It has been described that CPPs, even at low concentrations, are capable of crossing the cell membrane without damaging it and without the need to use a specific receptor. The different mechanisms by which CPPs are able to cross different biological barriers to one are not fully understood. As can be seen in Fig. 5.4, one of the CPP entry mechanisms is direct penetration. In this sense, when interacting CPP with the membrane causes a temporary stable or transient destabilization of the membrane [101], which allows the penetration of the peptide. This can be mediated in different mechanisms, such as pore formation, or narrowing of the lipid bilayer. The latter mainly produced by high concentrations of CPP. Another entry mechanism is the endocytosis mediated, or not, by clartin/caveolin. When CPPs are linked to NPs, endocytosis is mainly the mechanism that occurs for cell penetration. Endocytosis can also be facilitated by the interaction of CPP with some receptor on the cell membrane [102–104]. As for the CPPs, the most widely used for the functionalization of NPs in dementia are TAT, ApoE, or polycationic peptides. Some peptides such as APOE have anti-inflammatory activity, a useful property for the treatment of AD and other types of dementia [105–107].

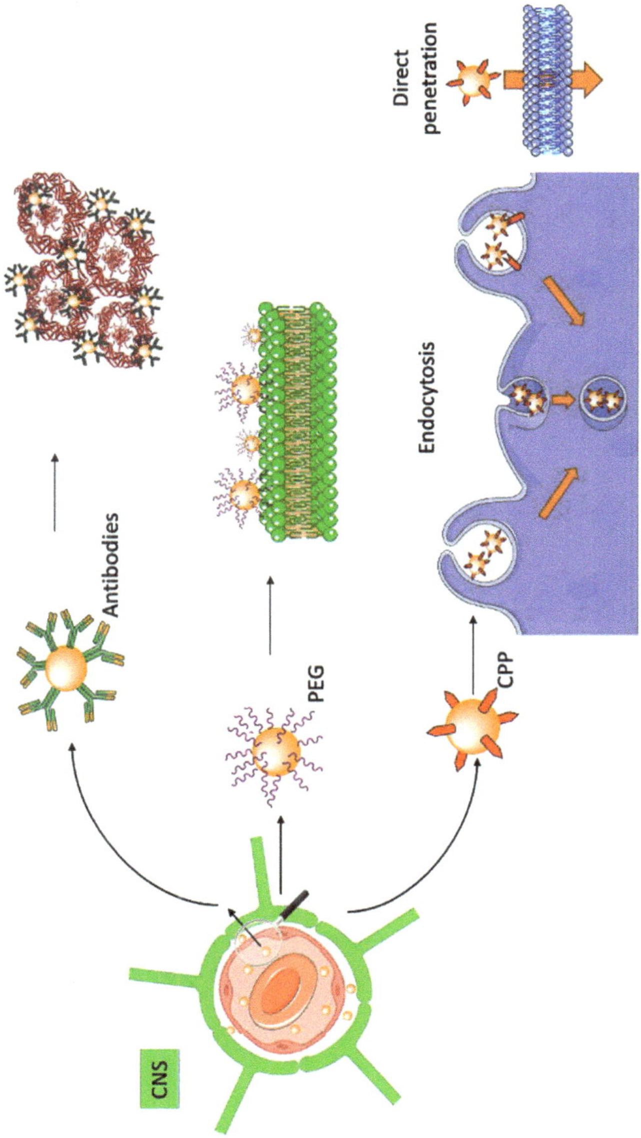

FIG. 5.4 Functionalization strategies used for polymeric NPs.

Moreover, another strategy is the binding on NPs surface of antibodies. These, unlike the CPP, will guide and transport the NPs in a way against a target. This strategy is especially used in the functionalization of NPs for the treatment of AD. These antibodies are used against Aβ-amyloid plaques. As is the case of the research carried out by Carradori et al. who functionalized polymeric NPs with an antibody against Aβ1-42 and with PEG. These NPs successfully achieved the improvement in memory of the AD animal model used [108].

5.6 Conclusions

Currently, the efficacy of treatments for dementia is still limited, despite the high incidence and mortality of these diseases. In this area, biodegradable NPs for controlled drug release are of crucial relevance. Moreover, the formation of NPs from biodegradable polymers is highlighted in order to encapsulate different types of drugs. These polymers are broken down into biocompatible metabolites, and constitute a promising therapeutic tool for drug delivery, improving the efficacy and safety of dementia treatments. Both polymers and polymeric NPs can be functionalized and thus being able to customize NPs for a specific type of dementia.

As a conclusion, although important advances have been made, it is crucial to continue the investigation in the field of nanomedicine in order to develop novel and effective treatments as well as diagnostic tools for all types of dementia.

Acknowledgements

A.C. aknowledges the support of the Spanish Ministry of Science, Innovation and Universities under the grant Juan de la Cierva (FJC2018-036012-I), and project grant PID2021-122473OA-I00. ESL acknowledges the support of the Programme of Requalification of the Spanish University System.

References

[1] Yetisgin A, Cetinel S, Zuvin M, Kosar A, Kutlu O. Therapeutic nanoparticles and their targeted delivery applications. Molecules 2020;25(9):1–31.

[2] Karthivashan G, Ganesan P, SY P, Kim JS, Choi DK. Therapeutic strategies and nano-drug delivery applications in management of ageing Alzheimer's disease. Drug Deliv 2018;25(1):307–20.

[3] Diagnosis D, Shakeri S, Ashrafizadeh M, Zarrabi A, Roghanian R. Multifunctional polymeric nanoplatforms for brain. Biomedicines 2020;8(1):13.

[4] Al-Ahmady ZS. Selective drug delivery approaches to lesioned brain through blood brain barrier disruption. Expert Opin Drug Deliv 2018;15(4):335–49.

[5] Chevalier R. Penetration assessment of dietary supplements and drugs through the blood-brain barrier for potential treatment of Parkinson's disease. bioRxiv 2018:1–16. doi:10.1101/362541.

[6] Banks WA. From blood-brain barrier to blood-brain interface: new opportunities for CNS drug delivery. Nat Rev Drug Discov 2016;15(4):275–92.

[7] Masoudi Asil S, Ahlawat J, Guillama Barroso G, Narayan M. Nanomaterial based drug delivery systems for the treatment of neurodegenerative diseases. Biomater Sci 2020;8(15): 4088–107.
[8] Worl Health Organization. The top 10 causes of death [Internet]. Worl Health Organization. [cited 2021 Feb 6]. Available from: https://www.who.int/news-room/fact-sheets/detail/the-top-10-causes-of-death.
[9] Chapman DP, Williams SM, Strine TW, Anda RF, Moore MJ. Dementia and its implications for public health. Prev Chronic Dis 2006;3(2):1–13.
[10] Organization WH, International AD A public health priority. Organization WH, Iternational AD, eds. 2012. p. 112.
[11] Arvanitakis Z, Leurgans SE, Fleischman DA, Schneider JA, Rajan KB, Pruzin JJ, et al. Memory complaints, dementia, and neuropathology in older blacks and whites. Ann Neurol 2018;83(4):718–29.
[12] Patel MM, Patel BM. Crossing the blood–brain barrier: recent advances in drug delivery to the brain. CNS Drugs 2017;31(2):109–33.
[13] Saeedi M, Eslamifar M, Khezri K, Dizaj SM. Applications of nanotechnology in drug delivery to the central nervous system. Biomed Pharmacother 2019;111(December 2018):666–75.
[14] Cholertona B, Larsond EB, Baker L, Craft S, Crane PK, Millard SP, et al. Neuropathologic correlates of cognition in a population-based sample. Bone 2012;23(1):1–7.
[15] World Health Organization. Dementia [Internet]. World Health Organization. 2020 [cited 2020 Jan 26]. Available from: https://www.who.int/news-room/fact-sheets/detail/dementia
[16] McKhann GM, Knopman DS, Chertkow H, Hyman BT, Jack CR, Kawas CH, et al. The diagnosis of dementia due to Alzheimer's disease: recommendations from the National Institute on Aging-Alzheimer's Association workgroups on diagnostic guidelines for Alzheimer's disease. Alzheimer's Dement 2011;7(3):263–9.
[17] Arvanitakis Z, Shah RC, Bennett DA. Diagnosis and management of dementia: review. JAMA - J Am Med Assoc 2019;322(16):1589–99.
[18] Palmer K, Bäckman L, Winblad B, Fratiglioni L. Early symptoms and signs of cognitive deficits might not always be detectable in persons who develop Alzheimer's disease. Int Psychogeriatr 2008;20(2):252–8.
[19] Bature F, Guinn BA, Pang D, Pappas Y. Signs and symptoms preceding the diagnosis of Alzheimer's disease: a systematic scoping review of literature from 1937 to 2016. BMJ Open 2017;7(8):e015746.
[20] Ridha BH, Barnes J, Bartlett JW, Godbolt A, Pepple T, Rossor MN, et al. Tracking atrophy progression in familial Alzheimer's disease: a serial MRI study. Lancet Neurol 2006;5(10):828–34.
[21] Kansagara D, Freeman M. A systematic evidence review of the signs and symptoms of dementia and brief cognitive tests available in VA. Methods 2010:1–55.
[22] Sandilyan MB, Dening T. Signs and symptoms of dementia. Nurs Stand 2015;29(41):42–51.
[23] Rasmussen, J.; Langerman, H. Alzheimer's disease–why we need early diagnosis. Degenerative neurological and neuromuscular disease, 2019; 9, 123.
[24] Bellou V, Belbasis L, Tzoulaki I, Middleton LT, Ioannidis JPA, Evangelou E. Systematic evaluation of the associations between environmental risk factors and dementia: an umbrella review of systematic reviews and meta-analyses. Alzheimer's Dement 2017;13(4):406–18.
[25] Dening TBSM. Dementia: definitions and types DENING. Nurs Stand 2015;29(37):37–42.
[26] Derreberry TM, Holroyd S. Dementia in women. Med Clin North Am 2019;103(4):713–21.
[27] Sacuiu SF. Dementias. Handb Clin Neurol 2016;138:123–51.

[28] Moreno Cervantes C, Mimenza Alvarado A, Aguilar Navarro S, Alvarado Ávila P, Gutiérrez Gutiérrez L, Juárez Arellano S, et al. Factors associated with mixed dementia vs Alzheimer disease in elderly Mexican adults. Neurol (English Ed) 2017;32(5):309–15.

[29] Scheltens P, Blennow K, Breteler MMB, de Strooper B, Frisoni GB, Salloway S, et al. Alzheimer's disease. Lancet 2016;388(10043):505–17.

[30] Naseri NN, Wang H, Guo J, Sharma M, Luo W. The complexity of tau in Alzheimer's disease. Neurosci Lett 2019;705:183–94.

[31] Bondi MW, Edmonds EC, Salmon DP, Jolla L, Diego S, Jolla L. Alzheimer's disease: past, present, and future. J Clin Invest 2017;23:818–31.

[32] Lane CA, Hardy J, Schott JM. Alzheimer's disease. Eur J Neurol 2018;25(1):59–70.

[33] Weller J, Budson A. Current understanding of Alzheimer's disease diagnosis and treatment. F1000Research 2018;7(0):1–9.

[34] Soria Lopez JA, González HM, Léger GC. Alzheimer's disease. Handb Clin Neurol 2019;167:231–55.

[35] Deture MA, Dickson DW. The neuropathological diagnosis of Alzheimer's disease. Mol Neurodegener 2019;14(1):1–18.

[36] Sanford AM. Lewy body dementia. Clin Geriatr Med 2018;34(4):603–15.

[37] Bonanni L, Franciotti R, Pizzi SD, Thomas A, Onofrj M. Lewy body dementia. Neurodegener Dis Clin Asp Mol Genet Biomarkers 2018:297–312.

[38] Capouch SD, Farlow MR, Brosch JR. A review of dementia with Lewy bodies' impact, diagnostic criteria and treatment. Neurol Ther 2018;7(2):249–63.

[39] Series H, Esiri M. Vascular dementia: a pragmatic review. Adv Psychiatr Treat 2012; 18(5):372–80.

[40] Vinters HV, Zarow C, Borys E, Whitman JD, Tung S, Ellis WG, et al. Review: vascular dementia: clinicopathologic and genetic considerations. Neuropathol Appl Neurobiol 2018; 44(3):247–66.

[41] Devenney EM, Ahmed RM, Hodges JR. Frontotemporal dementia. In: Devenney EM, editor. 1st ed. Handbook of clinical neurology, 167. Amsterdam, Netherlands: Elsevier B.V.; 2019. p. 279–99.

[42] Rojas-Prats E, Tosat-Bitrián C, Martínez-González L, Nozal V, Pérez DI, Martínez A. Increasing brain permeability of PHA-767491, a cell division cycle 7 kinase inhibitor, with biodegradable polymeric nanoparticles. Pharmaceutics 2021 Jan 28;13(2):180.

[43] Arts NJM, Walvoort SJW, Kessels RPC. Korsakoff's syndrome: a critical review. Neuropsychiatr Dis Treat 2017;13:2875–90.

[44] Su S, Kang PM. Systemic review of biodegradable nanomaterials in nanomedicine. Nanomaterials 2020;10(4):656.

[45] Rao JP, Geckeler KE. Polymer nanoparticles: preparation techniques and size-control parameters. Prog Polym Sci 2011;36(7):887–913.

[46] Marin E, Briceño MI, Caballero-George C. Critical evaluation of biodegradable polymers used in nanodrugs. Int J Nanomed 2013;8:3071–91.

[47] Gómez-Gaete C. Nanopartículas Poliméricas: Tecnología Y Aplicaciones Farmacéuticas (Polymeric nanoparticles: technologie and pharmaceutical applications). Rev Farm Chile 2014;7(2):7–16.

[48] Zielinska A, Carreiró F, Oliveira AM, Neves A, Pire B, Venkatesh DN, et al. Polymeric nanoparticles: production, characterization, toxicology and ecotoxicology. Molecules 2020;25(16):3731. doi: 10.3390/molecules25163731.

[49] Nazila K, Yameen B, Wu J, Farokhzad OC. Nanoparticles: mechanisms of controlling drug release. Chem Rev 2016;116(4):2602–63.

[50] Rai R, Alwani S, Badea I. Polymeric nanoparticles in gene therapy: new avenues of design and optimization for delivery applications. Polymers (Basel) 2019;11(4):745.

[51] Karlsson J, Vaughan HJ, Green JJ. Biodegradable polymeric nanoparticles for therapeutic cancer treatments. Annu Rev Chem Biomol Eng 2018;9:105–27.

[52] Idrees H, Zaidi SZJ, Sabir A, Khan RU, Zhang X, Hassan SU. A review of biodegradable natural polymer-based nanoparticles for drug delivery applications. Nanomaterials 2020;10(10):1–22.

[53] Anwunobi AP, Emeje MO. Recent applications of natural polymers in nanodrug delivery. J Nanomed Nanotechnol 2011;s4(01):2–7.

[54] Manek E, Darvas F, Petroianu GA. Use of biodegradable, chitosan-based nanoparticles in the treatment of Alzheimer's disease. Molecules 2020;25(20):1–26.

[55] Jana S, Maiti S. Chitosan-based nanoparticulate systems for oral drug delivery. In: Andronescu E, Grumezescu A, editors. Nanostructures for oral medicine. Amsterdam, Netherlands: Elsevier; 2017. p. 607–38.

[56] Wasiak I, Kulikowska A, Janczewska M, Michalak M, Cymerman IA, Nagalski A, et al. Dextran nanoparticle synthesis and properties. PLoS One 2016;11(1):1–17.

[57] Foerster F, Bamberger D, Schupp J, Weilbächer M, Kaps L, Strobl S, et al. Dextran-based therapeutic nanoparticles for hepatic drug delivery. Nanomedicine 2016;11(20):2663–77.

[58] Venkatesan J, Anil S, Singh SK, Kim SK. Preparations and applications of alginate nanoparticles. In: Venkatesan J, Anil S, Kim S-K, editors. Seaweed polysaccharides: isolation, biological and biomedical applications. Amsterdam, Netherlands: Elsevier; 2017. p. 251–68.

[59] Choukaife H, Doolaanea AA, Alfatama M. Alginate nanoformulation: influence of process and selected variables. Pharmaceuticals 2020;13:1–35.

[60] Yang DH, Kim HJ, Park K, Kim JK, Chun HJ. Preparation of poly-l-lysine-based nanoparticles with pH-sensitive release of curcumin for targeted imaging and therapy of liver cancer in vitro and in vivo. Drug Deliv 2018;25(1):950–60.

[61] Hamid Akash MS, Rehman K, Chen S. Natural and synthetic polymers as drug carriers for delivery of therapeutic proteins. Polym Rev 2015;55(3):371–406.

[62] Casalini T, Rossi F, Castrovinci A, Perale G. A perspective on polylactic acid-based polymers use for nanoparticles synthesis and applications. Front Bioeng Biotechnol 2019;7:1–16.

[63] Sharma S, Parmar A, Kori S, Sandhir R. PLGA-based nanoparticles: a new paradigm in biomedical applications. TrAC - Trends Anal Chem 2016;80:30–40.

[64] Essa D, Kondiah PPD, Choonara YE, Pillay V. The design of poly(lactide-co-glycolide) nanocarriers for medical applications. Front Bioeng Biotechnol 2020;8(February):1–20.

[65] Guarino V, Gentile G, Sorrentino L, Ambrosio L. Polycaprolactone: synthesis, properties, and applications. In: Mark HF, editor. Encyclopedia of polymer science and technology. Hoboken, New Jersey, U.S.: John Wiley & Sons, Inc; 2017:1–36.

[66] Devalapally H, Shenoy D, Little S, Langer R, Amiji M. Poly(ethylene oxide)-modified poly(beta-amino ester) nanoparticles as a pH-sensitive system for tumor-targeted delivery of hydrophobic drugs: part 3. Therapeutic efficacy and safety studies in ovarian cancer xenograft model. Cancer Chemother Pharmacol 2007;59(4):477–84.

[67] Iqbal S, Qu Y, Dong Z, Zhao J, Rauf Khan A, Rehman S, et al. Poly (β-amino esters) based potential drug delivery and targeting polymer; an overview and perspectives (review). Eur Polym J 2020;141:110097.

[68] Wilson B. Brain targeting PBCA nanoparticles and the blood-brain barrier. Nanomedicine 2009;4(5):499–502.

[69] Koczera P, Appold L, Shi Y, Liu M, Dasgupta A. PBCA-based polymeric microbubbles for molecular imaging and drug delivery. Control Release 2017;259:128–35.

[70] Krishnan A, Chuturgoon A. Integrative nanomedicine for new therapies. Krishnan A, Chuturgoon A, editors. Switzerland: Spinger; 2020. p. 1–1.
[71] Aalinkeel R, Kutscher HL, Singh A, Cwiklinski K, Khechen N, Schwartz SA, et al. Neuroprotective effects of a biodegradable poly(lactic-co-glycolic acid)-Ginsenoside Rg3 nanoformulation: a potential nanotherapy for Alzheimer's disease? J Drug Target 2018;26(2):182–93.
[72] Barbara R, Belletti D, Pederzoli F, Masoni M, Keller J, Ballestrazzi A, et al. Novel curcumin loaded nanoparticles engineered for blood-brain barrier crossing and able to disrupt Abeta aggregates. Int J Pharm 2017;526(1–2):413–24.
[73] Fan S, Zheng Y, Liu X, Fang W, Chena X, Liao W, et al. Curcumin-loaded PLGA-peg nanoparticles conjugated with b6 peptide for potential use in Alzheimer's disease. Drug Deliv 2018;25(1):1044–55.
[74] Sánchez-López E, Ettcheto M, Egea MA, Espina M, Cano A, Calpena AC, et al. Memantine loaded PLGA PEGylated nanoparticles for Alzheimer's disease: in vitro and in vivo characterization. J Nanobiotechnol 2018;16(1):1–16.
[75] Kavirajan H, Schneider LS. Efficacy and adverse effects of cholinesterase inhibitors and memantine in vascular dementia: a meta-analysis of randomised controlled trials. Lancet Neurol 2007;6(9):782–92.
[76] Loureiro JA, Gomes B, Fricker G, Coelho MAN, Rocha S, Pereira MC. Cellular uptake of PLGA nanoparticles targeted with anti-amyloid and anti-transferrin receptor antibodies for Alzheimer's disease treatment. Colloids Surfaces B Biointerfaces 2016;145:8–13.
[77] Joshi AS, Singh V, Gahane A, Thakur AK. Biodegradable nanoparticles containing mechanism based peptide inhibitors reduce polyglutamine aggregation in cell models and alleviate motor symptoms in a Drosophila model of Huntington's disease. ACS Chem Neurosci 2019;10(3):1603–14.
[78] Zeng J, Martin A, Han X, Shirihai OS, Grinstaff MW. Biodegradable PLGA nanoparticles restore lysosomal acidity and protect neural pc-12 cells against mitochondrial toxicity. Ind Eng Chem Res 2019;58(31):13910–7.
[79] Roy Chowdhury S, Mondal S, Muthuraj B, Balaji SN, Trivedi V, Krishnan Iyer P. Remarkably efficient blood-brain barrier crossing polyfluorene-chitosan nanoparticle selectively tweaks amyloid oligomer in cerebrospinal fluid and Aβ1-40. ACS Omega 2018;3(7):8059–66.
[80] Wilson B, Samanta MK, Santhi K, Kumar KPS, Ramasamy M, Suresh B. Chitosan nanoparticles as a new delivery system for the anti-Alzheimer drug tacrine. Nanomed Nanotechnol Biol Med 2010;6(1):144–52.
[81] Jaruszewsk KM, Ramakrishnan S, Poduslo JF, Kandimalla KK. Chitosan enhances the stability and targeting of immuno-nanovehicles to cerebro-vascular deposits of Alzheimer's disease amyloid protein. Bone 2011;72(2):132–5.
[82] Xue Y, Wang N, Zeng Z, Huang J, Xiang Z, Guan YQ. Neuroprotective effect of chitosan nanoparticle gene delivery system grafted with acteoside (ACT) in Parkinson's disease models. J Mater Sci Technol 2020;43:197–207.
[83] Mahmoudi M, Saeidian H, Mirjafary Z, Mokhtari J. Preparation and characterization of memantine loaded polycaprolactone nanocapsules for Alzheimer's disease. J Porous Mater 2021;28:205–212–2012.
[84] Liu Z, Jiang M, Kang T, Miao D, Gu G, Song Q, et al. Lactoferrin-modified PEG-co-PCL nanoparticles for enhanced brain delivery of NAP peptide following intranasal administration. Biomaterials 2013;34(15):3870–81.
[85] Mulik RS, Mönkkönen J, Juvonen RO, Mahadik KR, Paradkar AR. ApoE3 mediated poly(butyl) cyanoacrylate nanoparticles containing curcumin: study of enhanced activity of

curcumin against beta amyloid induced cytotoxicity using in vitro cell culture model. Mol Pharm 2010;7(3):815–25.
[86] Joshi SA, Chavhan SS, Sawant KK. Rivastigmine-loaded PLGA and PBCA nanoparticles: preparation, optimization, characterization, in vitro and pharmacodynamic studies. Eur J Pharm Biopharm 2010;76(2):189–99.
[87] Roney CA, Arora V, Kulkarni PV, Antich PP, Bonte FJ. Nanoparticulate radiolabelled quinolines detect amyloid plaques in mouse models of Alzheimer's disease. Int J Alzheimers Dis 2009;2009:1–8.
[88] Kulkarni PV, Roney CA, Antich PP, Bonte FJ, Raghu AV, Aminabhavi TM. Quinoline-n-butylcyanoacrylate-based nanoparticles for brain targeting for the diagnosis of Alzheimer's disease. Wiley Interdiscip Rev Nanomed Nanobiotechnol 2010;2(1):35–47.
[89] Siegemund T, Paulke BR, Schmiedel H, Bordag N, Hoffmann A, Harkany T, et al. Thioflavins released from nanoparticles target fibrillar amyloid β in the hippocampus of APP/PS1 transgenic mice. Int J Dev Neurosci 2006;24(2–3):195–201.
[90] Sun D, Li N, Zhang W, Zhao Z, Mou Z, Huang D, et al. Design of PLGA-functionalized quercetin nanoparticles for potential use in Alzheimer's disease. Colloids Surfaces B Biointerfaces 2016;148:116–29.
[91] Jeon SG, Cha MY, il KJ, Hwang TW, Kim KA, Kim TH, et al. Vitamin D-binding protein-loaded PLGA nanoparticles suppress Alzheimer's disease-related pathology in 5XFAD mice. Nanomed Nanotechnol Biol Med 2019;17:297–307.
[92] Radwan RR, Abdel Ghaffar AM, Ali HE. Gamma radiation preparation of chitosan nanoparticles for controlled delivery of memantine. J Biomater Appl 2020;34(8):1150–62.
[93] Dinesh Raja A, Mohambed M, Joji S, Sankar C, Mishra B. Design and evaluation of chitosan nanoparticles as novel drug carriers for the delivery of donepezil. Iran J Pharm Sci 2012;8(3):155–64.
[94] Sava V, Fihurka O, Khvorova A, Sanchez-Ramos J. Enriched chitosan nanoparticles loaded with siRNA are effective in lowering Huntington's disease gene expression following intranasal administration. Nanomed Nanotechnol Biol Med 2020;24:1–18.
[95] Nagpal K, Singh SKK, Mishra DNN. Optimization of brain targeted chitosan nanoparticles of Rivastigmine for improved efficacy and safety. Int J Biol Macromol 2013 Aug;59:72–83.
[96] Krishna KV, Saha RN, Dubey SK. Biophysical, biochemical, and behavioral implications of ApoE3 conjugated donepezil nanomedicine in a Aβ1-42Induced Alzheimer's disease rat model. ACS Chem Neurosci 2020;11(24):4139–51.
[97] D'souza AA, Shegokar R. Polyethylene glycol (PEG): a versatile polymer for pharmaceutical applications. Expert Opin Drug Deliv 2016;13(9):1257–75.
[98] Sánchez-López E, Esteruelas G, Ortiz A, Espina M, Prat J, Muñoz M, et al. Article dexibuprofen biodegradable nanoparticles: one step closer towards a better ocular interaction study. Nanomaterials 2020;10(4):1–24.
[99] Thi TTH, Pilkington EH, Nguyen DH, Lee JS, Park KD, Truong NP. The importance of poly(ethylene glycol) alternatives for overcoming PEG immunogenicity in drug delivery and bioconjugation. Polymers (Basel) 2020;12(2):298.
[100] Brasseur R, Divita G. Happy birthday cell penetrating peptides: already 20 years. Biochim Biophys Acta - Biomembr 2010;1798(12):2177–81.
[101] Madani F, Lindberg S, Langel Ü, Futaki S, Gräslund A. Mechanisms of cellular uptake of cell-penetrating peptides. J Biophys 2011 Apr 7;2011:1–10.
[102] Guidotti G, Brambilla L, Rossi D. Cell-penetrating peptides: from basic research to clinics. Trends Pharmacol Sci 2017;38(4):406–24.

[103] Xie J, Bi Y, Zhang H, Dong S, Teng L, Lee RJ, et al. Cell-penetrating peptides in diagnosis and treatment of human diseases: from preclinical research to clinical application. Front Pharmacol 2020;11(May):1–23.

[104] Borrelli A, Tornesello AL, Tornesello ML, Buonaguro FM. Cell penetrating peptides as molecular carriers for anti-cancer agents. Molecules 2018;23(2):295.

[105] Silva S, Almeida AJ, Vale N. Combination of cell-penetrating peptides with nanoparticles for therapeutic application: a review. Biomolecules 2019;9(1):22.

[106] Wong KH, Riaz MK, Xie Y, Zhang X, Liu Q, Chen H, et al. Review of current strategies for delivering Alzheimer's disease drugs across the blood-brain barrier. Int J Mol Sci 2019;20(2):381.

[107] Veloria JR, Li L, Breen GAM, Goux WJ. Novel cell model for tauopathy induced by a cell-permeable tau-related peptide. ACS Chem Neurosci 2017;8(12):2734–45.

[108] Carradori D, Balducci C, Re F, Brambilla D, Le Droumaguet B, Flores O, et al. Antibody-functionalized polymer nanoparticle leading to memory recovery in Alzheimer's disease-like transgenic mouse model. Nanomed Nanotechnol Biol Med 2018;14(2):609–18.

Chapter 6

Solid lipid nanoparticles-based drug delivery for dementia

Nilufer Yuksel, Zerrin Sezgin Bayindir, Gulin Amasya
Department of Pharmaceutical Technology, Faculty of Pharmacy, Ankara University, Ankara, Turkey

6.1 Introduction

6.1.1 Statistics

Dementia is one of the main causes of older people's disability and dependence on others around the world. There will be an increase in the incidence of dementia in the next century, along with the increase in life expectancy as a result of the improvement in economic conditions and the developments in medicine and health. Although dementia affects the elderly, it is not a normal part of the aging process [1-3]. According to the WHO's observation of dementia, almost 10 million new cases of dementia occur each year, with one case occurring every 3 seconds. Worldwide, 50 million people have dementia, and it is stated that this number will triple by 2050 and the majority will be in low- and middle-income countries. Accordingly, while its social cost was 818 billion US dollars in 2015, it is estimated to be 2 trillion US dollars in 2030. WHO recognizes dementia as a public health priority and established the Global Dementia Observatory platform to facilitate monitoring and sharing of information on dementia policies, service delivery, epidemiology, and research [3].

6.1.2 Definitions, etiology, and pathophysiology

Dementia is a neurodegenerative syndrome that leads to a progressive deterioration of a person's cognitive functions, resulting in a persistent decrease in memory, thinking, behavior, and social activities [4-6]. Dementia is etiologically associated with various heterogeneous diseases and accordingly, approximately a hundred types of reversible and irreversible dementia are known. Reversible dementia accounts for approximately 9–11% of cases [5]. The causes of reversible dementia are drug and alcohol toxicity, depression, vitamin deficiencies, metabolic diseases, normal pressure hydrocephalus, intracranial tumors, traumatic brain injuries, central nervous system (CNS) infections.

Nanomedicine-Based Approaches for the Treatment of Dementia. https://doi.org/10.1016/B978-0-12-824331-2.00008-X
Copyright © 2023 Elsevier Inc. All rights reserved.

Reversible dementia might be reversed by treating the underlying causes. The causes of irreversible dementia are mainly Alzheimer's disease (AD), which constitutes approximately 60–80% of cases, vascular dementia, which constitutes 18–20% of cases, Lewy body disease, which constitutes 15–20% of cases, and frontotemporal dementia, Parkinson's disease, Huntington's disease, multiple sclerosis, and mixed dementias, which are seen in lower percentages [5,6]. The mixed dementia is a coexistence of two or more types of dementia, for example, AD and another related type of dementia, frequently vascular dementia [7].

Aside from vascular dementia, other types of dementia involve a pathological accumulation of a native protein. In AD, the extracellular amyloid plaques by oligomerization of beta-amyloid (Aβ) proteins and intracellular neurofibrillary tangles by aggregation of hyperphosphorylated tau protein in the medial temporal lobe structures and cortical areas of the brain are the key proteins. Dementia with Lewy bodies includes the formation of the alpha-synuclein protein in the form of Lewy bodies. In frontotemporal lobar dementia, the accumulated proteins are TDP-43 [TAR (transactive response) DNA-binding-protein-43] and, the specific proteins of AD and dementia with Lewy bodies in a frontotemporal distribution [8]. Significant changes in the metabolism of the affected brain areas, neuroinflammation signs, and synaptic loss occur. While these neuropathological phenomena cause irreversible neuronal damage and death over time, there is also a continuous decline in memory, thinking, cognition, social skills, and behavior. These processes are thought to begin 20–30 years before the onset of clinical symptoms [1,4,8].

Genes also affect the risk of developing both early (<65 years) and late-onset (>65 years) dementia. Chromosome 14 defects account for the early onset of familial AD occurring between 30 and 60 years. The responsible genes are the amyloid precursor protein (APP) gene and two presenilin genes (PSEN-1 and PSEN-2). These genes are involved in the pathway of enzymatic cleavage of the Aβ peptide from APP, its conversion into insoluble aggregates in the form of dimers, oligomers, and fibers, thereby forming Aβ plaques. Another gene is the apolipoprotein E (APOE) on chromosome 19. It is involved in the lipid metabolism pathway. The isoform e4 of APOE may increase the risk of late-onset AD by inducing the accumulation of Aβ plaques [4,9-11].

Vascular dementia occurs as a result of vascular changes such as thickening of the capillary basement membrane and accumulation of collagen in the vascular endothelium. These changes cause vascular atrophy at the vascular ends as well as a reduction in the number of terminal vessels, thus affecting the cerebral microvasculature and reducing the cerebral blood flow. The risk factors are hypertension, cardiac disease, diabetes, dyslipidemia, obesity, and a sedentary lifestyle [7,12]. Neuroinflammation and oxidative stress are also stated to be the factors involved in the pathogenesis of both AD and vascular dementia [13,14].

6.1.3 Pharmacotherapy

Currently, there is no treatment available to stop the progression of irreversible dementia and prevent brain cell loss. Many of the available drugs are used for the treatment of AD, the most common form of dementia, and these drugs delay the progression of symptoms and improve the quality of life of the dementia patient [15]. Symptomatic treatment is based on the observed neurotransmitter system disorders (including cholinergic and glutamatergic transmissions). Today, only acetylcholine esterase inhibitors (donepezil, rivastigmine, galantamine) and N-methyl D-aspartate receptor antagonists (memantine) are used as approved antidementia drugs [1,2,4,7,15]. Intensive efforts are underway to develop disease-modifying therapeutic agents that cause permanent changes in the clinical progression of the disease, thus stopping or delaying the progression of the disease, by interfering with the pathophysiological mechanisms underlying the disease process, especially in the early stage [2,16]. Besides, improving the drug formulations is as important as the discovery of new dementia drugs. Usage of nanotechnology to develop better dosage forms in dementia treatment has brought new hopes for a cure.

6.2 Nano-based drug delivery systems in dementia

Nano-based drug delivery systems (nano-DDSs) are nanoparticulate drug carriers that could be targeted to the site of action providing controlled drug delivery to overcome obstacles such as poor drug solubility, absorption, crossing the barriers, bioavailability and therapeutic efficacy, fluctuations in plasma concentrations, the incidence of adverse effects and dosing frequency. Physicochemical properties such as molecular weight, charge, polarity, solubility, lipophilicity, and hydrophilicity of drug candidates play an important role in the therapeutic success or failure of drug candidates. Nano-DDSs can significantly modulate the properties of candidate drugs and increase their therapeutic potential [17].

Approved drugs for dementia are administered orally in repeated doses (except for rivastigmine; which is also available as a transdermal patch). Patients experience gastrointestinal problems such as nausea, vomiting, and diarrhea. In addition, general side effects such as dizziness, sleeplessness, fatigue, muscle cramps, urinary incontinence, and even weight loss occur [4,18]. Nano-DDSs are intensively studied in the treatment of dementia because of their benefits such as reducing the side effects of these drugs and thus increasing the patient's quality of life, as well as successful transport from the blood–brain barrier (BBB), long-term and steady-state release of drugs from the carrier system, reduced interpatient variability and suitability for personalized pharmacotherapy. Nano-DDSs are also the most suitable means for the application of candidate peptide and protein drugs for the treatment of dementia while maintaining their stability both in vivo and in vitro [1,17,19,20]. Furthermore, nano-DDSs in which both a diagnostic agent and a drug are loaded simultaneously, have the potential to be applied as theranostics. Nano-DDSs can be decorated with targeting moieties to selectively bind to receptors or carriers expressed in the BBB, thus improving CNS selectivity and permeability [12,18,19]. Depending on the materials used and their morphologies, nano-DDSs are classified as polymeric nanoparticles (nanospheres and nanocapsules, polymeric micelles, polymersomes, dendrimers), inorganic nanoparticles (silica nanoparticles, quantum dots, gold nanoparticles, carbon nanotubes, iron oxide nanoparticles), and lipid-based nanoparticles (nanoemulsions, liposomes, solid- and nanostructured lipid nanoparticles) [12,17,20,21]. In this chapter, the potential for use of solid lipid nanoparticles and nanostructured lipid nanoparticles in the treatment of dementia will be evaluated.

6.3 Solid lipid nanoparticles as drug delivery systems

Lipid nanoparticles, which are in the class of colloidal drug delivery systems, were discovered simultaneously by two different research groups in the early 1990s. While the German group (Prof. R.H Muller, Free University of Berlin, Germany) used the high-pressure homogenization (HPH) method for lipid nanoparticle manufacturing; Prof. Maria Gasco (Turin University, Italy) and her team developed the microemulsion technique [22,23]. These first-generation nanoparticles, whose basic ingredients were water, solid lipid, and surfactant, were called "solid lipid nanoparticles" (SLNs). Nowadays, it is possible to obtain lipid nanoparticles with many different physicochemical features by controlling the excipients as well as conducting numerous production methods.

SLNs are rigid particles in a 50–1000 nm size range. While biocompatible and biodegradable lipids in solid form at both body and room temperature are used to form the SLN structure, surfactants as the second essential ingredient are added to the formulation for stabilization of the nanoparticles. The nanostructured lipid carriers (NLC), which are generally called as the second-generation SLNs, are obtained by replacing some of the solid lipid used in the production of SLNs with lipids in liquid form at room temperature. However, despite the presence of liquid lipid, it should be emphasized that the particles are still in solid form [24]. Structural rearrangement of the lipid matrix in liquid lipid presence offers huge advantages as enhancing drug loading capacity and preventing drug leakage during storage. Because the structure of SLN, consisting of pure solid lipid or solid lipid mixtures, shows an excellent crystal lattice when nanoparticles are produced and recrystallized. Solid and liquid lipid blends, as in NLC structure, create imperfections in the lipid matrix and allow to form spaces where active substances can be trapped. Thus, drug encapsulation can be enhanced [25,26].

Another important point is lipid modifications that occur in the SLN structure over time. During the formation of the lipid core of SLNs, it first crystallizes in the least ordered and metastable α-form. But over time it gets transformed gradually into a more regular and more stable β form. However, the transition to a more ordered β form leads to the elimination of the defects that trap the

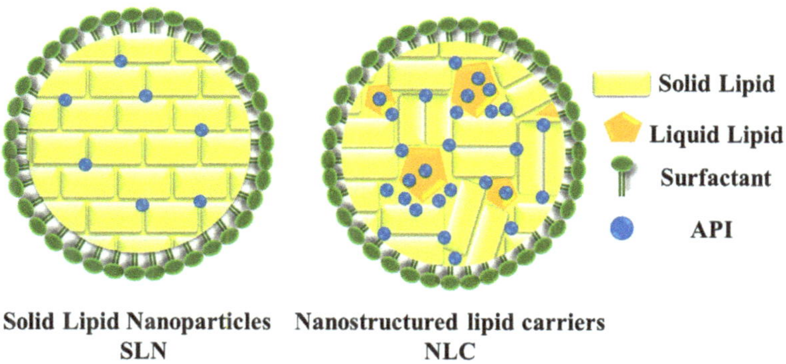

FIG. 6.1 Schematic diagram of the lipid nanoparticles (SLNs and NLCs).

drug molecules and may cause the drug leakage from the SLN during storage [27,28]. Hence, it can be said that the superiority of NLCs over SLNs is due to their structural defects. The schematic diagram of SLN and NLC structures is shown in Fig. 6.1.

Both SLNs and NLCs are remarkable systems when compared with other nanocarriers prepared using materials with different and specific characteristics. In this sense, lipid nanoparticles are dominant systems that combine the superiorities of nanoemulsions, vesicle systems, and polymeric nanoparticles, as emphasized by Muller et al. [29]. Just like polymeric ones, lipid nanoparticles have a solid core of biodegradable materials with definite properties such as colloidal size and large surface area. Lipid nanoparticles are suitable carriers for both lipophilic and hydrophilic drugs as well as genetic materials like DNA and siRNA. However, lipid nanoparticles are one step ahead of polymeric nanoparticles since lipid nanoparticles do not require organic solvents during their production steps. On the other hand, lipid nanoparticle structures are constructed by natural physiological lipids, which are also structural components of our cells. Therefore, SLNs and NLCs are less toxic than polymeric nanoparticles [30]. The solid matrix of lipid nanoparticles offers a clear advantage in terms of drug release profile if compared to nanoemulsions prepared with vegetable oils or medium-chain fatty acids, which are also included in the structure of NLCs. When solid lipid is used as a carrier instead of oil droplet, relatively controlled/sustained release can be achieved, since the mobility of the drug molecule will be limited [27]. Liposomes which are spherical soft vesicles having an inner aqueous cavity surrounded by a lipid bilayer membrane are capable of storing both hydrophilic and lipophilic active molecules. However, the major weakness of liposomes has been the physical and chemical stability issue of the system. At the same time, the cost of production is high due to the expensive components used in their structure and the complexity of the production technologies [31]. Lipid nanoparticles can be produced by ordinary homogenization techniques and are obtained using relatively cheaper raw materials

Table 6.1 Advantages and disadvantages of the lipid nanoparticles (SLNs and NLCs).

Advantages	Disadvantages
• Most lipids being biodegradable, excellent biocompatibility of SLNs&NLCs	• Low drug loading capacity of SLNs
• Improve stability of active molecules	• Polymorphic transition of lipids
• Controlled and/or targeted drug release	• Drug expulsion during storage
• Water-based production technology (avoidance of organic solvents)	• Thermal degradation of heat sensitive-drugs during manufacture
• Conventional homogenization techniques for production	• Drug burst release profile with core-shell model drug incorporation model (drug-enriched shell)
• Encapsulation of hydrophilic and lipophilic drugs	• SLNs&NLCs are obtained in the form of an aqueous dispersion and must be reformulated for the final product.
• The ease of scale-up	• Particle growth and gelation tendency
• The application of common sterilization methods	
• More reasonable/cheaper components	
• Wide range of administration route	
• Suitable for surface modification	

than liposomes. Besides, production technologies of lipid nanoparticles allow large-scale operation and can be adapted to industrial production [32-34]. The summary of clear advantages and disadvantages of lipid nanoparticles is listed in Table 6.1 [29,30,35,36].

6.3.1 Composition of SLN

The major component of lipid nanoparticles is lipids which are in a solid state at room temperature. To obtain the NLC structure, the solid lipids are replaced partly by the liquid lipids. It has been reported that the total solids content of the NLC structure can be up to 95% [37]. Since the structure of the lipid matrix is composed of water and surfactant apart from lipids, the physicochemical properties of lipid nanoparticles are strictly dependent on the type of lipid and surfactant. On the other hand, the composition of the excipients also has an impact on the in vivo performance of lipid nanoparticles [38,39]. The term "lipid" comprises the compound of mainly hydrocarbon nature that is insoluble in water but soluble in organic solvents such as chloroform, ethers, and alcohols. Fatty acids are considered as the structural units of lipids. Lipids can be mainly divided into three categories as triglycerides, phospholipids, and steroids, according to the additional groups like alcohol or phosphate besides the fatty acid [40,41]. A glycerol backbone esterified with three fatty acids forms the triglyceride molecule. Tristearin, tripalmitin, and trimyristin are the most preferred triglycerides in the production of lipid nanoparticles while stearic acid is the most frequently used fatty acid as highlighted by Gordillo-Galeano and Mora-Huertas [30]. Partial glycerides, such as glyceryl behenate, glyceryl monostearate (GMS), and glyceryl distearate which are the esters of fatty acids and with unesterified hydroxyl groups, are among the solid lipids included in the lipid nanoparticle composition. It should also be noted that triglycerides are the main component of dietary fats of vegetable and animal origin and all the above-mentioned lipids are physiological substances with generally recognized as safe status [42]. Fatty acids can also be classified as saturated and unsaturated depending on the presence of double bonds. Unsaturated fatty acids, which usually contain double bonds, are liquid at room temperature. Therefore, they are often included in the NLC structure and oleic acid which is a monounsaturated omega-9 fatty acid and medium-chain triglycerides containing 6–12 carbon atoms are the most frequently used liquid lipids [30,43].

The other essential component to form lipid nanoparticle structure is surfactants which provides sterical stabilization by reducing the interfacial energy between the lipid and the aqueous phase. Surfactants can be divided into three groups depending on their charges as ionic, nonionic, and amphoteric. Poloxamers, polysorbates, or their mixtures, which are nonionic surfactants, are the most preferred ones in the preparation of lipid nanoparticles, while soybean, egg, or hydrogenated soybean lecithin are used as amphoteric stabilizing agents [30,44]. Cationic lipid nanoparticles are highly effective nanocarriers of genetic materials. For this purpose, quaternary ammonium salts and stearylamine can be used as cationic surfactants to impart a positive charge to the lipid nanoparticle [39]. The selection of the type and the concentration of the surfactants are important to optimize the nanoparticle characteristics such as the size, entrapment efficiency, and the physical stability of the dispersion during storage and it depends on the administration route of the lipid nanoparticles [45,46].

In addition to the basic components of lipid nanoparticles, different compounds can also be included in their structures to provide mucoadhesive properties, improve cellular uptake or bioavailability, prolong circulation time, drug targeting to specific tissues or organs [35,47].

6.3.2 Methods of SLN preparation

Although many different techniques are used in the production of SLNs and NLCs, these methods can be simply divided into two groups as high-energy-based and low-energy-based methods. While the required energy to achieve particle size reduction is supplied by different types of equipments such as the homogenizer, sonicator, or microwave in the high-energy-based methods, lipid nanoparticles are usually formed spontaneously with low-energy-based methods and it is not necessary to use complex equipment. On the other hand, there are also methods based on the use of organic solvents [30,46,48]. Regardless of the type of production method, the basic principle in the preparation of lipid nanoparticles is to melt/dissolve the lipids and homogenize with an aqueous medium to form nanosized lipid droplets.

6.3.2.1 High-pressure homogenization method

HPH method ranks first in lipid nanoparticles production as the most reliable and efficient method [45]. The basic principle of this method is mechanically induced movements of fluid due to high pressure. Particle size reduction can be obtained by the formation of turbulence, shear stress, and cavitation while the fluid is forced to pass through a narrow gap [49]. The shear forces required for size reduction or homogenization are generated by high pressure. One of the most important reasons why HPH is preferred in the pharmaceutical industry is the feasibility for industrial needs such as low cost and large-scale production with higher reproducibility [50,51]. Furthermore, the ability to obtain nanostructures without using any acceptable organic solvents makes it environmentally friendly technology. The process parameters of this method are limited to different pressures and the number of cycles [29]. Submicron-sized particles may occur in the presence of the main forces as shear: deformation of product flow and contact with channel walls at high velocity. Small particles can be obtained with narrow particle size distribution at the end of the process and also with repeatability and scalability [45,52].

There are two main approaches including hot and cold homogenization for the HPH method. Hot homogenization operates at an average temperature of 5°C above the melting point of the lipid while cold homogenization is a modified method for the drugs affected by the applied temperature under hot homogenization conditions and lipid is used in solid form [27,53,54]. Besides, cold homogenization is preferred to overcome problems such as distribution of the active substance in the aqueous phase during hot homogenization and the difficulty of lipid recrystallization of the nanoemulsion due to the supercooled melts. It can also be adopted for loading hydrophilic active substances into the lipid matrix [27,29]. However, in order to obtain suitable particle size and narrow size distribution, more cycles and high pressure are required compared to the hot homogenization method [30]. Hot and cold homogenization approaches are schematized in Fig. 6.2.

6.3.2.2 Ultrasonication method

Although the production steps of the ultrasonication method are the same as HPH method; ultrasonic probe is used instead of high-pressure homogenizer in

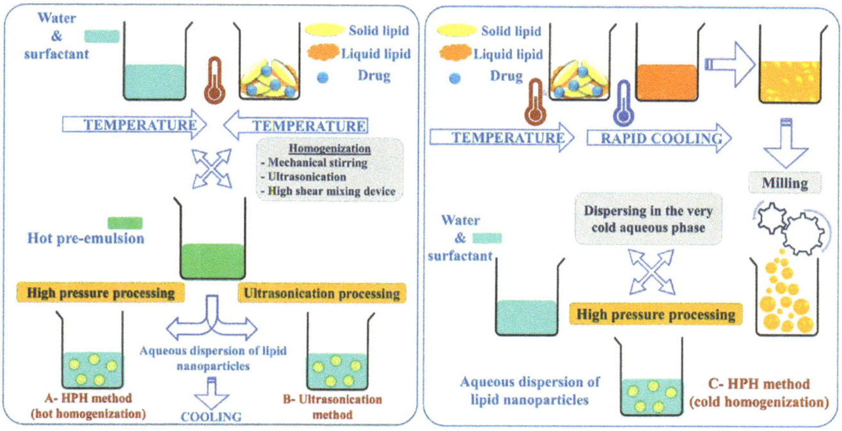

FIG. 6.2 Steps of high-energy-based lipid nanoparticle productions (high-pressure homogenization [hot and cold homogenization] and ultrasonication method).

the final stage of the SLN production as presented in Fig. 6.2. The high energy required for the formation of SLN is provided by sound waves. The reduction in droplet size in hot emulsion is associated with acoustic cavitation, which is the formation and collapse of bubbles in the liquid irradiated with intense ultrasound. While sonication time and amplitude are critical process parameters of the method, possible metal contamination is the most important disadvantage of this method [25].

Methods such as "microwaves" or "supercritical fluid" used in the production of SLN also require high energy input, however these are not widespread production methods for lipid nanoparticles.

6.3.2.3 *Microemulsion method*

Microemulsions are clear, thermodynamically stable, and optically isotropic systems consisting of oil, water, surfactant, and cosurfactant mixture [55]. In the microemulsion technique, which is the first patented method used in the production of lipid nanoparticles, a stable microemulsion is essentially formed. Then, microemulsion is diluted to precipitate lipid nanoparticles. The spontaneous formation of microemulsions is originated from the high surfactant/lipid ratio and does not require the use of complex instruments [33]. This method does not also require high input of energy. Schematic diagram of microemulsion method is given in Fig. 6.3.

The phase inversion temperature method and the membrane contactor method are another low-energy input production technique to fabricate lipid nanoparticles.

6.3.2.4 *Solvent emulsification–evaporation method*

The most widely used method in which organic solvent is included is the solvent emulsification–evaporation method to produce lipid nanoparticles. The

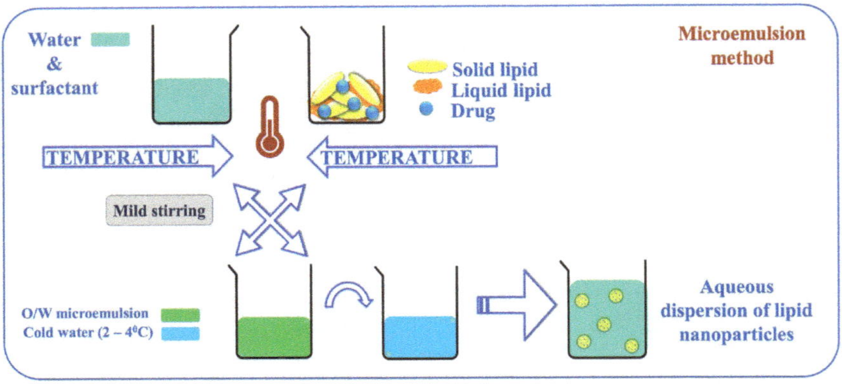

FIG. 6.3 Steps of low-energy-based lipid nanoparticle production (microemulsion method).

difference of the solvent emulsification–evaporation method from the above-mentioned SLN production technique is that to dissolve lipid in a water-immiscible solvent such as chloroform, toluene, cyclohexane, or ethyl acetate instead of melting the lipid. Hence, the method involves emulsifying the lipid solution in the aqueous solution of surfactant followed by evaporation of the solvent. On the other hand, it is also possible to modify the method to obtain w/o/w double emulsion for drugs. Although this method is suitable for loading the drugs that deteriorate at high temperature, the use of organic solvents is the major drawback of the method [27,33,46].

6.3.3 Characterization of SLN

Nano drug delivery systems offer keen opportunities over conventional pharmaceutical formulations in terms of treatment of the diseases as well as diagnosis since the unique particle size enables the system to interact with the biological environment. Therefore, various parameters need to be assessed by specific methods in terms of product quality, stability, and drug release management. The most important parameters to consider for an adequate characterization of SLNs and NLCs can be listed as particle size and distribution, particle morphology and surface properties, stability, drug release properties, as well as biological properties such as in vitro cell viability [36,56,57].

Particle size, polydispersity index (PDI), and zeta potential are key properties of lipid nanoparticles, as these variables may be relevant to their therapeutic potential as in other nano drug delivery systems. While particle size and size distribution directly affect the release profile, the biodistribution and cellular uptake of drug, zeta potential indicates the stability of colloidal system [58,59]. Among the laser light scattering methods, dynamic light scattering (DLS) or often known as photon correlation spectroscopy is the most widely used method for defining the particle size and the size distribution of lipid nanoparticles. The PDI is the indicator of particle size distribution uniformity and, it is should be as small as possible for monodisperse particles [36,46,56]. Both the formulation and the process parameters such as lipid type and ratio, surfactant concentration, homogenization cycle/pressure or sonication time can significantly influence the particle size and size distribution of lipid nanoparticles. The zeta potential is critical for the physical stability of lipid nanoparticles against particle aggregation. The zeta potential of lipid nanoparticles is usually estimated from the determination of electrophoretic mobility by the photon correlation spectroscopy technique [30,56,58]. In addition to DLS analysis, microscopic techniques such as transmission electron microscopy (TEM), scanning electron microscopy, and atomic force microscopy are also used for characterization, as they allow the visualization of particle morphology. Thus, it is also possible to verify the DLS data. TEM is the most frequently used technique for both SLNs and NLCs due to its simplicity and direct information on the particle shape can be obtained. But, lipid nanoparticles need to be stained to be easily visible with electron microscope because they do not have electron-dense enough. For this purpose ammonium molybdate, phosphotungstic acid, and uranyl acetate can be used as negative staining agents. Atomic force microscopy is preferred for determining the mean diameter of lipid particles and observing particle surface properties by obtaining topographic images [44,59,60].

Lipid crystallinity and modification are other important parameters that need to be studied to demonstrate the quality of lipid nanoparticles. The three-dimensional structure of lipid nanoparticles, whether SLN or NLC, can be considered as a solid spherical lipid matrix containing active substance and to be surrounded by surfactant as the stabilizing agent, as schematized in Fig. 6.1. Thus, the degree of lipid crystallinity and the modification of the lipid are the dominant factors influencing the drug incorporation into the lipid matrix as well as the release profiles of the drug from lipid nanoparticles. The heating and cooling processes involved in the production of lipid nanoparticles may affect the lipid crystallization and modification that form the core of the particle, as well as the storage conditions. In general, thermodynamically labile polymorphs of lipid molecules are known to have higher mobility, resulting in higher drug loading capacity. Lipid polymorphism refers to a rearrangement and can be defined as the time-dependent transition of lipid from a less stable to a more stable crystalline form. This crystal modification is observed especially in triglycerides as a transition from the least stable form α (alpha) to β′ (beta prime) and the most stable β (beta) form. Finally, the formation of the β form may cause the expulsion of the active molecule from the lipid matrix. Therefore, the polymorphic form of the lipid is one of the major factors that determine drug incorporation and release [27-29,42]. Differential scanning calorimetry (DSC) and X-ray diffraction are the two most commonly used techniques to determine the physical state and elucidate the crystal structure of lipid nanoparticles and structural information of the particles can be easily evaluated [61,62]. DSC is a highly sensitive technique used to determine different lipid modifications by utilizing different melting points and melting enthalpies. It is used for lipid nanoparticles to determine the changes in the melting and recrystallization behavior of lipid as a function of temperature. On the other hand, X-ray diffraction can identify certain crystalline compounds based on the principle that the intensity and location of the diffraction peaks are unique to each type of crystalline material, providing information on the crystallinity of both the lipid core and the active ingredient [56].

It is possible to incorporate many different drugs with different physicochemical characteristics including hydrophilic molecules into lipid nanoparticles. Therefore, determining drug incorporation which refers to the localization of the drug molecule in the lipid matrix is another essential factor for both the physicochemical properties and the in vivo performance of the delivery system. Solubility of the active molecule in the melted lipid, miscibility of drug melt and lipid melt, chemical and physical structure of lipid matrix, and the polymorphic state of lipid material are the parameters that determine the incorporation of the drug as stated by Müller et al. [29]. Drug loading capacity and drug encapsulation efficiency are key parameters that provide information about the amount of drug associated with nanoparticles as well as drug release patterns [33]. According to the localization of the active molecule incorporated in the lipid matrix, drug incorporation models can be categorized as the homogeneous matrix, drug-enriched shell, and drug-enriched core as presented in Fig. 6.4 [29].

The homogeneous matrix, known as the solid solution model is generally observed when the drug is in amorphous aggregates or homogeneously dispersed at the molecular level within the lipid matrix [30,36]. Hence, drug release occurs via diffusion from the lipid matrix and the prolonged release pattern of drug can be obtained. On the other hand, the core–shell model can be obtained in the form of a drug-enriched shell or a drug-enriched core when phase separation occurs during the cooling process. Drug-enriched shell model provides biphasic release behavior with burst release, since the drug is mainly located on the nanoparticle surface. Conversely, controlled and prolonged drug release is possible with drug-enriched core model due to the lipid shell that acts as a membrane and the expanded diffusional distance of the drug [33,35,42].

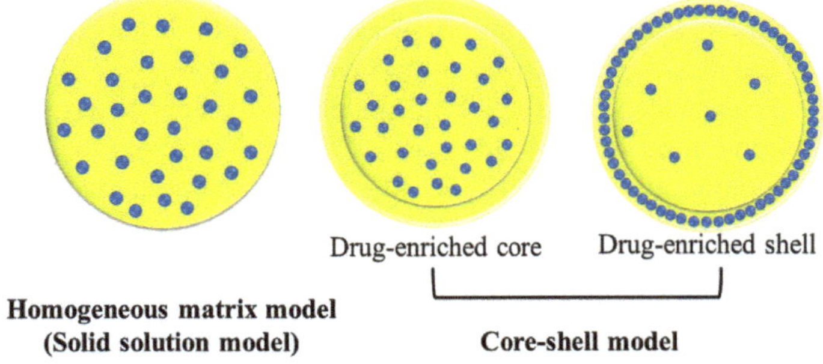

FIG. 6.4 Schematic representation of the incorporation models of drug into the lipid matrix.

6.3.4 Toxicological aspects of lipid nanoparticles

Although the distinctive physicochemical characteristics of nano-DDSs bring together many advantages, the primary challenge of the nanoparticles is to achieve nontoxic systems or at least nanoparticles with the lowest toxicity both for the environment and the organisms. An ideal drug delivery system should be degraded in the body or eliminated after complete drug release in order to avoid or minimize toxicity [34]. In this sense, Müller et al. proposed a "nanotoxicological classification system" considering the particle size as well as the material properties used in the production of nanoparticles. According to this system, four classes were established based on the particle size (>100 nm or not) and biodegradability of the nanoparticles. As stated previously, the lipids, the main component of lipid nanoparticles, are dietary fats of vegetable or animal origin and there are physiological pathways that allow their degradation in the body. Hence, SLNs and NLCs are classified in Class I (no or low risk) or III (medium risk) when evaluated in terms of particle size. It can be indicated that the toxicological profile of lipid nanoparticles is related to the particle size, since the surface area and reactivity increase as the particle size decreases [63]. However, toxicity levels of lipid nanoparticles vary depending on the degradation rate of the lipid used. Besides, the surfactant may affect the toxicological character of the lipid nanoparticles. Doctorovota et al. [39] reported that anionic and nonionic surfactants have lower toxicity than cationic surfactants and amphoteric surfactants exhibit low toxicity.

6.4 Penetration of SLN to the central nervous system

6.4.1 Barriers in the brain

Cellular and molecular barriers in the brain provide a stable environment for the proper functioning of the CNS regulating the exchange of molecules between the internal environment of the brain and the external blood flow environment. On the other hand, the treatment of neurological diseases is often difficult or hampered by the fact that only minimal amounts of therapeutic agents can penetrate through fully functioning brain barriers. The development of realistic strategies to ensure the controlled release of drugs into the CNS requires an in-depth understanding of the molecular mechanisms for the formation and maintenance of these barriers [64-66].

The BBB is the barrier between the lumen of cerebral blood vessels and the brain parenchyma. The blood–cerebrospinal fluid (CSF) barrier is the barrier between the choroid plexus blood vessels and the CSF. Tight junctions (TJs) between endothelial cells in the BBB and between epithelial cells in the blood–CSF barrier form physical barriers (Fig. 6.5A and B). Other endothelial cells in BBB are astrocytes surrounding endothelial cells with foot processes and pericytes in the basement membrane between these two cells. In the blood–CSF barrier, the blood vessels of the choroid plexus are fenestrated and form

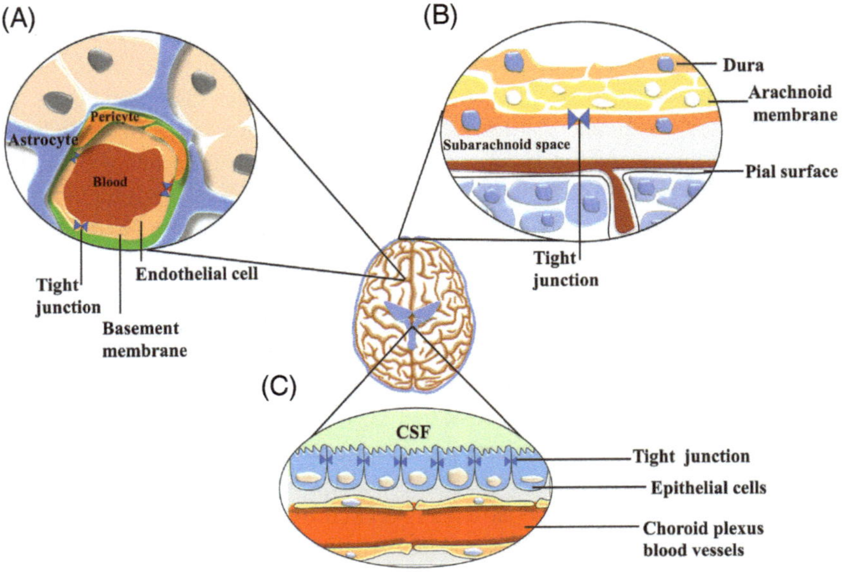

FIG. 6.5 Schematic representation of the structure of brain barriers. (A) Blood–brain barrier; (B) blood–cerebrospinal fluid barrier; (C) meningeal or arachnoid barrier.

a nonrestrictive barrier, while epithelial cells have apical TJs that prevent the intercellular passage of molecules. Another barrier is the meningeal or arachnoid barrier covering the CNS and composed of the dura, arachnoid, and pial membranes (Fig. 6.5C). In this barrier, there are TJs between the inner cells of the avascular arachnoid epithelium. The blood vessels in the subarachnoid and pial membrane have TJs, as in the cerebral vessels; but astrocytes and pericytes are absent. Due to avascular structure and relatively small surface area, this barrier is not an important route for the entry of solutes from blood to the brain [64,67].

TJs, located most apical of the lateral plasma membrane in the epithelium and endothelium, contain transmembrane proteins (connexin, occludin, tricellulin, and claudin family proteins) that form TJ strands, as well as cytoplasmic attachment proteins (membrane-associated guanylate kinase proteins) and cytoskeletal (actin binding) proteins. The expression and regulation of proteins in TJs are the main requirement for the proper functions of the brain barriers. Some drugs and pretreatments may affect the expression of these proteins and therefore, the barrier permeability. TJs significantly reduce the permeation of ions and other small hydrophilic molecules via the paracellular pathway [65,66,68]. Moreover, at the apical side of endothelial cells in BBB, there are ABC transporters such as P-gp (P-glycoprotein, ABCB1), ABCG2 (also breast cancer resistance protein), and MRP4 (multidrug resistance protein 4, ABCC4) that cause the small molecules to back into lumen (Fig. 6.6A). Nutrients are uptaken from the blood via facilitated carrier transporters such as glutamate (excitatory amino acid transporter 1, Eaat1, SLC1A3) and D-glucose (glucose

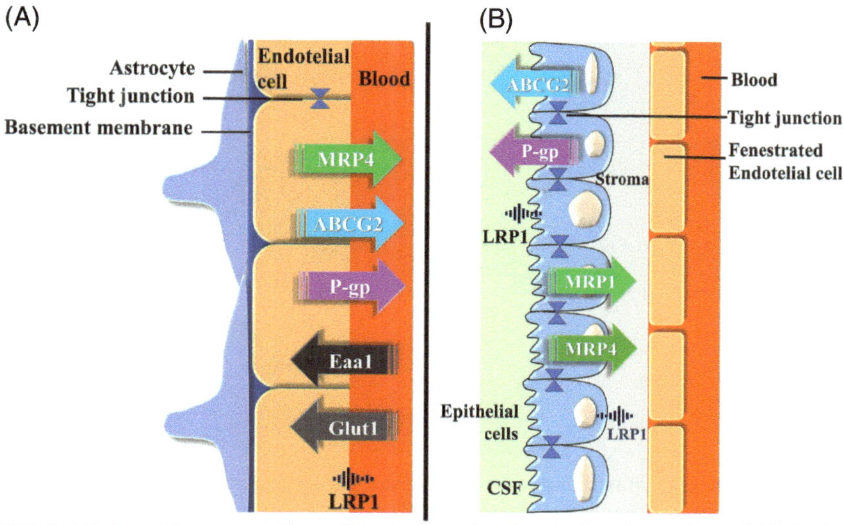

FIG. 6.6 Schematic presentation of the transporters located at the surface of (A) brain endothelial cells in capillaries, (B) choroid plexus epithelial cells.

uptake transporter 1, Glut1, SLC2A1). LRP1 (low-density lipoprotein receptor-related protein 1 receptor, APOER) mediates receptor-mediated transcytosis (RMT) to brain endothelial cells; it is one of several target receptors located on the apical side of the BBB that can be exploited for drug targeting to the brain. In the blood–CSF barrier, fenestrated endothelial capillary cells allow the passage of proteins from the choroid plexus, providing nutrients for CSF production. In choroid plexus epithelial cells, which have TJs, MRP (ABCC) transporters are located in the blood direction, while P-gp and ABCG2 transporters are located in the direction of CSF (Fig. 6.6B). It has been hypothesized that the choroid plexus supplies the drug to the CSF and that this is a "back door" for drug access to the brain parenchyma [69].

6.4.2 Uptake mechanisms in the brain

The endogenous transport pathways across the BBB are shown schematically in Fig. 6.7. Only small lipid molecules with the molecular weight <600 Da, chain length <6 amino acids have the ability of passive diffusion (transcellular pathway). Adsorptive-mediated transcytosis (AMT) is an endocytic process for the positively charged molecules enabling localized electrostatic disruption of the cell membrane phospholipids. In this way, the positively charged proteins could be adsorbed on the negatively charged cerebral endothelial cell surfaces. The receptors expressed on the luminal and abluminal sides of the BBB transport-specific endogenous peptides from the blood to the brain and from the brain to the blood, thus contributing to brain homeostasis. RMT involves the binding of receptor-specific ligands to the receptors on the luminal surface of endothelial cells and then internalizing them as

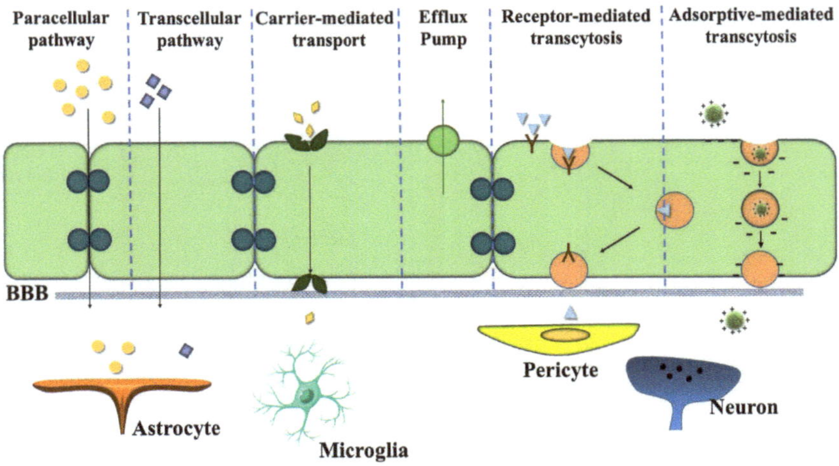

FIG. 6.7 Schematic illustrations of endogenous transport pathways across the BBB. Derived with permission from reference [122].

receptosomes, intracellular vesicular trafficking and exocytosis steps. A variety of macromolecules and proteins, such as leptin, insulin, transferrin, and apolipoproteins can be transported to the cerebral endothelium by RMT. In carrier-mediated transport, inward carriers, for example, solute carrier transporters bind substrates at the luminal surface and then release them into the endothelial cytoplasm for subsequent export by carriers located at the abluminal membrane. It functions via the transport proteins on endothelium which act as carriers for the delivery of brain-necessary substances, such as glucose, amino acids, purine bases, nucleosides, small peptides, monocarboxylates, and choline. Contrarily, outward carriers (efflux pumps, ABC transporters) such as P-gp (P-glycoprotein, ABCB1), ABCG2 (also breast cancer resistance protein), and MRP4 (multidrug resistance protein 4, ABCC4) prevent the compounds which are the substrates of efflux transporters, to enter into the brain. While this process contributes brain homeostasis by blocking the brain entry of toxic substances, it is one of the main obstacles for drug delivery [64,65,69-74].

Elucidation of uptake mechanisms in the brain has guided the development of strategies for drug targeting to the brain. Penetration of drugs into the CNS is related to their properties such as molecular size, lipophilicity, binding to plasma proteins, and affinity for transport systems. Paracellular transport of drugs is precluded by TJs; modulation of TJs can increase the permeation of polar substances from the BBB through the strategies such as opening TJs as a result of shrinkage of endothelial cells with the use of osmotic agents (mannitol) or reversibly disassembling TJ proteins with the use of permeation enhancers (aromatic substances like borneol) [65,75]. The transcellular pathway by passive diffusion is limited to lipid-soluble substances. For this reason, chemically increasing the lipid solubility of drugs has been investigated as a classical approach to increase brain penetration. However, in this case, the penetration of the drug through all in vivo biological membranes also increases and the drug is rapidly removed from the blood. Transcranial drug delivery through intracerebral implantation, intracerebroventricular infusion, and convection-enhanced diffusion of the drug into the brain parenchyma is another approach to bypass brain barriers. However, this invasive strategy carries risks of brain trauma or infection and does not appear to be suitable for repeated treatments. Another route is disruption of the BBB by intracarotid arterial infusion of hyperosmolar vasoactive agents, solvents, alkylating agents, immune adjuvants, and cytokines. However, it is inevitable to observe toxic side effects in chronic drug administration in these applications [70,71,76]. Another noninvasive drug delivery route for bypassing the BBB is intranasal (i.n.) administration. The drug after i.n. administration deposits on the olfactory mucosa spread around the olfactory bulb's subarachnoid space and then, is transported to the CSF. Besides, the conjugation with transport proteins or a permeation-enhancing agent to cross the arachnoid membrane is found to be beneficial [70,77,78].

Effective treatment cannot be provided for many CNS diseases such as treatment-resistant dementia, dementia-related diseases, autism, fragile X syndrome, liposomal storage disease, inherited ataxias, and blindness. However, the genes underlying many of these diseases are known, but release into the brain is a rate-limiting problem in gene therapy or enzyme-replacement therapy. None of the classical approaches mentioned above provide a general solution to the BBB problem [70]. This has led to the development of approaches directed to carrier-mediated transport, AMT, and RMT for brain penetration of drugs.

Many solute carrier (solute carrier transporter) transporters expressed in the BBB are potential portals for the entry of drugs into the brain. For example: GLUT1 glucose transporter type 1; MCT1 monocarboxylic; acid transporter type 1; LAT1 large neutral amino acid transporter type 1; CAT1 cationic amino acid transporter type 1; CNT2 concentrative nucleoside transporter type 2. If the drugs are structured as the substrate for carriers or the moieties that are specific for these carriers are linked chemically to the drugs, those drugs could cross CNS in the same way as nutrients. For instance, L-DOPA, nifluminic acid, valproate, baclofen, melphalan can be transported by the LAT1 carrier. Glycosylated peptides and drugs could be substrates for GLUT-1 glucose transporters [65,70]. Another pathway to brain entry is the inhibition of active efflux transporters in the brain barriers. Many drugs are substrates of P-gp and P-gp inhibitors could be used as "codrugs" to increase the brain penetration of such drugs. However, the fact that the inhibitors have their pharmacological effects, careful evaluation requires in terms of risk-benefit.

In the RMT process, receptor-specific endogenous ligands or peptidomimetic mAbs are considered molecular Trojan horses. Molecular Trojan horses ferry drugs, recombinant proteins, mAbs, RNA, DNA, and nonviral gene drugs which could not penetrate BBB due to their high molecular weights, and pass them to the brain via RMT. Two general technologies are employed to prepare formulations according to this approach. The first is the conjugation of the drug with RMT-targeting moiety and the second is nanoparticle drug delivery systems decorated with RMT-targeting ligand. RMT-targeting drug delivery has attracted great attention as a valid and effective way to treat CNS diseases. Target receptors in drug release based on RMT are mainly transferrin, insulin, low-density lipoprotein. However, RMT systems are not specific to the brain and there is also peripheral organ uptake. Therefore, there is a need to identify new BBB RMT systems such as the receptors, FC5 antibody, and the viral coat peptide RVG29 [20,71,72,74,79-81].

Lipid nanoparticles (SLNs and NLCs) are nanocarriers that have the potential to overcome BBB by accumulating in the CNS due to their lipophilic structure and by endocytic mechanism. The use of cationic lipids in the preparation of lipid nanoparticles may be a strategy to increase the bioadhesion of these nanoparticles in the nasal cavity by facilitating the electrostatic interaction of these nanoparticles with mucus and mediating their migration from the BBB into the cell via the AMT pathway. Coating the surface of lipid nanoparticles with surfactants is another strategy for passing through the BBB. Surfactant-coated lipid nanoparticles can pass through the BBB via RMT by selectively adsorbing apolipoproteins to their surfaces in blood. Similarly, targeting the BBB can be achieved by decorating the surface of lipid nanoparticles with ligands specific to other receptors in the BBB [76,82,83].

6.5 Application SLN in dementia

Several studies have been conducted to utilize the phenomenon of brain-targeted drug delivery via SLNs to treat AD. Different drugs and lipid compositions were used for this purpose. The most widely documented administration routes are i.n., oral and intra venous (i.v.) injection. Although most studies concentrated on SLN formulations of approved dementia drugs, there are some other reports on drugs, which are not indicated yet. The development of SLNs is widely studied for improving drug stability, modifying drug release and providing brain-targeted drug delivery, which may result in dose reduction.

Donepezil (DPL) is a Food and Drug Administration-approved cholinesterase inhibitor drug prescribed for mild to moderate AD [84]. The marketed forms of DPL are orally administered tablets and capsules with high bioavailability. However, these forms cause various gastrointestinal (anorexia, diarrhea, nausea, etc.) and hepatotoxic side effects due to the need of frequent drug administration. Additionally, the high aqueous solubility of DPL limits its passage to brain. Therefore, the need for brain-targeted DPL delivery led researchers to work on DPL-loaded SLNs [84-86]. In a study by Yasir et al. [86], DPL-loaded GMS-based SLNs were prepared and optimized by Box–Behnken design for i.n. DPL delivery. Formulations with improved physical stability (shelf life of approximately 2 years) were obtained. Upon i.n. application, SLNs exhibited superior pharmacokinetic and biodistribution properties on Wistar rats compared to i.n. and i.v. DPL solution. Brain-targeted drug delivery was shown in rabbits by scintigraphy images. Olfactory route was found to be the possible pathway for direct drug transport upon i.n. SLN administration. The improved brain drug delivery was also attributed to increased nasal retention time provided by the occlusiveness of the SLN forming lipids and permeability enhancing effects of Tween 80 (polysorbate 80) which was used as a surfactant. APOE-targeted Dynasan 116-based SLN formulations were shown to improve DPL uptake in both cultured human brain endothelial cells and neurons. Accordingly, ApoE ligand improved SLN penetration across a coculture BBB model composed of primary rat brain endothelial cells, pericytes, and astrocytes [84]. This study emphasizes that for improved BBB transport the SLN size should be less than 200 nm and should be neutral or negatively charged. Improved recognition between ApoE on SLNs and low-density lipoprotein receptors overexpressed on the BBB was shown and possible transport pathways were discussed by Neves et al. [87,88]. In another study carried out by Mendes et al. [89] enhanced transdermal transport of DPL via NLCs was shown and suggested as an alternative for the treatment of AD.

Rivastigmine inhibits both acetylcholinesterases (AChE) and butrylcholinesterases and it is used to treat dementia. The patient compliance of conventional oral rivastigmine formulations is low due to cognitive impairment and other adverse effects such as anorexia, vomiting, and nausea. This is primarily attributed to poor oral bioavailability of rivastigmine which is a hydrophilic agent but highly degraded due to first pass metabolism. Several studies were conducted to improve the poor transport of rivastigmine to brain through their encapsulation into lipid nanoparticles. A transdermal patch formulation was developed to administer rivastigmine carrying NLCs to treat dementia. Optimum NLC formulation with a particle size of 134.60 ± 15.10 nm and surface charge of −11.80 ± 2.24 mV was obtained using Box–Behnken design. The nanoparticles composed of castor oil and GMS were prepared by HPH technique and integrated in transdermal patches. Slow and prolonged drug release was obtained from the patches resulting in extended T_{max} and increased AUC in rats compared to conventional Exelon patch [90]. To eliminate the risk of therapy related neurodegenaration due to synthetic surfactants in NLC composition, a natural/safer biosurfactant (Ryoto sugar ester) was used to prepare rivastigmine containing NLCs [91]. The results on drug diffusion through nasal mucosa exhibited improved diffusion and aldicarb assay on *C. elegans* model revealed increased acetylcholine concentration via NLCs. Besides, the nanoformulations provided significant retention of memory in Wistar rats at Morris water maze test. Shah et al. [92] developed rivastigmine containing Compritol 888 ATO (glyceryl dibehenate) SLN formulations by combining homogenization and ultrasonication techniques for brain-targeted drug delivery via i.n. administration. A quality by design-based formulation development strategy was used to obtain SLNs for better drug delivery through BBB. Therefore, the quality target product profile was high encapsulation efficiency, small size, and PDI. Ex vivo diffusion studies on goat nasal mucosa revealed enhanced drug diffusion via optimum SLN formulation compared to drug solution due to the lipophilic nature of SLNs.

This improvement was also attributed to drug solubilization within the lipidic matrix and/or the formation of amorphous dispersion as confirmed by DSC results and small particle size. The histopathological studies have shown that SLNs were safe; the structure of the epithelial layer was preserved, and nasociliary damage or cell necrosis was not observed.

Tacrine (TAC) is the first Food and Drug Administration-approved treatment for AD. It acts as an AChE inhibitor and improve the memory and cognition of AD patients. TAC has low bioavailability and exhibits a short plasma half-life. TAC is discontinued in the United States due to serious side effects such hepatotoxicity, nausea, vomiting, shivering. In order to compensate these side effects, model amphipathic peptide-conjugated NLC-based TAC formulations were studied. Compritol 888 ATO and Transcutol HP (diethylene glycol monoethyl ether) were used as solid and liquid lipids and NLCs were obtained by hot high shear homogenization technique. The safety of TAC-loaded NLCs was demonstrated by the low toxicity level against SH-SY5Y cells. However, since toxicity is increased in the case of model amphipathic peptide-conjugated NLC, it has been suggested to examine its efficacy in low-dose therapy as an alternative therapy [93].

Galantamine hydrobromide (GH) is another AChE inhibitor used in AD. However it causes serious cholinergic side effects. Although its gastrointestinal absorption is at high level, its hydrophilic nature limits the brain-targeted accumulation. Misra et al. [94] obtained twofold improvement on oral GH bioavailability in rabbits after loading it into SLNs. Authors explain this by improved tissue binding via intact absorption of GH-loaded SLNs and consequent drug release. The SLN formulations were also found to be more effective in reversing cognitive deficit in isoproterenol-induced rats after oral administration.

Lassera et al. [95] performed a very interesting study that aimed to synthesize lipoyl-memantine as codrug for treating AD. In this study, stealth SLN formulation of lipoyl-memantine was prepared to improve the oral bioavailability of the drug. The optimized formulation with a diameter of 170 nm was found to be stable under in vitro conditions and toxicologically safe. The drug release in simulated gastric fluid—SGF and simulated intestinal fluid—SIF within the initial 4 hour was maintained at a level of 20% indicating the ability of SLN to carry the remaining entrapped drug to CNS.

Resveratrol (RSV), a naturally occurring polyphenolic compound, can activate nuclear factor (erythroid-derived 2)-like 2 (Nrf2) and exert neuroprotective activity [96]. RSV has been demonstrated to have beneficial effects in animal models of AD. However, the bioavailability of RSV is low due to its poor solubility, low stability, and short biological half-life. Incorporation of RSV into SLNs composed of stearic acid, lecithin, and taurocholate provided sixfold higher drug accumulation in brain upon intraperitoneal administration compared to pure RSV. Amelioration of vascular dementia-induced oxidative stress and cognitive deficits via Nrf2/HO-1 pathway was shown [97]. Different research groups reported improved RSV permeability through BBB by modifying SLN formulations with APOE, OX26 (antitransferrin receptor antibody IgG2a), and D-α-tocopheryl polyethyleneglycol succinate [98-100].

Curcumin has been reported as a natural neuroprotective agent with high antioxidant activity. Recent studies suggest its potential in the treatment of dementia. Despite its potential, curcumin has poor bioavailability and cannot effectively penetrate to biological membranes. Curcumin was encapsulated in SLNs to overcome these restrictions and its potential against homocysteine-induced oxidative stress in vascular dementia was shown by Prathipati et al. [101]. The biochemical, neurochemical, and histological assessments proved the effectiveness of SLNs. There are several other studies showing brain-targeted delivery of curcumin leading improved pharmacokinetic and pharmacodynamic parameters via SLNs [102-106]. In addition, NLCs were found to be significantly more effective on improving brain accumulation of curcumin compared to SLNs [107]. This was partly attributed to smaller particle size and flexibility of NLCs due to liquid lipids in its structure that prolonged systemic circulation time and improved intracellular transport through BBB. Kuo et al. [108] prepared dual phase SLN formulations carrying nerve growth factor, rosmarinic acid, curcumin, and quercetin. The SLN was composed of five different lipids (beeswax, cacao butter, glyceryl dibehenate, tricaprin, cardiolipin) and the system was further conjugated with transferrin. SLNs effectively decreased the drugs cytotoxicity on BBB due to controlled drug release and improved drugs infiltration to the BBB. The system was suggested for rescuing degenerated neurons in AD.

Apart from the active substances mentioned here, it is stated that the use of different active substance groups (antidepressants, anxiolytics, antipsychotics, sleep inducers, antioxidants) may provide benefits for the treatment of symptoms related to the disorders that occur in the progression of dementia. In this context, drugs that target proteolytic enzymes involved in the formation of Aβ plaques, tau protein and APOE, neuroinflammation regulators, immunotherapeutics targeting Aβ protein are also evaluated [4]. SLN-based strategies for using such drugs for dementia treatment are summarized in Table 6.2.

6.6 Conclusion and final remarks

There are several medications available to treat different types of dementia, but they are not capable of preventing or reversing the disease progression. Other than the approved medications, the intensive research on a wide range of biological substances, such as proteins, peptides, growth factors, and nucleic acids, revealed their efficacy in slowing the progression of AD, the most common type of dementia, and restoring damaged cells [18]. However, there is no new dementia drug on the market yet. The success of new drugs highly depends on providing a suitable delivery system that ensures the drug stability, prolong its residence time in the blood, cross barriers, and selectively accumulate at the site of action. It is apparent that "one-size-fits-all" approach is not valid for dementia

Table 6.2 Lipid nanoparticle-based formulations for treatment of dementia.

Admin-stra-tion Route	Active Molecule	Excipients	Prepa-ration Method	Characteristics a. Particle size b. Zeta potential c. Encapsulation efficiency	Outcomes	Refs.
Oral	Sesamol	Tween 80 Soy lecithin Compritol 888 ATO*	Micro-emulsion technique	40–70 nm N.A.* 75.9±2.91 %	Cognitive deficits were restored in wistar rats with intracerebroventricular (ICV) streptozotocin (STZ) induced-cognitive impairment and oxidative stress parameters (catalase, superoxide dismutase and reduced glutathion) were better regulated via sesamol-SLN. Its impact at a dose of 16 mg/kg was found to be essentially identical to that of rivastigmine.	[109]
	Chrysin	Stearic acid Lecithin Taurocholate	Micro-emulsion technique	240.0 ± 4.79 nm −40.4 ± 2.54 mV 86.29 ± 3.42 %	The extend of neuronal damage in hippocampal region of rats due to amyloid-β25–35 (Aβ25–35) injection was successfully reduced upon SLN injection. The effective dose was reduced and SLNs suggest improved bioavailability.	[110]
	Nimodip-ine	Poloxamer 188 Soya lecithin Palmitic acid	High pressure homogenisation method	116.0 ± 21 nm −10.0 ± 4.8 mV 93.66 ± 9.7 %	The oral bioavailability of nimodipine in wistar rats was increased 2.08-fold compared to pure drug solution. The improvement was attributed to lymphatic transport of drug loaded SLNs.	[111]
	Pome-granate extract	Tween 80 Stearic acid Lecithin Cholesterol Chitosan	Solvent evaporation method	297.5 nm N.A. 45 %	The cognitive functions and antioxidant levels were significantly increased in AlCl 3-induced AD rat model via pomegranate extract loaded SLNs. The histopathological observations has shown the restoration of the cortex structure and neurons.	[112]

Admin-stra-tion Route	Active Molecule	Excipients	Prepa-ration Method	Characteristics a. Particle size b. Zeta potential c. Encapsulation efficiency	Outcomes	Refs.
Intra-perito-neal	Erythro-poietin	Tween 80 Transcutol®P * Capmul® MCM * Glyceryl monostearate	Double emulsion solvent evapo-ration method	219.9 ± 15.6 nm - 22.4 ± 0.8 mV 41.4 ± 3.6 IU/mg of SLN	Morris water maze test on the beta-amyloid-induced AD-like animal model revealed significant restoration of cognitive deficit via SLNs. Significant decrease of ADP/ATP ratio, Aβ plaque deposition and improved antioxidant activity were obtained compared to control group.	[113]
	Cycloas-tragenol	Poloxamer-188 Propylene glycol Stearic acid	Solvent evapo-ration method	347.98 nm -14.12 9 mV 82.9 %	Significant cognitive improvement was obtained on STZ induced vascular dementia in zebrafish model. The behavioral tests, analysis of blood and brain biomarkers support this data.	[114]
	Nicotin-amide	Stearic acid Phospholipon® 90G* Phosphatidyl-serine	Micro-emulsion technique	124 ± 0.8 nm –46.1 ± 0.65 mV 41.3 ± 0.41 %	Phosphatidylserine functionalized SLNs were shown to be non-toxic on human neuroblastoma cells. In biodistribution studies, improved brain accumula-tion via SLNs was shown upon i.p. injection of SLNs carrying fluorescent market. In vivo experiments based on Morris water maze test revealed improved memory and decreased tau hyperphosphorylation.	[115]

(Continued)

Table 6.2 Cont'd

Admin-stra-tion Route	Active Molecule	Excipients	Prepa-ration Method	Characteristics a. Particle size b. Zeta potential c. Encapsulation efficiency	Outcomes	Refs.
Intrave-nous	Quercetin	Tween 80 Compritol 888 ATO*	Micro-emulsion technique	159 nm 21.05 mV 85.73 %	Chronic treatment with quercetin loaded SLNs provided better behavioral improvement in rats with aluminium-induced dementia. The antioxidant potential of the compound was increased, glutathione and nitrite levels were preserved in brain. Tween 80 coating on SLNs was found to cause particle coalescence leading decreased brain uptake.	[116]
Intrana-sal	Tarenflur-bil	Tween 20 Soya lecithin Glyceryl monostearate Stearic acid	Emulsifi-cation and solvent evapo-ration method	175.32 ± 10.32 nm −23.13 ± 2.32 mV 57.81 ± 5.32%	Tissue distribution studies revealed improvement on the poor permeation of tarenflurbil through BBB upon i.n. administration to Sprague Dawley rats. The drug targeting efficiency % and drug transport % were 183.15 and 45.41 respectively, which proves the effectiveness of SLN delivery via olfactory pathway upon i.n. administration.	[117]
Trans-dermal SLN	Huperzine A	Glyceryl monostearate Capmul® MCM* Transcutol®P* Tween 80 Tri-ethanolamine	Micro-emulsion technique	119.1 ± 6.94 nm −20 ± 5.81 mV 60.05 ± 5.84 %	Drug carrying NLCs were loaded into gels and improved drug permeation across skin was obtained. The formulations did not cause any skin irritation in draize patch test at albino rabbits and upon transdermal application to scopolamine induced amnesia mice significant improvement in cognitive functions was observed compared to control group.	[118]

Admin-stra-tion Route	Active Molecule	Excipients	Prepa-ration Method	Characteristics a. Particle size b. Zeta potential c. Encapsulation efficiency	Outcomes	Refs.
NA	α-Bisabolol	Tween 80	Hot	139.5 nm	α-Bisabolol loaded SLNs effectively inhibit AChE and revealed antioxidant activity. Neuro-2a cells were protected from Aβ induced neurotoxicity as indicated by MTT test. Besides, thioflavin T assay, fluorescent microscope and FT-IR analysis revealed the inhibition of Aβ aggregation.	[119]
		Lecithin	homog-enization method			
		Cholesterol		-31.7 mV		
				98.44 %		
	Quercetin	Tween 80	Hot	234±18 nm	The safety of transferrin functionalized quercetin NLCs were shown by LDH assay on hCMEC/D3 cells. Enhanced permeability was also shown in the same cell line. Studies on in vitro model of Alzheimer's disease with Aβ(1–42) peptide revealed the neuropro-tective effects of NLCs compared to pure drug .	[120]
		Cetyl palmitate	homog-enization method			
		Miglyol-812*		–32±8 mV		
				77±11 %		

**N.A.: Not available; Compritol 888 ATO : glyceryl dibehenate; Phospholipon® 90G: natural and hydrogenated lecithin fractions and phospholipids from soybean, rapeseed (canola) or sunflower; Capmul® MCM:glyceryl mono-dicaprylate; Transcutol®P: purified diethylene glycolmonoethyl ether; Miglyol-812: medium-chain triglyceride.*

treatment due the complexity of underlying causes and symptoms [19]. In such diseases, it is necessary to determine the pathophysiology on an individual basis and to apply targeted treatments. In recent years, brain-targeted delivery of SLN for the treatment of neurodegenerative diseases including dementia has become a common approach. There is an increasing focus on formulating different drugs with different lipids to improve the in vivo treatment efficacy. Many of these studies revealed excellent data on supporting the success of SLNs in terms of bioavailability improvement and BBB transport enhancement leading better neuronal damage reduction, cognitive deficits restoration compared to free drugs. It is apparent that if addressed properly SLNs will provide significant benefits over conventional dosage forms. The high level of control over the design of lipid nanoparticles such as their size, charge, lipophilicity, surface functionality enables these systems as ideal carriers in brain-targeted personalized drug delivery to treat dementia [20]. Unfortunately, many of the products of these studies have not been commercialized due to several existing challenges. Limited drug loading capacity, drug release during storage, polydisperse size distribution due to inadequate preparation methods are several problems [121]. One of the major issue relevant to SLN-based drug delivery involves the cytotoxic potential of these systems in chronic prolong applications due to accumulation in other body organs [45]. The safety concerns should be further evaluated with detailed standardized in vivo studies. Studies on the use of advanced approaches such as theranostic SLNs and/or ligand decorated SLNs with improved brain penetration are negligible in dementia and this area is open to research and development. Nonetheless, clinical applications of SLNs should be considered as a personalized medicine matter. Studies to be carried out on this topic will accelerate the transfer of lipid nanoparticulate drug delivery systems to clinical studies for a more effective treatment of dementia. Besides, the pharmaceutical industry should closely follow the recent developments on lipid nanoparticle-based drug delivery initiated by academia and urgently adopt their manufacturing technologies to this rapidly growing and promising technology.

References

[1] Noetzli M, Eap CB. Pharmacodynamic, pharmacokinetic and pharmacogenetic aspects of drugs used in the treatment of Alzheimer's disease. Clin Pharmacokinet 2013;52(4):225–41.

[2] Cummings J, Feldman HH, Scheltens P. The "rights" of precision drug development for Alzheimer's disease. Alzheimers Res Ther 2019;11(76):1–14. doi:10.1186/s13195-019-0529-5.

[3] WHO. https://apps.who.int/gho/data/node.dementia. (Accessed 26.06.2021).

[4] Plascencia-Villa G, Perry G. Alzheimer's disease pharmacology. In: Kenakin T, editors. Comprehensive Pharmacology, 1. 1st ed. UK: Elsevier; 2022. p. 34–63.

[5] Rone-Adams S, Stern DF, Olivier TW, Blodgett MG. Understanding dementia: etiology, communication, and exercise intervention. Strength Cond J 2013;35(4):88–98.

[6] Bansal N, Parle M. Dementia: an overview. J Pharm Technol Res Manage 2014;2(1):29–45. doi:10.15415/jptrm.2014.21003.

[7] Custodio N, Montesinos R, Lira D, Herrera-Pérez E, Bardales Y, Valeriano-Lorenzo L. Mixed dementia: a review of the evidence. Dementia Neuropsychol 2017;11:364–70.

[8] Cunningham EL, McGuinness B, Herron B, Passmore AP. Dementia. Ulster Med J 2015;84(2):79–87.

[9] Harvey RJ, Ellison D, Hardy J, Hutton M, Rogues PK, Collinge J, Fox NC, Rossor MN. Chromosome 14 familial Alzheimer's disease: the clinical and neuropathological characteristics of a family with a leucine ->serine (L250S) substitution at codon 250 of the presenilin 1 gene. J Neurol Neurosur Ps 1998;64(1):44–9.

[10] Nazarko L. Dementia: prevalence and pathophysiology. Br J Healthcare Assist 2019;13(6):266–70.

[11] Peng X, Xing PQ, Li XH, Qian Y, Song FH, Bai ZX, Han GC, Lei HX. Towards personalized intervention for Alzheimer's disease. Genom Proteom Bioinf 2016;14(5):289–97.

[12] Siafaka PI, Mutlu G, Okur NU. Alzheimer's disease and its related dementia types: a review on their management via nanotechnology based therapeutic strategies. Curr Alzheimer Res 2020;17(14):1239–61.

[13] Cordaro M, Cuzzocrea S, Di Paola R. Vascular dementia and aliamides: a new approach for the future. J Transl Sci 2018;5:1–4.

[14] Luca M, Luca A, Calandra C. The role of oxidative damage in the pathogenesis and progression of Alzheimer's disease and vascular dementia. Oxid Med Cell Longev 2015;2015:1–8.

[15] Duong S, Patel T, Chang F. Dementia: what pharmacists need to know. Can Pharm J 2017;150(2):118–29.

[16] Cummings J, Fox N. Defining disease modifying therapy for Alzheimer's disease. JPAD - J Prev Alzheim 2017;4(2):109–15.

[17] Karthivashan G, Ganesan P, Park SY, Kim JS, Choi DK. Therapeutic strategies and nano-drug delivery applications in management of ageing Alzheimer's disease. Drug Deliv 2018;25(1):307–20.

[18] Wen MM, El-Salamouni NS, El-Refaie WM, Hazzah HA, Ali MM, Tosi G, Farid RM, Blanco-Prieto MJ, Billa N, Hanafy AS. Nanotechnology-based drug delivery systems for Alzheimer's disease management: technical, industrial, and clinical challenges. J Control Release 2017;245:95–107.

[19] De Matteis L, Martin-Rapun R, de la Fuente JM. Nanotechnology in personalized medicine: a promising tool for Alzheimer's disease treatment. Curr Med Chem 2018;25(35):4602–15.

[20] Mitchell MJ, Billingsley MM, Haley RM, Wechsler ME, Peppas NA, Langer R. Engineering precision nanoparticles for drug delivery. Nat Rev Drug Discov 2021;20(2):101–24.

[21] Anselmo AC, Mitragotri S. Nanoparticles in the clinic. Bioeng Transl Med 2016;1(1):10–29.

[22] Gasco MR. Method for producing solid lipid microsphere having a narrow size distribution. United States Patent US5250236A. United States Patent and Trademark Office. 5 Oct. 1993.

[23] Lucks JS, Müller RH Medication vehicles made of solid lipid particles (solid lipid nanospheres - SLN). Canada Patent CA2119253A1. Canada Patent and Trademark Office.18 Sept. 1991.

[24] Muller RH, Petersen RD, Hornmoss A, Pardeike J. Nanostructured lipid carriers (NLC) in cosmetic dermal products. Adv Drug Deliver Rev 2007;59(6):522–30.

[25] Kumar S, Randhawa JK. High melting lipid based approach for drug delivery: solid lipid nanoparticles. Mater Sci Eng C-Mater 2013;33(4):1842–52.

[26] Salvi VR, Pawar P. Nanostructured lipid carriers (NLC) system: a novel drug targeting carrier. J Drug Deliv Sci Technol 2019;51:255–67.

[27] Mehnert W, Mader K. Solid lipid nanoparticles -- production, characterization and applications. Adv Drug Deliv Rev 2001;47(2-3):165–96.

[28] Pink DL, Loruthai O, Ziolek RM, Wasutrasawat P, Terry AE, Lawrence MJ, Lorenz CD. On the structure of solid lipid nanoparticles. Small 2019;15(45):1–10.
[29] Muller RH, Mader K, Gohla S. Solid lipid nanoparticles (SLN) for controlled drug delivery -- a review of the state of the art. Eur J Pharm Biopharm 2000;50(1):161–77.
[30] Gordillo-Galeano A, Mora-Huertas CE. Solid lipid nanoparticles and nanostructured lipid carriers: a review emphasizing on particle structure and drug release. Eur J Pharm Biopharm 2018;133:285–308.
[31] Daraee H, Etemadi A, Kouhi M, Alimirzalu S, Akbarzadeh A. Application of liposomes in medicine and drug delivery. Artif Cell Nanomed B 2016;44(1):381–91.
[32] Dingler A, Gohla S. Production of solid lipid nanoparticles (SLN): scaling up feasibilities. J Microencapsul 2002;19(1):11–6.
[33] Battaglia L, Gallarate M. Lipid nanoparticles: state of the art, new preparation methods and challenges in drug delivery. Expert Opin Drug Deliv 2012;9(5):497–508.
[34] Montoto SS, Muraca G, Ruiz ME. Solid lipid nanoparticles for drug delivery: pharmacological and biopharmaceutical aspects. Front Mol Biosci 2020;7:1–24.
[35] Uner M, Yener G. Importance of solid lipid nanoparticles (SLN) in various administration routes and future perspectives. Int J Nanomed 2007;2(3):289–300.
[36] Mishra V, Bansal KK, Verma A, Yadav N, Thakur S, Sudhakar K, Rosenholm JM. Solid lipid nanoparticles: emerging colloidal nano drug delivery systems. Pharmaceutics 2018;10(4):1–21.
[37] Pardeike J, Weber S, Haber T, Wagner J, Zarfl HP, Plank H, Zimmer A. Development of an itraconazole-loaded nanostructured lipid carrier (NLC) formulation for pulmonary application. Int J Pharm 2011;419(1-2):329–38.
[38] Nasirizadeh S, Malaekeh-Nikouei B. Solid lipid nanoparticles and nanostructured lipid carriers in oral cancer drug delivery. J Drug Deliv Sci Technol 2020;55:101458. doi:10.1016/j.jddst.2019.101458.
[39] Doktorovova S, Shegokar R, Souto EB. Role of excipients in formulation development and biocompatibility of lipid nanoparticles (SLNs/NLCs). In: Denisa Ficai D, Grumezescu AM, editors. Nanostructures for novel therapy. Netherlands: Elsevier; 2017. p. 811–43.
[40] Apostolou M, Assi S, Fatokun AA, Khan I. The effects of solid and liquid lipids on the physicochemical properties of nanostructured lipid carriers. J Pharm Sci 2021;110:2859–2872.
[41] Cole AS, Eastoe JE. Molecular architecture – the building materials, lipids. In: Cole AS, Eastoe JE, editors. Biochemistry and oral biology. UK: Butterworth-Heinemann; 1988. p. 100–8.
[42] Wissing SA, Kayser O, Muller RH. Solid lipid nanoparticles for parenteral drug delivery. Adv Drug Deliv Rev 2004;56(9):1257–72.
[43] Khosa A, Reddi S, Saha RN. Nanostructured lipid carriers for site-specific drug delivery. Biomed Pharmacother 2018;103:598–613.
[44] Geszke-Moritz M, Moritz M. Solid lipid nanoparticles as attractive drug vehicles: composition, properties and therapeutic strategies. Mater Sci Eng C-Mater 2016;68:982–94.
[45] Tapeinos C, Battaglini M, Ciofani G. Advances in the design of solid lipid nanoparticles and nanostructured lipid carriers for targeting brain diseases. J Control Release 2017;264:306–32.
[46] Subramaniam B, Siddik ZH, Nagoor NH. Optimization of nanostructured lipid carriers: understanding the types, designs, and parameters in the process of formulations. J Nanopart Res 2020;22(6):1–29. 141. doi:10.1007/s11051-020-04848-0.
[47] Paliwal R, Paliwal SR, Kenwat R, Kurmi BD, Sahu MK. Solid lipid nanoparticles: a review on recent perspectives and patents. Expert Opin Ther Pat 2020;30(3):179–94.

[48] Dhiman N, Awasthi R, Sharma B, Kharkwal H, Kulkarni GT. Lipid nanoparticles as carriers for bioactive delivery. Front Chem 2021;9:1–19.
[49] Muchow M, Maincent P, Muller RH. Lipid nanoparticles with a solid matrix (SLN, NLC, LDC) for oral drug delivery. Drug Dev Ind Pharm 2008;34(12):1394–405.
[50] Jenning V, Lippacher A, Gohla SH. Medium scale production of solid lipid nanoparticles (SLN) by high pressure homogenization. J Microencapsul 2002;19(1):1–10.
[51] Hu CB, Qian AR, Wang Q, Xu F, He Y, Xu J, Xia YC, Xia Q. Industrialization of lipid nanoparticles: from laboratory-scale to large-scale production line. Eur J Pharm Biopharm 2016;109:206–13.
[52] Ganesan P, Narayanasamy D. Lipid nanoparticles: different preparation techniques, characterization, hurdles, and strategies for the production of solid lipid nanoparticles and nanostructured lipid carriers for oral drug delivery. Sustain Chem Pharm 2017;6:37–56.
[53] Amasya G, Ergin AD, Cakirci OE, Ozcelikay AT, Bayindir ZS, Yuksel N. A study to enhance the oral bioavailability of s-adenosyl-l-methionine (SAMe): SLN and SLN nanocomposite particles. Chem Phys Lipids 2021;237:1–11.
[54] Shegokar R, Singh KK, Muller RH. Production & stability of stavudine solid lipid nanoparticles--from lab to industrial scale. Int J Pharm 2011;416(2):461–70.
[55] Simonazzi A, Cid AG, Villegas M, Romero AI, Palma SD, Bermúdez JM. Nanotechnology applications in drug controlled release. In: Grumezescu AM, editor. Drug Target Stimuli Sensitive Drug Delivery Systems. UK: Elsevier, William Andrew Publishing; 2018.
[56] Das S, Chaudhury A. Recent advances in lipid nanoparticle formulations with solid matrix for oral drug delivery. Aaps Pharmscitech 2011;12(1):62–76.
[57] Kumar A, Dixit CK. Methods for characterization of nanoparticles. UK: Elsevier, Woodh Pub Ser Biomed; 2017. p. 43–58.
[58] Heurtault B, Saulnier P, Pech B, Proust JE, Benoit JP. Physico-chemical stability of colloidal lipid particles. Biomaterials 2003;24(23):4283–300.
[59] Hallan SS, Sguizzato M, Esposito E, Cortesi R. Challenges in the physical characterization of lipid nanoparticles. Pharmaceutics 2021;13(4):1–31. 549. doi:10.3390/pharmaceutics13040549.
[60] Kuntsche J, Horst JC, Bunjes H. Cryogenic transmission electron microscopy (cryo-TEM) for studying the morphology of colloidal drug delivery systems. Int J Pharm 2011;417(1-2):120–37.
[61] Souto EB, Mehnert W, Muller RH. Polymorphic behaviour of Compritol (R) 888 ATO as bulk lipid and as SLN and NLC. J Microencapsul 2006;23(4):417–33.
[62] Bunjes H, Unruh T. Characterization of lipid nanoparticles by differential scanning calorimetry, X-ray and neutron scattering. Adv Drug Deliv Rev 2007;59(6):379–402.
[63] Muller RH, Gohla S, Keck CM. State of the art of nanocrystals -- special features, production, nanotoxicology aspects and intracellular delivery. Eur J Pharm Biopharm 2011;78(1):1–9.
[64] Saunders NR, Ek CJ, Habgood MD, Dziegielewska KM. Barriers in the brain: a renaissance?. Trends Neurosci 2008;31(6):279–86.
[65] He QG, Liu J, Liang J, Liu XP, Li W, Liu Z, Ding ZY, Tuo D. Towards improvements for penetrating the blood-brain barrier-recent progress from a material and pharmaceutical perspective. Cells - Basel 2018;7(4):1–21. 24. doi:10.3390/cells7040024.
[66] Bauer HC, Krizbai IA, Bauer H, Traweger A. You shall not pass"--tight junctions of the blood brain barrier. Front Neurosci - Switz 2014;8:1–21. 392. doi:10.3389/fnins.2014.00392.
[67] Abbott NJ, Patabendige AAK, Dolman DEM, Yusof SR, Begley DJ. Structure and function of the blood-brain barrier. Neurobiol Dis 2010;37(1):13–25.

[68] Piontek J, Winkler L, Wolburg H, Muller SL, Zuleger N, Piehl C, Wiesner B, Krause G, Blasig IE. Formation of tight junction: determinants of homophilic interaction between classic claudins. FASEB J 2008;22(1):146–58.

[69] Basseville A, Hall MD, Chau CH, Robey RW, Gottesman M, Figg WD, Bates SE. The ABCG2 multidrug transporter. In: George AM, editor. ABC transporters - 40 years on. Cham: Springer; 2016. p. 195–226.

[70] Pardridge WM. The blood-brain barrier: bottleneck in brain drug development. NeuroRx 2005;2(1):3–14.

[71] Bellettato CM, Scarpa M. Possible strategies to cross the blood-brain barrier. Ital J Pediatr 2018;44:127–61. 131. doi:10.1186/s13052-018-0563-0.

[72] Pulgar VM. Transcytosis to cross the blood brain barrier, new advancements and challenges. Front Neurosci - Switz 2019;12:1–9. 1019. doi:10.3389/fnins.2018.01019.

[73] Lombardo SM, Schneider M, Tureli AE, Tureli NG. Key for crossing the BBB with nanoparticles: the rational design. Beilstein J Nanotechnol 2020;11:866–83.

[74] Herda LM, Polo E, Kelly PM, Rocks L, Hudecz D, Dawson KA. Designing the future of nanomedicine: current barriers to targeted brain therapeutics. Eur J Nanomed 2014;6(3):127–39.

[75] Duan MM, Xing YM, Guo JQ, Chen H, Zhang R. Borneol increases blood-tumour barrier permeability by regulating the expression levels of tight junction-associated proteins. Pharm Biol 2016;54(12):3009–18.

[76] Kaur IP, Bhandari R, Bhandari S, Kakkar V. Potential of solid lipid nanoparticles in brain targeting. J Control Release 2008;127(2):97–109.

[77] Patel RB, Patel MR, Bhatt KK, Patel BG, Gaikwad RV. Microemulsion-based drug delivery system for transnasal delivery of Carbamazepine: preliminary brain-targeting study. Drug Deliv 2016;23(1):207–13.

[78] Teixeira MI, Lopes CM, Amaral MH, Costa PC. Current insights on lipid nanocarrier-assisted drug delivery in the treatment of neurodegenerative diseases. Eur J Pharm Biopharm 2020;149:192–217.

[79] Pardridge WM. Re-engineering biopharmaceuticals for delivery to brain with molecular Trojan horses. Bioconjugate Chem 2008;19(7):1327–38.

[80] Pardridge WM. Drug targeting to the brain. Pharm Res 2007;24(9):1733–44.

[81] Lajoie JM, Shusta EV. Targeting receptor-mediated transport for delivery of biologics across the blood-brain barrier. Annu Rev Pharmacol 2015;55:613–31.

[82] Fonseca-Santos B, Gremiao MPD, Chorilli M. Nanotechnology-based drug delivery systems for the treatment of Alzheimer's disease. Int J Nanomed 2015;10:4981–5003.

[83] Gobbi M, Re F, Canovi M, Beeg M, Gregori M, Sesana S, Sonnino S, Brogioli D, Musicanti C, Gasco P, Salmona M, Masserini ME. Lipid-based nanoparticles with high binding affinity for amyloid-beta(1-42) peptide. Biomaterials 2010;31(25):6519–29.

[84] Topal GR, Meszaros M, Porkolab G, Szecsko A, Polgar TF, Siklos L, Deli MA, Veszelka S, Bozkir A. ApoE-targeting increases the transfer of solid lipid nanoparticles with donepezil cargo across a culture model of the blood-brain barrier. Pharmaceutics 2021;13(1).

[85] Kopparam M, Kulkarni SV, Shivu S. Development, characterization and in vitro evaluation of donepezil solid lipid nanoparticles. Res J Pharm Technol 2020;13(7):3113–21.

[86] Yasir M, Sara UVS, Chauhan I, Gaur PK, Singh AP, Puri D, Ameeduzzafar. Solid lipid nanoparticles for nose to brain delivery of donepezil: formulation, optimization by Box-Behnken design, in vitro and in vivo evaluation. Artif Cell Nanomed B 2018;46(8):1838–51.

[87] Neves AR, Queiroz JF, Lima SAC, Reis S. Apo E-functionalization of solid lipid nanoparticles enhances brain drug delivery: uptake mechanism and transport pathways. Bioconjugate Chem 2017;28(4):995–1004.

[88] Neves AR, Queiroz JF, Weksler B, Romero IA, Couraud PO, Reis S. Solid lipid nanoparticles as a vehicle for brain-targeted drug delivery: two new strategies of functionalization with apolipoprotein E. Nanotechnology 2015;26(49):1–11. 495103. doi:10.1088/0957-4484/26/49/495103.

[89] Mendes IT, Ruela ALM, Carvalho FC, Freitas JTJ, Bonfilio R, Pereira GR. Development and characterization of nanostructured lipid carrier-based gels for the transdermal delivery of donepezil. Colloid Surface B 2019;177:274–81.

[90] Chauhan MK, Sharma PK. Optimization and characterization of rivastigmine nanolipid carrier loaded transdermal patches for the treatment of dementia. Chem Phys Lipids 2019;224:1–10. 104794. doi:10.1016/j.chemphyslip.2019.104794.

[91] Anand A, Arya M, Kaithwas G, Singh G, Saraf SA. Sucrose stearate as a biosurfactant for development of rivastigmine containing nanostructured lipid carriers and assessment of its activity against dementia in C-elegans model. J Drug Deliv Sci Technol 2019;49:219–26.

[92] Shah B, Khunt D, Bhatt H, Misra M, Padh H. Application of quality by design approach for intranasal delivery of rivastigmine loaded solid lipid nanoparticles: effect on formulation and characterization parameters. Eur J Pharm Sci 2015;78:54–66.

[93] Silva S, Marto J, Goncalves L, Almeida AJ, Vale N. Formulation, characterization and evaluation against SH-SY5Y cells of new tacrine and tacrine-MAP loaded with lipid nanoparticles. Nanomater - Basel 2020;10(10):1–14. 2089. doi:10.3390/nano10102089.

[94] Misra S, Chopra K, Sinha VR, Medhi B. Galantamine-loaded solid-lipid nanoparticles for enhanced brain delivery: preparation, characterization, in vitro and in vivo evaluations. Drug Deliv 2016;23(4):1434–43.

[95] Laserra S, Basit A, Sozio P, Marinelli L, Fornasari E, Cacciatore I, Ciulla M, Turkez H, Geyikoglu F, Di Stefano A. Solid lipid nanoparticles loaded with lipoyl-memantine codrug: preparation and characterization. Int J Pharm 2015;485(1-2):183–91.

[96] Chen JY, Zhu Q, Zhang S, OuYang DF, Lu JH. Resveratrol in experimental Alzheimer's disease models: a systematic review of preclinical studies. Pharmacol Res 2019;150:1–9. 104476. doi:10.1016/j.phrs.2019.104476.

[97] Yadav A, Sunkaria A, Singhal N, Sandhir R. Resveratrol loaded solid lipid nanoparticles attenuate mitochondrial oxidative stress in vascular dementia by activating Nrf2/HO-1 pathway. Neurochem Int 2018;112:239–54.

[98] Neves AR, Queiroz JF, Reis S. Brain-targeted delivery of resveratrol using solid lipid nanoparticles functionalized with apolipoprotein E. J Nanobiotechnol 2016;14:27.

[99] Loureiro JA, Andrade S, Duarte A, Neves AR, Queiroz JF, Nunes C, Sevin E, Fenart L, Gosselet F, Coelho MA, Pereira MC. Resveratrol and grape extract-loaded solid lipid nanoparticles for the treatment of Alzheimer's disease. Molecules 2017;22(2).

[100] Vijayakumar MR, Kumari L, Patel KK, Vuddanda PR, Vajanthri KY, Mahto SK, Singh S. Intravenous administration of trans-resveratrol-loaded TPGS-coated solid lipid nanoparticles for prolonged systemic circulation, passive brain targeting and improved in vitro cytotoxicity against C6 glioma cell lines. Rsc Adv 2016;6(55):50336–48.

[101] Prathipati B, Rohini P, Kola PK, Danduga RCSR. Neuroprotective effects of curcumin loaded solid lipid nanoparticles on homocysteine induced oxidative stress in vascular dementia. Curr Res Behav Sci 2021;2:1–11. 100029. doi:10.1016/j.crbeha.2021.100029.

[102] Ban C, Jo M, Park YH, Kim JH, Han JY, Lee KW, Kweon DH, Choi YJ. Enhancing the oral bioavailability of curcumin using solid lipid nanoparticles. Food Chem 2020;302:125328.

[103] Kakkar V, Singh S, Singla D, Kaur IP. Exploring solid lipid nanoparticles to enhance the oral bioavailability of curcumin. Mol Nutr Food Res 2011;55(3):495–503.

[104] Kakkar V, Singh S, Singla D, Sahwney S, Chauhan AS, Singh G, Kaur IP. Pharmacokinetic applicability of a validated liquid chromatography tandem mass spectroscopy method for orally administered curcumin loaded solid lipid nanoparticles to rats. J Chromatogr B 2010;878(32):3427–31.

[105] Kakkar V, Kaur IP. Evaluating potential of curcumin loaded solid lipid nanoparticles in aluminium induced behavioural, biochemical and histopathological alterations in mice brain. Food Chem Toxicol 2011;49(11):2906–13.

[106] Kakkar V, Mishra AK, Chuttani K, Kaur IP. Proof of concept studies to confirm the delivery of curcumin loaded solid lipid nanoparticles (C-SLNs) to brain. Int J Pharm 2013;448(2):354–9.

[107] Malvajerd SS, Azadi A, Izadi Z, Kurd M, Dara T, Dibaei M, Zadeh MS, Javar HA, Hamidi M. Brain delivery of curcumin using solid lipid nanoparticles and nanostructured lipid carriers: preparation, optimization, and pharmacokinetic evaluation. Acs Chem Neurosci 2019;10(1):728–39.

[108] Kuo YC, Lou YI, Rajesh R, Chen CL. Multiple-component dual-phase solid lipid nanoparticles with conjugated transferrin for formulating antioxidants and nerve growth factor against neuronal apoptosis. J Taiwan Inst Chem E 2020;110:140–52.

[109] Sachdeva AK, Misra S, Kaur IP, Chopra K. Neuroprotective potential of sesamol and its loaded solid lipid nanoparticles in ICV-STZ-induced cognitive deficits: behavioral and biochemical evidence. Eur J Pharmacol 2015;747:132–40.

[110] Vedagiri A, Thangarajan S. Mitigating effect of chrysin loaded solid lipid nanoparticles against amyloid beta(25-35) induced oxidative stress in rat hippocampal region: an efficient formulation approach for Alzheimer's disease. Neuropeptides 2016;58:111–25.

[111] Chalikwar SS, Belgamwar VS, Talele VR, Surana SJ, Patil MU. Formulation and evaluation of nimodipine-loaded solid lipid nanoparticles delivered via lymphatic transport system. Colloid Surface B 2012;97:109–16.

[112] Almuhayawi MS, Ramadan WS, Harakeh S, Al Jaouni SK, Bharali DJ, Mousa SA, Almuhayawi SM. The potential role of pomegranate and its nano-formulations on cerebral neurons in aluminum chloride induced Alzheimer rat model. Saudi J Biol Sci 2020;27(7):1710–6.

[113] Dara T, Vatanara A, Sharifzadeh M, Khani S, Vakilinezhad MA, Vakhshiteh F, Meybodi MN, Malvajerd SS, Hassani S, Mosaddegh MH. Improvement of memory deficits in the rat model of Alzheimer's disease by erythropoietin-loaded solid lipid nanoparticles. Neurobiol Learn Mem 2019;166:1–13. 107082. doi:10.1016/j.nlm.2019.107082.

[114] Rishitha N, Muthuraman A. Therapeutic evaluation of solid lipid nanoparticle of cycloastragenol in streptozotocin induced vascular dementia in danio rerio. In: De Caridi G, editor. Abnormalities of Vascular System. Las Vegas, NV, USA Open Access eBooks; 2019. p. 1–19. https://openaccessebooks.com/vascular-system.html. [Accessed 19 July 2022].

[115] Vakilinezhad MA, Amini A, Javar HA, Zarandi BFBB, Montaseri H, Dinarvand R. Nicotinamide loaded functionalized solid lipid nanoparticles improves cognition in Alzheimer's disease animal model by reducing Tau hyperphosphorylation. Daru 2018;26(2):165–77.

[116] Dhawan S, Kapil R, Singh B. Formulation development and systematic optimization of solid lipid nanoparticles of quercetin for improved brain delivery. J Pharm Pharmacol 2011;63(3):342–51.

[117] Muntimadugu E, Dhommati R, Jain A, Gopala V, Challa S, Shaheen M, Khan W. Intranasal delivery of nanoparticle encapsulated tarenflurbil: a potential brain targeting strategy for Alzheimer's disease. Eur J Pharm Sci 2016;92:224–34.

[118] Patel PA, Patil SC, Kalaria DR, Kalia YN, Patravale VB. Comparative in vitro and in vivo evaluation of lipid based nanocarriers of Huperzine A. Int J Pharm 2013;446(1-2):16–23.

[119] Sathya S, Shanmuganathan B, Manirathinam G, Ruckmani K, Devi KP. Alpha-bisabolol loaded solid lipid nanoparticles attenuates a beta aggregation and protects Neuro-2a cells from a beta induced neurotoxicity. J Mol Liq 2018;264:431–41.

[120] Pinheiro RGR, Granja A, Loureiro JA, Pereira MC, Pinheiro M, Neves AR, Reis S. Quercetin lipid nanoparticles functionalized with transferrin for Alzheimer's disease. Eur J Pharm Sci 2020;148:1–11. 105314. doi:10.1016/j.ejps.2020.105314.

[121] Akel H, Ismail R, Csoka I. Progress and perspectives of brain-targeting lipid-based nanosystems via the nasal route in Alzheimer's disease. Eur J Pharm Biopharm 2020;148:38–53.

[122] Chen Y, Liu L. Modern methods for delivery of drugs across the blood–brain barrier. Adv Drug Deliv Rev 2012;7:640–65.

Chapter 7

Liposome: A potential drug delivery vector to treat dementia

Mukta Agrawal[a], Upal Roy[b], Amit Alexander[c]
[a]School of Pharmacy & Technology Management, SVKM's Narsee Monjee Institute of Management Studies (NMIMS), Hyderabad, India, [b]Department of Health and Biomedical Sciences, University of Texas Rio Grande Valley College of Health Affairs One West University Blvd. Brownsville, Texas, [c]Department of Pharmaceutics, National Institute of Pharmaceutical Education and Research (NIPER), Guwahati, Assam, India

Abbreviations

2-PAM	Pralidoxime chloride
AChE	Acetylcholinesterase
AChEI	Acetylcholinesterase inhibitor
AD	Alzheimer's disease
APP	Amyloid precursor protein
Aβ	Amyloid β peptide
BBB	Blood–brain barrier
BSA	Bovine serum albumin
CL	Cardiolipin
CPP	Cell penetrating peptide
DMPC	1,2-dimyristoyl-sn-glycero-3-phosphocholine
EYPC	Egg yolk phosphatidylcholine
FDA	Food and Drug Administration
FTD	Frontotemporal Dementia
GI	Gastrointestinal
hCMEC	Human brain capillary endothelial cells
hIGF	Human insulin-like growth factor
LBD	Lewy Body Dementia
LDLR	Low-density lipoprotein receptors
Lf	Lactoferrin
MAb	Monoclonal antibody
mApoE	Modified apolipoprotein E
MPS	Mononuclear phagocyte system

Nanomedicine-Based Approaches for the Treatment of Dementia. https://doi.org/10.1016/B978-0-12-824331-2.00010-8
Copyright © 2023 Elsevier Inc. All rights reserved.

NGF	Nerve growth factor
NLC	Nano lipid carrier
NMDA	N-methyl D-aspartate
PA	Phosphatidic acid
PD	Parkinson's Disease
PEG	Poly ethylene glycol
PLGA	Poly (lactic-co-glycolic acid)
PS1	Presenilin
RES	Reticuloendothelial system
RGV	Rabies virus glycoprotein
RMT	Receptor-mediated transcytosis
S14G-HN	S14G-humanin
SLN	Solid lipid nanoparticles
Tf	Transferrin
V24P	Scavenger peptide
VHH-pa2H	Anti-amyloid single domain antibody fragment
WGA	Wheat germ agglutinin
WHO	World Health Organization

7.1 Introduction

Dementia is an umbrella term that represents a group of physiological conditions associated with a decline of regular brain functions. It is manifested by cognitive impairment, loss of memory, learning, communication, and thinking abilities. The clinical symptoms include amnesia, difficulty in performing routine activities, poor judgment, loss of social skills, emotional control, behavioral changes, unawareness about time, places and persons, etc. As per WHO, dementia is not a single disease, it is a syndrome or group of symptoms that arises from varying disease conditions or injuries which have a significant impact on brain functions. Among such disease conditions, Alzheimer's disease (AD) is one of the most prominent reasons or type of dementia [1].

The statistics of WHO, Alzheimer's Association, and other regulatory bodies reported, in the present time, more than 50 million people throughout the world are suffering from dementia form which around 60%–70% of cases are caused due to AD. As per the current global scenario, increasing aged population, and increasing life expectancy, by the year 2050 the number will be supposed to boost up to 135 million dementia cases [1,2].

AD and other disease-associated dementia remain the greater challenge for the human health care system for decades. After all such advancements in the medical and healthcare sector, no satisfactory improvement was observed. All the available approaches barely improve the cognitive functions and initial symptoms of the disease at its early stages. There is no single therapy to treat the root cause and slow down the disease progression [3,4].

7.2 Types of dementia

7.2.1 Alzheimer's disease-associated dementia

Alzheimer-associated dementia is the most common type of dementia worldwide, accounting for around 60%–80 % of all cases. Although, AD is a type and most prominent cause of dementia. Particularly, both the terms can be differentiated as dementia is a group of symptoms that appears due to decline of brain functioning while AD is a specific disorder caused due to progressive degeneration of neurons [5]. As per the reports of the Alzheimer's Association and WHO, AD is considered the sixth leading cause of death in the United States but recent studies suggested it as the third possible cause of death in the older population, just after cardiac diseases and cancer [6]. The characteristic features of AD involve progressive and irreversible loss of thinking, memory, and cognitive functions of the brain. It affects an individual's abilities of reasoning, remembering, and performing routine activities. Dementia usually seems with the mild stages of AD which get worsen with disease progression to severe stages when the person gets completely dependent upon others [7,8]. AD is a multifactorial disorder caused due to a combination of physiological changes in the brain. Amyloid plaque formation and tau hyperphosphorylation are the hallmarks of AD. Also, cholinergic imbalance, mitochondrial dysfunction, NMDA excitotoxicity, oxidative stress, neuroinflammation, etc., are other associated factors. The exact cause of such abnormalities are not known but some hypothesis and studies suggested aging, genetic factors, environmental stimulus, trauma, any injury, or stress might be the reason [9,10]. Till date, only five drug molecules are approved by USFDA for AD therapy including galantamine, donepezil, rivastigmine, tacrine (discontinued) (AChE inhibitors), and memantine (NMDA antagonist). All the available drugs are symptomatic and not effective in severe stages of the disease [11]. Hence, studies are going on to find some promising therapies to treat the disease in a better way using various novel approaches.

7.2.2 Vascular dementia

It is considered the second most prominent type of dementia after AD caused due to reduced blood flow in different regions of the brain. The blockage or narrowing of the brain blood vessels may occur due to any injury, trauma, stress, or disease condition which affects the blood and oxygen supply. This inadequate blood and oxygen supply causes damage of nerve cells and significantly affects the cognitive, thinking, and memory functions of the brain [12]. Statistics suggested vascular dementia accounts for 20%–25% of all dementia cases with a higher risk for the aged population. Neuronal injury and vascular damage are the primary pathophysiological factors of vascular dementia which might be due to calcium overload of neurons, cerebral ischemia, oxidative, and glutamatergic stress [13]. Alongside, amyloid accumulation, tau hyperphosphorylation, immune dysfunction, neuroinflammation, cholinergic abnormalities, etc., act as contributing factors to worsen the disease [14]. The heterogenic nature of the disease makes its diagnosis complex although the neurocognitive tests and MRI scan gives some idea about dementia, stroke, and brain injury. To date, there is no approved therapy for vascular dementia by USFDA. The treatment only focused on minimizing the symptoms and reducing the risk of vascular damage, stroke, hypertension by healthy lifestyle habits [15].

7.2.3 Lewy body dementia

Lewy body dementia (LBD) embodies both dementias associated with Parkinson's disease and Lewy bodies. It is another prevalent type of dementia, contributed around 10% of clinical dementia cases [16–18]. Aggregation and accumulation of alpha-synuclein, a synaptic protein is a key factor responsible for LBD. The disease is clinically characterized by progressive impairment of motor and cognitive functions, associated with rapid eye movement sleep disorder, fluctuating cognition, and recurrent visual hallucination [19]. The association of both the disease terms together is not clear which makes the diagnosis challenging. The diagnosis depends upon the development of symptoms including motor symptoms in comparison to cognitive impairment [20]. In spite of the available clinical evidence of pathological resemblance, distinct genetic characteristics have been observed between Lewy body and PD-associated dementia. Clinical features of LBD align with both the neurodegenerative diseases AD and PD.

7.2.4 Frontotemporal dementia

Dementia caused by damage in the neurons of the frontal and temporal lobes of the brain is termed frontotemporal dementia (FTD). The nerve cell death in these regions results in shrinking or atrophy of the frontal and temporal lobes which gradually cause a decline of the functions regulated by these regions like behavior and thinking abilities [21]. After AD and Lewy bodies, FTD is considered as a third prime cause of dementia, contributes around 5%–15% of total cases. It is one of the major types of early onset dementia which is mostly observed in a population younger than 65 years of age (10% less than 45 years; 60% 45–64 years and 30% more than 64 years) [22,23]. The sign and symptoms involved the progressive decline of behavior, language, and executive functions. The closely related symptoms often mislead the FTD with AD or other psychiatric disorders and make its diagnosis more challenging [22,24]. Till date, the only approved drug for the treatment of FTD is riluzole [25]. Hence, all the current therapies are concerned for managing the symptoms of neuropsychiatric disorders by using off-label existing drug moieties. Such symptomatic treatment does not exert a potential effect on FTD therapy. The symptomatic therapy utilizes serotonin reuptake inhibitors [25,26], dopaminergic [27], antipsychotic [28], and other drugs in FTD therapy. On the other hand, anti-AD drugs like AChEI (acetylcholinesterase inhibitor) and NMDA antagonists exert no effect or sometimes negative effect on cognitive functions [29].

7.2.5 Mixed dementia

The condition, where the brain experiences two or more dementia simultaneously due to different causative factors is termed mixed dementia. Dementia caused by amyloid plaque and neurofibrillary tangle formation associated with AD and vascular changes due to cerebrovascular disease presents a typical clinical prototype of mixed dementia. The coexistence of AD with abnormal protein deposition due to Lewy body and PD dementia is another commonly seen mixed dementia. In some instances, a person might experience dementia due to collective impact of all three pathological conditions, AD, cerebrovascular disease, and LBD. The complex pathophysiology and multifactorial origin make the diagnosis and treatment highly challenging for the physician. The currently practiced medicines are insufficient and only slightly improves the symptoms at initial phases [30]. The researchers found that in older age brain, dementia is mostly mixed type with two or more pathologies. Among which AD is the most common pathological factor which rarely appears alone. The sign and symptoms of mixed dementia may vary person-to-person, depending upon the type and region of damage. Usually, the symptoms are similar to AD or other prevalent causes of dementia. Often the symptoms indicate the presence of any specific kind of dementia which complicates the diagnosis. Comprehensive studies and research are needed to enhance the understanding of the disease prognosis and the relation between cognitive brain functions and underlying abnormalities [31].

7.3 Need of novel drug carrier

Exponential growth in the number of dementia cases has been observed in the past few years which is supposed to enhance with higher frequency in coming years. While the available treatment options are very limited with moderate potency and high cost. The existence of blood–brain barrier (BBB), highly complex, and isolated anatomy of the brain is the major factor to reduce the therapeutic potency of the drug [32]. The available therapies exert symptomatic action and are found effective in minimizing the symptoms only. Alongside, the poor pharmacokinetic profile of the available and investigational drugs like poor drug absorption, solubility, biodistribution, higher clearance, and degradation, etc., is another critical factors to be considered [33]. Thus, a promising drug carrier is needed to target the drug to the brain by circumventing the BBB and to improve the pharmacokinetic properties and therapeutic efficacy of the drug moieties. Nanocarriers also protect the bioactives from the harsh physiological environment, rapid degradation, and hepatic metabolism [34]. With the objective to improve brain delivery, various nanoparticulate systems like polymeric nanoparticles (chitosan, PLGA, dendrimers, etc.), lipid nanoparticles (liposomes, nanoemulsion, SLN, NLC, etc.), and colloidal carriers, etc., have been developed and investigated. Among these, liposome is one of the most popular and highly explored nanocarriages to approach the brain [32]. Detailed application and potential of liposome as a drug delivery vector in the treatment of dementia is discussed in subsequent sections.

7.4 Liposome

Liposome is a lipid-based vesicular system consisting of aqueous core surrounded by a single or multiple phospholipid bilayer. From its discovery in 1965 by Alec D. Bengham, liposomes have become one of the most popular drug delivery vectors because of their lipophilic and highly biocompatible nature. The phospholipid bilayer mimics the cell membrane which eases the permeation of drug-loaded carriers across the biological barriers [35]. Structurally, liposomes are composed of natural lipids, fatty acids, and their derivatives which makes them highly biocompatible and biodegradable [36]. The phospholipid forms a spherical nanosized vesicle by self-assembly of its molecules as a bilayer structure enclosing an aqueous core. The amphiphilic molecules get arranges in a manner that the hydrophobic tails face each other and hydrophilic head toward the outer environment. Such arrangement allows the encapsulation/entrapment of both the lipophilic and hydrophilic moieties [37]. Owing to their natural origin, liposomes are weakly immunogenic, biologically inert, and exert minimum systemic toxicity. It also protects the drug from enzymatic degradation and harsh physiological environment. Alongside, minimum toxicity profile, higher permeability, higher solubility, and surface flexibility make it a potential nanovectors for brain targeting [38]. Although, poor stability, limited drug loading ability, and susceptibility to the reticuloendothelial system (RES) limit its applications.

These lipidic vesicles are usually classified on the basis of their size (small, medium, and large vesicles), structural composition (unilamellar, oligolamellar, and multilamellar vesicles), and method of preparation. The unilamellar vesicles have a size range from 50 to 250 nm and consist of a single phospholipid bilayer. These are generally preferred for the delivery of hydrophilic drugs because of their large aqueous core. On the other hand, the multilamellar vesicles fall in a higher size range (around 1–5 μm) due to the presence of multiple concentric phospholipid bilayers enclosing comparatively smaller aqueous core. These are used for lipophilic drug moieties, entrapped in the lipid bilayers [39].

The selection of an appropriate liposomal carrier system based on its composition, size, surface functionalization, and targeting strategy is a crucial factor to achieve desired goals of drug delivery. The chain length, head group, type of phospholipid used, and the ratio of different components greatly affects the drug loading, stability, safety, and efficacy of the system [40]. Thus, various modifications have been made to improve the targeting ability and overcome the limitations of liposomes like surface functionalization, PEGylation (stealth liposome).

7.4.1 Strategies of brain targeting

7.4.1.1 Stealth liposome (PEGylated liposomes)

Surface PEGylation is a unique strategy to improve the stability and circulation time of the liposome. PEG is a widely used steric stabilizer that can be anchored to the surface of liposomes via different methods like physical adsorption, cross-linking, covalent bonding, and PEG-lipid conjugation. PEGylation of the lipid vesicles offers a number of biological and technological advantages like prolonged circulation time, higher stability, and protects the nanocarrier from RES and MPS (mononuclear phagocyte system) uptake and thus, improves distribution to the desired tissue/organ. Surface PEGylation prevents the aggregation of vesicles due to attractive Van der Waals forces by strong interbilayer repulsion [39]. Although some studies and observations of the marketed PEGylated liposomal formulation (DOXIL, Doxorubicin loaded PEGylated liposome) indicated that PEGylation neither assure the complete inertness nor fully circumvent the uptake by MPS and RES. The characteristic features of the PEG-grafted liposome depend upon the properties of PEG derivatives used and the mode of PEGylation. It also increases the size and molecular weight of the liposome [41]. Ordonez-Gutierrez et al. have reported the application of stealth liposome as immunoliposome to treat AD with anti-Aβ monoclonal antibody. Stealth liposome was used due to its excellent stability and physicochemical properties. In the engineered PEGylated liposome, PEG also acts as a linker to bind the developed IgG antibody (STAB-MAb) with the liposome surface. The prepared immune PEG liposomes were evaluated for Aβ targeting potency and ability to suppress the uptake of Aβ by hCMEC (human brain capillary endothelial cells) and enhance the uptake by macrophage cell lines. It was observed that immune PEG liposome considerably diminishes the Aβ oligomer uptake by hCMEC/D3 cells by binding with the Aβ monomer and oligomer present in plasma. Together, the Aβ liposomal conjugate also dramatically promotes the Aβ uptake and clearance by macrophages. The study also demonstrated that free STAB-MAb has some salutary effects on the brain health of aged animals. The therapeutic efficacy of STAB-MAb might be due to the antibody translocation and peripheral effects which could be improved with higher doses and shorter injection frequency. Although, higher doses and increased frequency also triggered the immune reactions. The study suggested, combined administration of STAB-MAb and immune PEG liposome could be an efficient strategy for AD therapy while further investigations are needed to understand its effect on other factors of AD and brain physiology [42]. Another piece of work by Rotman et al. also reported the use of PEGylated liposome for brain delivery of anti-amyloid antibody fragment in the mouse model to treat AD. The PEGylated liposome was surface-functionalized with glutathione which assured brain targeting and delivery across the BBB. Two types of glutathione-modified PEGylated liposomes were synthesized using two different phospholipids DMPC (1,2-dimyristoyl-sn-glycero-3-phosphocholine), EYPC (egg yolk phosphatidylcholine) and encapsulated with VHH-pa2H (anti-amyloid single domain antibody fragment). To study the brain targeting efficiency and biodistribution of the developed liposome system, the VHH-pa2H antibody was tagged with a radioactive agent, indium-111. Further, the radiolabeled antibody-loaded liposomes were given to the APP_{swe}/PS1dE9 double transgenic mice through IV bolus injection. The study revealed that both the formulations considerably increased the brain uptake of encapsulated antibody fragments (VHH-pa2H) as compared to the free VHH-pa2H injection. PEGylated liposomes prepared with EYPC demonstrated higher encapsulation and significantly greater brain concentration of VHH-pa2H than DMPC-based PEGylated liposomes [43]. A recent study utilized PEGylated nanoliposome for brain targeting of rosemary extract to treat AD-associated dementia. The PEGylated nanoliposome prolonged the release of encapsulated bioactives that were found directly proportional to the amount of PEG on the liposome surface. PEGylation enhanced the stability of the formulation and also promoted bond formation with BSA (bovine serum albumin). The binding with the serum protein affected the size and physicochemical properties of the liposome and increased its circulation time which prolonged the drug release [44]. In the same sequence, Kong et al. developed and investigated the brain targeting efficiency of Transferrin (Tf) modified PEGylated liposome to deliver a neuroprotective agent osthole across BBB using APP/PS1 transgenic mice. The therapeutic efficiency of the osthole is hindered due to its poor solubility and permeability across BBB. In vitro cell line studies indicated that the Tf-PEG-liposome significantly enhanced uptake across in vitro BBB cell line models; APP-SH-SY5Y and hCMEC/D3 cells. The stealth liposome was also found safe and exerts protective effects on the brain cell lines. The developed nanocarrier increased the concentration of drugs in the brain region which might be due to prolonged circulation time of stealth lipid and targeting potency of Tf modification [45]. The available studies supported the hypothesis that PEGylated or stealth liposomes prolonged the circulation time in physiological fluid and offer an effective carrier system for brain targeting of bioactives.

7.4.1.2 Surface-modified liposome

Surface functionalization can add significant values to the liposome in terms of its physicochemical properties, stability, release behavior, and targeting efficiencies. The liposome surface has been modified with the number of biomolecules like different polymers, ligands, targeting agents antibodies, etc., to add desired features to this lipidic carrier system. For example, Tf [46–48], lactoferrin (Lf) [49], glutathione [43] modification facilitates brain targeting of liposome; PEG modification prolonged circulation time and protects the liposome from physiological degradation [45] while glyco-conjugation promote cell permeation by mimicking the biological membrane [48]. mApoE (apolipoprotein E) and phosphatidic acid (PA) modified bifuntionalized liposome (mApoE-PA-lip) were designed to deliver across BBB for the treatment of AD. In vivo studies confirmed the efficiency of mApoE-PA-lip to transport across the BBB and increased bioavailability of the encapsulated drug in the brain [50]. It considerably reduced the Aβ plaque and enhanced the memory function in the AD mouse model. mApo-PA-lip have a higher affinity to Aβ peptide and hence it effectively binds, inhibits the aggregation, and destabilize the already formed Aβ aggregates. At the same time, it did not have any inverse effect on the BBB integrity or associated cell lines like endothelial cells, neuroblastoma, etc. These might be the plausible mechanism responsible for memory improvements [51]. The surface-functionalized liposomes provided ease of internalization by in vitro BBB cell lines via receptor-mediated endocytosis [50]. Previously, Conti et al. demonstrated the Aβ binding affinity and sequestering ability of mApoE-PA-lip in biological fluids. The nanocarrier has a higher Aβ binding affinity and considerably sequesters the Aβ from the plasma or CSF obtained from the patients of AD or Down's syndrome which have higher Aβ content [52]. In another similar attempt, a multifunctional liposome was prepared by surface functionalization of liposome with Tf, mAb, and ApoE for enhanced brain targeting [53]. The multifunctional liposome remarkably inhibited the Aβ plaque formation in the hCMEC/D3 in vitro cell model due to Aβ inhibiting potency of ApoE peptide [54]. While Tf and mAb facilitated the BBB permeation. In vivo imaging after administration of different doses of the multifunctional liposome to APP/PS1 double transgenic mice and WT mice indicated a considerable difference in the brain DiR signals. The study showed the brain uptake is dose dependent and also affected by surface functionalization [53]. Interaction between multiple ligands can alter the functionalities of surface modifiers in the case of multifunctional nanocarriers. Multifunctionalization are usually preferred to accomplish multiple objectives like crossing the BBB, Aβ binding affinity to facilitate its degradation, targeting particular regions of brain or cell organelles, etc. Thus, it is essential to preserve the individual functionality of the ligands. The selection of ligand is a crucial step to avoid the possible interactions and to get desired functionalization [55]. Another interesting finding suggested that the multifunctional liposome are prone to be taken up by the spleen, liver, or other macrophage-rich organs and also reduce the stealth nature of the liposome. This behavior will ultimately reduce the brain concentration of the multifunctional liposomes as compared to single functionalized ones [56]. Although studies have proven that the presence of curcumin at the liposome surface suppresses the macrophages, alleviates their number, and minimizes the uptake by the liver and spleen [57] along with its therapeutic benefits [58].

7.4.1.3 Liposome for direct nose-to-brain drug delivery

The intranasal route of drug administration offers a direct, alternative, and attractive approach to reach the brain by evading the BBB and other limitations of oral and parenteral administration. Most of the experimental drugs intended for neurodegenerative disorder or dementia are of herbal origin, derivatives of natural compounds, protein, or peptides that belong to the category of BCS class II or IV. These drug moieties are highly susceptible to gastrointestinal (GI) degradation, undergo extensive hepatic metabolism, rapid clearance, and experience bioavailability issues due to poor volume of distribution and the presence of various physiological barriers like BBB. Poor bioavailability and therapeutic efficacy call for a higher dose and increased dosing frequencies which seem to be inconvenient for dementia patients. Besides the parenteral route is painful, uncomfortable, and needs expert assistance for dose administration. It was found suitable for hospitalized patients and for conditions where immediate actions are desired [59]. In this context, the nose-to-brain delivery route overcomes such limitations and considerably increases drug bioavailability to the brain region. The nasal cavity is directly connected to the brain via olfactory and trigeminal neurons. The olfactory mucosa of the nasal cavity is enriched with olfactory sensory nerve endings which assist the sense of olfaction while the respiratory region is supplied with trigeminal neurons [7]. The drug administered through the intranasal route directly enters the olfactory bulb and other regions of the brain via cellular transport through olfactory and trigeminal nerve channels. Nowadays, this route has become popular among researchers and scientists exploring the treatment of neurological disorders owing to various advantages including sidestep BBB, protection of the drug from first-pass metabolism, enzymatic degradation, etc., as mentioned above. Despite this, the intranasal route also has some limitations like mucociliary clearance, poor retention time, and enzymatic degradation [51]. Various novel approaches like permeation enhancers to enhance nasomucosal permeation [60], mucoadhesive system to improve nasal retention time [61], and novel drug carrier systems or nanoparticulate systems are used to improve the associated limitations of the intranasal route [62,63]. The lipidic nature of liposomes makes them suitable drug carriers for intranasal administration. The natural lipid base is highly compatible, nonirritating to the nasal mucosa, promotes nasomucosal permeation, and also protects the therapeutic moiety from enzymatic degradation [32]. Li et al. developed a flexible liposome for direct nose-to-brain delivery of galantamine [64]. It is a well-known, USFDA-approved drug for the treatment of AD-associated dementia which exerts symptomatic effects. It is a reversible AChE inhibitor that potentially improves memory function and is also found to minimize the Aβ aggregation and toxicity in the brain [65]. Although, the oral and parenteral administration limits its bioavailability in the brain, thus hinders therapeutic efficiency, and is also associated with severe GI and systemic side effects [66]. Flexible liposomes are advantageous over conventional liposomes in terms of higher elasticity and better cellular permeability due to their fluidic membranes [67]. The composition involves the use of an edge activator along with the phospholipid and water contents which contributes to the flexibility and fluidity of the phospholipid membrane. The intranasal administration of galantamine-loaded flexible liposome demonstrated greater AChE inhibition and considerably higher pharmacokinetic profile in the brain region in contrast to the oral administration. The flexible liposomes did not exert any toxic effects on the PC-12 cell line and also possess minimum cytotoxicity [64].

Another successful attempt was made for the nose-to-brain delivery of cell penetrating peptide (CPP) modified rivastigmine-loaded liposomes to treat AD by Zhen-Yang et al. Akin to galantamine, rivastigmine is also an approved AChE inhibitor marketed as an oral tablet or capsule for AD therapy. The drug is highly susceptible to GI environment, enzymatic degradation, hepatic metabolism, rapid clearance, and exerts GI irritation and adverse effects. The brain bioavailability and therapeutic efficacy are also hindered after oral administration due to the aforementioned factors [68]. Intranasal administration of rivastigmine-loaded liposomes substantially increased the concentration and distribution in different brain regions including the cortex and hippocampus (highly affected areas of the brain in AD). An obvious evasion of GI degradation, irritation, and systemic toxicity was noted with the intranasal administration as it sidesteps the GI exposure of the drug. Surface modification with CPP greatly enhanced the cellular permeation and transport through the olfactory mucosal pathway [69]. Narayan et al. reported the use of intranasal PEGylated liposomes for brain targeting of risperidone to treat schizophrenia. The PEGylated liposome administered through the intranasal route demonstrated higher nasomucosal uptake and enhanced drug concentration in the brain region than plasma [70]. Further, Upadhyay et al. have also utilized the intranasal liposomes for effective brain delivery of an antischizophrenic drug, quetiapine fumarate. The drug is highly lipophilic and suffers from poor bioavailability issues in the brain. The ex vivo diffusion studies through sheep nasal mucosa showed that the liposome notably increased drug diffusion with a higher rate of diffusion. It was also found to exert no or minimum possible irritation/toxicity to the nasal mucosa [71]. Such findings are in line with the hypothesis that liposome presents a highly compatible and minimally toxic lipid-based nanocarrier system for intranasal administration of any therapeutic moiety to the brain.

Another interesting piece of work highlighted the design and brain targeting efficiency of a mixed cationic liposome for intranasal delivery of 2-PAM (pralidoxime chloride, a cholinesterase reactivator). 2-PAM is used to treat acute poisoning or brain damage due to chemical or organophosphorus agents exposure which particularly affects AChE [72]. The positive surface charge on the cationic liposome facilitates cellular uptake, nasal permeation, and brain targeting owing to its higher affinity to negatively charged nasal mucosa and epithelial cells [73,74]. 2-PAM loaded cationic liposomes considerably increased the nasal permeation, brain concentration of bioactive, and hence higher therapeutic efficacy [72]. All these studies are clearly in agreement with our initial proposition that intranasal liposomes offer great advantages of brain targeting over oral and parenteral routes.

7.4.2 In-line research: liposome-based therapies

7.4.2.1 Protein and peptide delivery

Protein and peptide-based therapeutics like nerve growth factor (NGF), brain fibroblast growth factors, human insulin-like growth factor, neuroprotective protein, erythropoietin, V24P (scavenger peptide), S14G-HN (S14G-humanin), H102 peptide, etc., found prevalent application in the treatment of dementia [62]. Although their large molecular size, lipophilic nature, and stability issues create hurdles in brain delivery of protein and peptide-based therapies and thus, these are given through the parenteral route in the conventional system. Among various novel drug carriers, liposomes emerged as a promising carrier for protein and peptide delivery owing to their lipidic nature and ability to carry larger lipophilic compounds. The larger molecules of protein/peptide can be easily intercalated into the phospholipid bilayer of multilamellar vesicles [75]. Kuo et al. reported the use of RMP-7 (cereport) and Tf modified liposome for brain targeting of NGF. The preclinical investigations on human astrocyte regulated HBMECs and Aβ-insulted SK-N-MC cells demonstrated significantly higher permeability and neuroprotective effects [76]. As an expansion of work, the same group of authors studied the brain targeting efficiency of wheat germ agglutinin and CL (cardiolipin) conjugated liposome for dual delivery of NGF and curcumin. The studies demonstrated higher BBB permeability and better neuroprotective effects of NGF [77]. In another piece of work, Bana et al. investigated the effects of mApoE and PA conjugated liposome against Aβ aggregation. It was found that mApoE and PA conjugated liposome efficiently crossed the BBB and caused Aβ disaggregation [51]. All the studies proved liposomes as a potential candidate for brain delivery of protein and peptides.

7.4.2.2 Gene delivery

In the past few years, gene therapy appears as a promising approach to repair and treat genetic hallmarks associated with AD. Usually, gene therapy is referred to as a process to repair abnormal genes by replacing them with the normal gene in the genome [78]. Although the success of gene therapy greatly relies on the efficacy and potency of a suitable vector system. The selection of a potential vector is highly desirable to overcome the limitations associated with gene therapy like specific targeting to the desired site, improving its half-life, membrane permeability, protection from physiological environment, and enhancing the stability of the therapeutic gene [79]. The ultimate goal is to deliver the gene fragment/therapeutic gene to the nucleus so that the therapeutic protein could be synthesized by transcription or translation. Thus, the vector with an ability to deliver the gene across various extracellular and intracellular barriers is highly desirable for gene therapy [80]. The presence of various barrier functions like BBB, BCSFB, etc., lends more challenges to gene therapy for AD. In this context, novel, nonviral vectors like liposomes gain much attention over viral vectors in terms of easy preparation techniques, safety profile, lower immunogenicity, reduced cost, and compatibility with a broad range of plasmid size [81]. Dos Santos Rodrigues et al. developed a dual functionalized liposome, modified with transferrin, and penetratin as a vector for gene (β-galactosidase) delivery across the BBB [82]. Transferrin promoted the transport of the gene-carrier system across BBB via receptor-mediated transcytosis (RMT). RMT is usually a saturable process that is why the dual-targeting strategy was adopted to overcome the saturation of transferrin receptors [83]. The second surface modifier, penetratin facilitates cellular transport through the protein transduction domain [84]. The dual targeting strategy provided a higher degree of cell uptake, internalization, and effective targeting to the desired site. The effective neural transfection was studied on a triple cell coculture BBB model. In vivo investigation of β-galactosidase expression indicated the dual-targeted liposome significantly enhanced brain accumulation of the gene-loaded cargo and induced gene expression [85]. In all, higher neuronal transfection and enhanced transport across BBB presented the multifunctional liposome as a potential vector for gene delivery.

In another similar piece of work, the same group of authors reported brain targeting of a different gene ApoE2 via penetratin and transferrin conjugated PEGylated liposomes to treat AD [85]. ApoE2 exerts a neuroprotective effect by regulating the clearance of Aβ through microglia, neurons, or BBB. Alongside, greater affinity to Aβ, lower affinity toward LDLR (low-density lipoprotein receptors), and greater conformational stability present ApoE2 as a potential candidate to exert a disease-modifying effect as compared to the E3 and E4 isoforms [86]. The liposomal vector significantly targeted encapsulated ApoE2 and enhanced its bioavailability in the brain [85]. In the same sequence, pApoE2 (ApoE2 encoding plasmid DNA) is delivered to the brain through mannose and CPP including RGV (rabies virus glycoprotein) and penetratin conjugated liposome. Mannose is a GLUT-1 substrate that facilitates brain targeting via carrier-mediated transcytosis through GLUT-1 transporter protein [87,88]. On the other hand, CPP promoted translocation of the developed system across BBB through direct transport (penetratin) and ACh (acetylcholine) receptor-mediated transcytosis (RGV) [89]. The target-modified liposome demonstrated considerably higher gene transfection in the mice brain without any sign of adverse effect or toxicity [90].

7.5 Conclusion

Treatment of neurological disorders always being a very challenging and critical area of research due to the complex anatomy of the brain and physiological barriers. Phospholipid bilayer of liposome enables its transport across BBB and makes it highly biocompatible as compared to various polymeric and inorganic nanoparticles. Its amphiphilic nature resulted from the unique structural composition including phospholipid bilayer and aqueous core allows the encapsulation/entrapment of a wide variety of therapeutics such as hydrophilic drugs, lipophilic moieties, and large molecules like protein, peptide, etc. Alongside, higher surface flexibility and modification with target-acting ligands facilitate drug targeting to the desired site of action and enhance the bioavailability, thus overall therapeutic efficacy. Various studies have proven liposomes exert minimum toxicities and compatibility issues. Owing to such advantages, it has been widely explored for the delivery of therapeutics to treat AD and other kinds of dementia. These are also found useful in gene, protein, and peptide delivery to inhibit pathophysiological hallmarks of the disease like Aβ aggregation, tau hyperphosphorylation, etc., and improve nerve functioning. In all, we can say that liposome offers a great advantage as a novel drug carrier system for brain targeting to treat dementia and other associated disorders. Although, more scientific efforts are needed to establish a promising strategy after exhaustive clinical investigations.

Acknowledgment

The author wants to acknowledge National Institute of Pharmaceutical Education and Research, Guwahati, India, and College of Health Professions at University of Texas Rio Grande Valley, Texas, USA, to provide necessary support.

Funding

NIH/NINDS (R15NS108815) and NIH/NIAID (R01AI147731).

Conflict of Interest

None.

References

[1] WHO. Dementia. World Health Organization; 2021. https://www.who.int/news-room/fact-sheets/detail/dementia#:~:text=In%20July%202021%2C%20WHO%20released,their%20carers%20can%20meaningfully%20participate. (Accessed on 11.12.21).

[2] Cummings J, Aisen PS, DuBois B, Frölich L, Jack Jr CR, Jones RW, et al. Drug development in Alzheimer's disease: the path to 2025. Alzheimer's Res Therapy 2016;8:39.

[3] Agatonovic-Kustrin S, Kettle C, Morton DW. A molecular approach in drug development for Alzheimer's disease. Biomed Pharmacother 2018;106:553–65.

[4] Mauricio R, Benn C, Davis J, Dawson G, Dawson LA, Evans A, et al. Tackling gaps in developing life-changing treatments for dementiaAlzheimer's & Dementia (New York, NY)5; 2019:241–53.

[5] Alzheimer's Association Dementia vs. Alzheimer's disease: what is the difference? Alzheimer's Association, Chicago; 2021. alz.org/alzheimers-dementia/difference-between-dementia-and-alzheimer-s.

[6] NIA. Alzheimer's disease fact sheet. National Institute on Aging by NIH; 2021. https://www.nia.nih.gov/health/alzheimers-disease-fact-sheet. (Accessed 21 December 2021).
[7] Alexander A, Saraf S. Nose-to-brain drug delivery approach: a key to easily accessing the brain for the treatment of Alzheimer's disease. Neural Regeneration Res 2018;13(12):2102–4.
[8] Agrawal M, Prathyusha E, Ahmed H, Dubey SK, Kesharwani P, Singhvi G, et al. Biomaterials in treatment of Alzheimer's disease. Neurochem Int 2021;145:105008.
[9] Agrawal M, Saraf S, Saraf S, Antimisiaris SG, Hamano N, Li SD, et al. Recent advancements in the field of nanotechnology for the delivery of anti-Alzheimer drug in the brain region. Expert Opinion Drug Del 2018;15(6):589–617.
[10] Dubey SK, Ram MS, Krishna KV, Saha RN, Singhvi G, Agrawal M, et al. Recent expansions on cellular models to uncover the scientific barriers towards drug development for alzheimer's disease. Cell Mol Neurobiol 2019;39(2):181–209.
[11] Alexander A, Agrawal M, Uddin A, Siddique S, Shehata AM, Shaker MA, et al. Recent expansions of novel strategies towards the drug targeting into the brain. Int J Nanomed 2019;14:5895–909.
[12] Bir SC, Khan MW, Javalkar V, Toledo EG, Kelley RE. Emerging concepts in vascular dementia: a review. J Stroke Cerebrovascular Diseases 2021;30(8):105864.
[13] Kalaria RN. The pathology and pathophysiology of vascular dementia. Neuropharmacology 2018;134(Pt B):226–39.
[14] Sinha K, Sun C, Kamari R, Bettermann K. Current status and future prospects of pathophysiology-based neuroprotective drugs for the treatment of vascular dementia. Drug Discovery Today 2020;25(4):793–9.
[15] Tariq S, Barber PA. Dementia risk and prevention by targeting modifiable vascular risk factors. J Neurochem 2018;144(5):565–81.
[16] Chouliaras L, Kumar GS, Thomas AJ, Lunnon K, Chinnery PF, O'Brien JT. Epigenetic regulation in the pathophysiology of lewy body dementia. Prog Neurobiol 2020;192:101822.
[17] Taylor JP, McKeith IG, Burn DJ, Boeve BF, Weintraub D, Bamford C, et al. New evidence on the management of lewy body dementia. Lancet Neurol 2020;19(2):157–69.
[18] Kane JPM, Surendranathan A, Bentley A, Barker SAH, Taylor JP, Thomas AJ, et al. Clinical prevalence of lewy body dementia. Alzheimer's Res Therapy 2018;10(1):19.
[19] McKeith IG, Boeve BF, Dickson DW, Halliday G, Taylor JP, Weintraub D, et al. Diagnosis and management of dementia with lewy bodies: fourth consensus report of the dlb consortium. Neurology 2017;89(1):88–100.
[20] Chin KS, Yassi N, Churilov L, Masters CL, Watson R. Prevalence and clinical associations of tau in lewy body dementias: a systematic review and meta-analysis. Parkinsonism Relat Disord 2020;80:184–93.
[21] Benussi L, Ciani M, Tonoli E, Morbin M, Palamara L, Albani D, et al. Loss of exosomes in progranulin-associated frontotemporal dementia. Neurobiol Aging 2016;40:41–9.
[22] Young JJ, Lavakumar M, Tampi D, Balachandran S, Tampi RR. Frontotemporal dementia: latest evidence and clinical implications. Therapeutic Adv Psychopharmacol 2018;8(1):33–48.
[23] Olney NT, Spina S, Miller BL. Frontotemporal dementia. Neurologic Clinics 2017; 35(2):339–74.
[24] Bang J, Spina S, Miller BL. Frontotemporal dementiaLancet (London)386; 2015:1672–82.
[25] Panza F, Lozupone M, Seripa D, Daniele A, Watling M, Giannelli G, et al. Development of disease-modifying drugs for frontotemporal dementia spectrum disorders. Nat Rev Neurol 2020;16(4):213–28.

[26] Lozupone M, La Montagna M, D'Urso F, Piccininni C, Sardone R, Dibello V, et al. Pharmacotherapy for the treatment of depression in patients with Alzheimer's disease: a treatment-resistant depressive disorder. Expert Opin Pharmacother 2018;19(8):823–42.

[27] Huey ED, Garcia C, Wassermann EM, Tierney MC, Grafman J. Stimulant treatment of frontotemporal dementia in 8 patients. J Clin Psychiatry 2008;69(12):1981–2.

[28] Panza F, Solfrizzi V, Seripa D, Imbimbo BP, Santamato A, Lozupone M, et al. Progresses in treating agitation: a major clinical challenge in Alzheimer's disease. Expert Opin Pharmacother 2015;16(17):2581–8.

[29] Moretti R, Torre P, Antonello RM, Cattaruzza T, Cazzato G, Bava A. Rivastigmine in frontotemporal dementia: an open-label study. Drugs Aging 2004;21(14):931–7.

[30] Custodio N, Montesinos R, Lira D, Herrera-Pérez E, Bardales Y, Valeriano-Lorenzo L. Mixed dementia: a review of the evidence. Dementia Neuropsychologia 2017;11(4):364–70.

[31] Fierini F. Mixed dementia: neglected clinical entity or nosographic artifice? J Neurol Sci 2020;410:116662.

[32] Agrawal M, Ajazuddin TDK, Saraf S, Saraf S, Antimisiaris SG, et al. Recent advancements in liposomes targeting strategies to cross blood-brain barrier (BBB) for the treatment of Alzheimer's disease. J Controlled Release 2017;260:61–77.

[33] Rip J. Liposome technologies and drug delivery to the CNS. Drug Discovery Today Technologies 2016;20:53–8.

[34] Saraf S, Gupta A, Alexander A, Khan J, Jangde M, Saraf S. Advancements and avenues in nanophytomedicines for better pharmacological responses. J Nanosci Nanotechnol 2015;15(6):4070–9.

[35] Large DE, Abdelmessih RG, Fink EA, Auguste DT. Liposome composition in drug delivery design, synthesis, characterization, and clinical application. Adv Drug Deliv Rev 2021;176:113851.

[36] Alavi M, Karimi N, Safaei M. Application of various types of liposomes in drug delivery systems. Adv Pharmaceutical Bull 2017;7(1):3–9.

[37] Has C, Sunthar P. A comprehensive review on recent preparation techniques of liposomes. J Liposome Res 2020;30(4):336–65.

[38] Antimisiaris SG, Marazioti A, Kannavou M, Natsaridis E, Gkartziou F, Kogkos G, et al. Overcoming barriers by local drug delivery with liposomes. Adv Drug Deliv Rev 2021;174:53–86.

[39] Immordino ML, Dosio F, Cattel L. Stealth liposomes: review of the basic science, rationale, and clinical applications, existing and potential. Int J Nanomed 2006;1(3):297–315.

[40] Guimarães D, Cavaco-Paulo A, Nogueira E. Design of liposomes as drug delivery system for therapeutic applications. Int J Pharm 2021;601:120571.

[41] Immordino ML, Brusa P, Arpicco S, Stella B, Dosio F, Cattel L. Preparation, characterization, cytotoxicity and pharmacokinetics of liposomes containing docetaxel. J Controlled Release 2003;91(3):417–29.

[42] Ordóñez-Gutiérrez L, Posado-Fernández A, Ahmadvand D, Lettiero B, Wu L, Antón M, et al. ImmunoPEGliposome-mediated reduction of blood and brain amyloid levels in a mouse model of alzheimer's disease is restricted to aged animals. Biomaterials 2017;112:141–52.

[43] Rotman M, Welling MM, Bunschoten A, de Backer ME, Rip J, Nabuurs RJ, et al. Enhanced glutathione PEGylated liposomal brain delivery of an anti-amyloid single domain antibody fragment in a mouse model for Alzheimer's disease. J Controlled Release 2015;203:40–50.

[44] Shalabalija D, Mihailova L, Crcarevska MS, Karanfilova IC, Ivanovski V, Nestorovska AK, et al. Formulation and optimization of bioinspired rosemary extract loaded PEGylated nanoliposomes for potential treatment of Alzheimer's disease using design of experiments. J Drug Delivery Sci Technol 2021;63:102434.

[45] Kong L, Li XT, Ni YN, Xiao HH, Yao YJ, Wang YY, et al. Transferrin-modified osthole PEGylated liposomes travel the blood-brain barrier and mitigate alzheimer's disease-related pathology in APP/PS-1 mice. Int J Nanomed 2020;15:2841–58.
[46] Johnsen KB, Moos T. Revisiting nanoparticle technology for blood-brain barrier transport: unfolding at the endothelial gate improves the fate of transferrin receptor-targeted liposomes. J Controlled Release 2016;222:32–46.
[47] Olsman M, Sereti V, Mühlenpfordt M, Johnsen KB, Andresen TL, Urquhart AJ, et al. Focused ultrasound and microbubble treatment increases delivery of transferrin receptor-targeting liposomes to the brain. Ultrasound Med Biol 2021;47(5):1343–55.
[48] Chen ZL, Huang M, Wang XR, Fu J, Han M, Shen YQ, et al. Transferrin-modified liposome promotes α-mangostin to penetrate the blood-brain barrier. Nanomed: Nanotechnol, Biol, Med 2016;12(2):421–30.
[49] De Luca MA, Lai F, Corrias F, Caboni P, Bimpisidis Z, Maccioni E, et al. Lactoferrin- and antitransferrin-modified liposomes for brain targeting of the NK3 receptor agonist senktide: preparation and in vivo evaluation. Int J Pharm 2015;479(1):129–37.
[50] Binda A, Panariti A, Barbuti A, Murano C, Dal Magro R, Masserini M, et al. Modulation of the intrinsic neuronal excitability by multifunctional liposomes tailored for the treatment of Alzheimer's disease. Int J Nanomed 2018;13:4059–71.
[51] Bana L, Minniti S, Salvati E, Sesana S, Zambelli V, Cagnotto A, et al. Liposomes bi-functionalized with phosphatidic acid and an apoe-derived peptide affect aβ aggregation features and cross the blood-brain-barrier: implications for therapy of Alzheimer disease. Nanomed: Nanotechnol, Biol, Med 2014;10(7):1583–90.
[52] Conti E, Gregori M, Radice I, Da Re F, Grana D, Re F, et al. Multifunctional liposomes interact with abeta in human biological fluids: therapeutic implications for alzheimer's disease. Neurochem Int 2017;108:60–5.
[53] Papadia K, Giannou AD, Markoutsa E, Bigot C, Vanhoute G, Mourtas S, et al. Multifunctional LUV liposomes decorated for BBB and amyloid targeting - B. in vivo brain targeting potential in wild-type and APP/PS1 mice. Eur J Pharm Sci 2017;102:180–7.
[54] Kim J, Basak JM, Holtzman DM. The role of apolipoprotein e in Alzheimer's disease. Neuron 2009;63(3):287–303.
[55] Papadia K, Markoutsa E, Mourtas S, Giannou AD, La Ferla B, Nicotra F, et al. Multifunctional LUV liposomes decorated for BBB and amyloid targeting. A. in vitro proof-of-concept. Eur J Pharm Sci 2017;101:140–8.
[56] Lombard M, Naoumov NV, Bomford A, Williams R, Hynes M, Dervan P, et al. Optimizing the immunohistochemical signal from the transferrin receptor in liver tissue. Histochem J 1989;21(4):223–7.
[57] Amano C, Minematsu H, Fujita K, Iwashita S, Adachi M, Igarashi K, et al. Nanoparticles containing curcumin useful for suppressing macrophages in vivo in mice. PLoS One 2015;10(9):e0137207.
[58] Mahmud M, Piwoni A, Filipczak N, Janicka M, Gubernator J. Long-Circulating curcumin-loaded liposome formulations with high incorporation efficiency, stability and anticancer activity towards pancreatic adenocarcinoma cell lines in vitro. PLoS One 2016;11(12):e0167787.
[59] Doody RS, Raman R, Farlow M, Iwatsubo T, Vellas B, Joffe S, et al. A phase 3 trial of semagacestat for treatment of Alzheimer's disease. N Engl J Med 2013;369(4):341–50.
[60] Wu Y, Yang W, Wang C, Hu J, Fu S. Chitosan nanoparticles as a novel delivery system for ammonium glycyrrhizinate. Int J Pharm 2005;295(1-2):235–45.
[61] Wilson B, Samanta MK, Santhi K, Kumar KP, Ramasamy M, Suresh B. Chitosan nanoparticles as a new delivery system for the anti-Alzheimer drug tacrine. Nanomed: Nanotechnol, Biol, Med 2010;6(1):144–52.

[62] Agrawal M, Saraf S, Saraf S, Antimisiaris SG, Chougule MB, Shoyele SA, et al. Nose-to-brain drug delivery: an update on clinical challenges and progress towards approval of anti-Alzheimer drugs. J Controlled Release 2018;281:139–77.
[63] Lockman PR, Mumper RJ, Khan MA, Allen DD. Nanoparticle technology for drug delivery across the blood-brain barrier. Drug Dev Ind Pharm 2002;28(1):1–13.
[64] Li W, Zhou Y, Zhao N, Hao B, Wang X, Kong P. Pharmacokinetic behavior and efficiency of acetylcholinesterase inhibition in rat brain after intranasal administration of galanthamine hydrobromide loaded flexible liposomes. Environ Toxicol Pharmacol 2012;34(2):272–9.
[65] Matharu B, Gibson G, Parsons R, Huckerby TN, Moore SA, Cooper LJ, et al. Galantamine inhibits beta-amyloid aggregation and cytotoxicity. J Neurol Sci 2009;280(1-2):49–58.
[66] Scharre DW, Shiovitz T, Zhu Y, Amatniek J. One-week dose titration of extended release galantamine in patients with Alzheimer's disease. Alzheimer's Dementia 2008;4(1):30–7.
[67] Elsayed MM, Abdallah OY, Naggar VF, Khalafallah NM. Deformable liposomes and ethosomes: mechanism of enhanced skin delivery. Int J Pharm 2006;322(1-2):60–6.
[68] Venkatesh K, Bullock R, Akbaş A. Strategies to improve tolerability of rivastigmine: a case series. Curr Med Res Opin 2007;23(1):93–5.
[69] Yang ZZ, Zhang YQ, Wang ZZ, Wu K, Lou JN, Qi XR. Enhanced brain distribution and pharmacodynamics of rivastigmine by liposomes following intranasal administration. Int J Pharm 2013;452(1-2):344–54.
[70] Narayan R, Singh M, Ranjan O, Nayak Y, Garg S, Shavi GV, et al. Development of risperidone liposomes for brain targeting through intranasal route. Life Sci 2016;163:38–45.
[71] Upadhyay P, Trivedi J, Pundarikakshudu K, Sheth N. Direct and enhanced delivery of nanoliposomes of anti schizophrenic agent to the brain through nasal route. Saudi Pharmaceutical J 2017;25(3):346–58.
[72] Pashirova TN, Zueva IV, Petrov KA, Lukashenko SS, Nizameev IR, Kulik NV, et al. Mixed cationic liposomes for brain delivery of drugs by the intranasal route: the acetylcholinesterase reactivator 2-PAM as encapsulated drug model. Colloids Surfaces B, Biointerfaces 2018;171:358–67.
[73] Ingvarsson PT, Rasmussen IS, Viaene M, Irlik PJ, Nielsen HM, Foged C. The surface charge of liposomal adjuvants is decisive for their interactions with the calu-3 and A549 airway epithelial cell culture models. Eur J Pharmaceutics Biopharmaceutics 2014;87(3):480–8.
[74] Bonaccorso A, Musumeci T, Serapide MF, Pellitteri R, Uchegbu IF, Puglisi G. Nose to brain delivery in rats: effect of surface charge of rhodamine B labeled nanocarriers on brain subregion localization. Colloids Surfaces B, Biointerfaces 2017;154:297–306.
[75] Jash A, Ubeyitogullari A, Rizvi SSH. Liposomes for oral delivery of protein and peptide-based therapeutics: challenges, formulation strategies, and advances. J Materials Chem B 2021;9(24):4773–92.
[76] Kuo YC, Chou PR. Neuroprotection against degeneration of sk-N-mc cells using neuron growth factor-encapsulated liposomes with surface cereport and transferrin. J Pharm Sci 2014;103(8):2484–97.
[77] Kuo YC, Lin CY, Li JS, Lou YI. Wheat germ agglutinin-conjugated liposomes incorporated with cardiolipin to improve neuronal survival in Alzheimer's disease treatment. Int J Nanomed 2017;12:1757–74.
[78] Gonçalves GAR, Paiva RMA. Gene therapy: advances, challenges and perspectives. Einstein (Sao Paulo, Brazil) 2017;15(3):369–75.
[79] Naldini L. Gene therapy returns to centre stage. Nature 2015;526(7573):351–60.
[80] Yin H, Kanasty RL, Eltoukhy AA, Vegas AJ, Dorkin JR, Anderson DG. Non-viral vectors for gene-based therapy. Nat Rev Genet 2014;15(8):541–55.

[81] Tapeinos C, Battaglini M, Ciofani G. Advances in the design of solid lipid nanoparticles and nanostructured lipid carriers for targeting brain diseases. J Controlled Release 2017;264:306–32.
[82] Dos Santos Rodrigues B, Oue H, Banerjee A, Kanekiyo T, Singh J. Dual functionalized liposome-mediated gene delivery across triple co-culture blood brain barrier model and specific in vivo neuronal transfection. J Controlled Release 2018;286:264–78.
[83] Srinivasarao M, Low PS. Ligand-targeted drug delivery. Chem Rev 2017;117(19):12133–64.
[84] Bashyal S, Noh G, Keum T, Choi YW, Lee S. Cell penetrating peptides as an innovative approach for drug delivery; then, present and the future. J Pharmaceutical Investigation 2016;46(3):205–20.
[85] Dos Santos Rodrigues B, Kanekiyo T, Singh J. ApoE-2 brain-targeted gene therapy through transferrin and penetratin tagged liposomal nanoparticles. Pharm Res 2019;36(11):161.
[86] Huang YA, Zhou B, Wernig M, Südhof TC. ApoE2, apoe3, and apoe4 differentially stimulate app transcription and aβ secretion. Cell 2017;168(3):427–41e21.
[87] Umezawa F, Eto Y. Liposome targeting to mouse brain: mannose as a recognition marker. Biochem Biophys Res Commun 1988;153(3):1038–44.
[88] Tsuji A. Small molecular drug transfer across the blood-brain barrier via carrier-mediated transport systems. NeuroRx 2005;2(1):54–62.
[89] Jin GZ, Chakraborty A, Lee JH, Knowles JC, Kim HW. Targeting with nanoparticles for the therapeutic treatment of brain diseases. J Tissue Eng 2020;11:2041731419897460.
[90] Arora S, Layek B, Singh J. Design and validation of liposomal apoe2 gene delivery system to evade blood-brain barrier for effective treatment of alzheimer's disease. Mol Pharmaceutics 2021;18(2):714–25.

Chapter 8

Micelles-based drug delivery for dementia

Oly Katari, Sheetal Yadav, Junia Akhtar, Sanyog Jain

Centre for Pharmaceutical Nanotechnology, Department of Pharmaceutics, National Institute of Pharmaceutical Education and Research (NIPER), S.A.S. Nagar, Punjab, India

Abbreviations

Aβ	Amyloid β-protein
AD	Alzheimer's disease
APP	Amyloid precursor protein
BBB	Blood–brain barrier
CLA	Conjugated linoleic acid
Ca^{+2}	Calcium
CNS	Central Nervous System
COX	Cyclooxygenase
DLB	Dementia with Lewy bodies
DMF	N,N-dimethylformamide
DMSO	Dimethylsulfoxide
DQA	Dequalinium
FTD	Frontotemporal dementia
GSK-3β	Glycogen synthase kinase-3β
HT	hydroxytyrosol
IL	Interleukin
i.n.	Intranasal
i.v.	Intravenous
MgO	Magnesium oxide
mRNA	Messenger RNA
miRNA	microRNA
MSC	Mesenchymal stromal cells
pDNA	plasmid DNA
PEG	Poly(ethylene glycol)
PEG-PCL	Polyethylene glycol-polycaprolactone
PMO	Poly-2-(2-methoxy ethoxy)-ethyl methacrylate-*co*-oligo(ethylene glycol) methacrylate

Nanomedicine-Based Approaches for the Treatment of Dementia. https://doi.org/10.1016/B978-0-12-824331-2.00002-9

Copyright © 2023 Elsevier Inc. All rights reserved.

POEG	Polyoligo(ethylene glycol) methacrylates
PS1	Presenilin-1
PSA-ODC	Polysialic acid with octadecylamine
RAGE	Receptor for advanced glycation end-products
ROS	Reactive oxygen species
shRNA	Short hairpin RNA
siRNA	Small interfering RNA
TNF	Tumour necrosis factor
TPP	Triphenylphosphonium
VaD	Vascular dementia

8.1 Introduction

With the increase in population, dementia stands as an alarming global health issue in the 21st century. Presently, around 47 million people are living with the disease and the number is expected to increase threefolds by 2050 [1]. The reason behind its occurrence is not restricted to any specific physiological change, rather involves a number of neuropathological and cerebrovascular mechanisms. A lack of proper diagnosis or underdetection further augments the progression of the disease. Till now, an accurate diagnosis is only carried out postmortem, and hence, there lies an urgent necessity in performing a proper detection as a measure to provide early intervention in dementia [2]. Over the years, dementia has occurred in several forms and subsequently, they have been categorized into different types. Alzheimer's disease (AD), dementia with Lewy bodies (DLB), frontotemporal dementia (FTD), Parkinson's disease dementia, vascular dementia (VaD), and mixed dementia are the different types of dementia out of which AD and DLB are the most common ones [3–5]. For all the dementia types, aging plays a very crucial role. More than 50% of the patients suffering from AD are above 85 years of age. Although there lie some common characteristics between the different dementias, their symptoms vary to great extents from one another. The brain damage occurring in most of the types is due to a phenomenon of protein misfolding while VaD involves neuronal death due to lack of blood supply [6].

In recent years, the understanding of underlying disease-causing mechanisms has reached new heights. Yet, an affordable, effective, and noninvasive treatment is still missing when a neurodegenerative disease like dementia is concerned. This caused the researchers to investigate different molecules effective against the occurrence of symptoms as well as come up with active preventive measures. A number of therapeutic agents such as curcumin, quercetin, etc., are known to be effective in different neurodegenerative diseases. However, their efficacy is limited by various factors like low solubility, inability to cross blood–brain barrier (BBB), and ultimately leading to lower bioavailability at the target site [7]. This led to the exploration of the potential of nanotherapeutics in delivering a drug to the brain. These nanocarriers can be tailored by surface modification with certain targeting agents for an effective BBB translocation. Also, the utilization of surfactants to coat the nanocarrier surface enhances the tendency of these nanosystems to interact with endothelial cells, thus paving their way to the brain [8]. Scientists have already been successful in developing various polymeric (polymeric nanoparticles, micelles) and lipid nanocarriers (liposomes, nanostructured lipid carriers, solid lipid nanoparticles, etc.) intended for brain-related disorders. The application of micelles in dementia has seen a sudden surge in recent years. They have the potential to overcome bioavailability problems of the drugs as well as enhance their efficacy in the brain [9]. Micelles are amphiphilic molecules that spontaneously self-assemble at particular concentration and temperature conditions. Their size ranges from 5 to 50 nm [10]. They consist of both hydrophilic/polar and hydrophobic/nonpolar parts, where the hydrophilic heads face outwards and the hydrophobic tail form the core. The amphiphilic block copolymers have a tendency to assemble with one another in order to minimize the interfacial area of the hydrophobic blocks for decreased free energy [11]. Copolymers such as distearyl-sn-glycero-3-phosphoethanolamine-N-methoxy poly(ethylene glycol), poly(ethylene glycol)-b-poly(lactic acid), and poly(styrene)-poly(acrylic acid) have been found effective against neurodegenerative diseases [12]. Micelles can easily deliver low water-soluble drugs, protect the drug from the outer environment, and provide a sustained release of the drug [13]. The cellular uptake of micelles is often determined or enhanced by the nature of the copolymers used. Apart from surface modification, the micellar size and surface charge play a very vital role in determining the targeting ability of these nanosystems [14]. Particle size in the nanometer range can pose extra benefits of enhanced drug absorption and bioavailability, while macro-range particles exhibit lower volume of distribution [15]. Again, a positively charged system is prone to be taken up by the liver and spleen, however, a negative or neutral charged system tends to have an extended blood circulation time [16]. Interestingly, the micelles not only deliver drugs to the target site but also effectively carry genetic materials within their structure. Therefore, the probability of rejection of these materials by the immune systems gets minimized. Within just a few years of research, micelles have successfully come a long way in dementia management and soon they will be available for clinical translations as well.

8.2 Interaction of micelles with β-amyloid

Among the different types mentioned earlier, the most common cause of dementia is AD. It is characterized by amyloid β-protein (Aβ)-induced formation of extracellular senile plaques and intraneuronal tangles in the brain. It also involves hyperphosphorylation of tau protein [17]. Aβ is a hydrophobic peptide that natively exists as disordered monomers but spontaneously interacts with each other to form neurotoxic β-sheeted aggregates [18]. At the initial stage, the Aβ peptide shows α-helical conformation when present in the cell membrane. It is further broken down into small fragments (mainly Aβ-40 and Aβ-42 residues) by the action of enzyme secretase on amyloid precursor protein (APP). These residues then come in close vicinity to one another and form aggregates of β-sheet [19].

In the past few years, extensive researches have been carried out to explore the mechanism-based approaches in inhibiting Aβ aggregate formation. Therefore, the possible pathways by which micelles interact with Aβ to slow down AD progression are being interpreted. It has been found that PEGylated phospholipid nanomicelles hindered the formation of β-sheet conformation from α-helical form of Aβ-42 (Fig. 8.1; Scheme 1) [20]. Two different pathways were postulated from the outcomes of this study. The first mechanism involves the interaction of micelles with native Aβ-42 (α-helical form) where the hydrophobic domain of the peptide gets accommodated in the hydrophobic core of the micelles. Consequently, the resultant complex becomes highly stable, thus averting β-sheet formation as well as self-aggregation. Unlike the previous mechanism, the second pathway involves only monomers of the PEGylated micelles. The hydrophobic acyl chains of this monomer prevent further accumulation of early Aβ-42 aggregates, that is, protofibrils and oligomers, by protecting the hydrophobic domains of these aggregates. This reduces the chances of further amyloid plaque formation [20]. The involvement of reactive oxygen species (ROS) was found to be crucial in avoiding Aβ-induced neurotoxicity

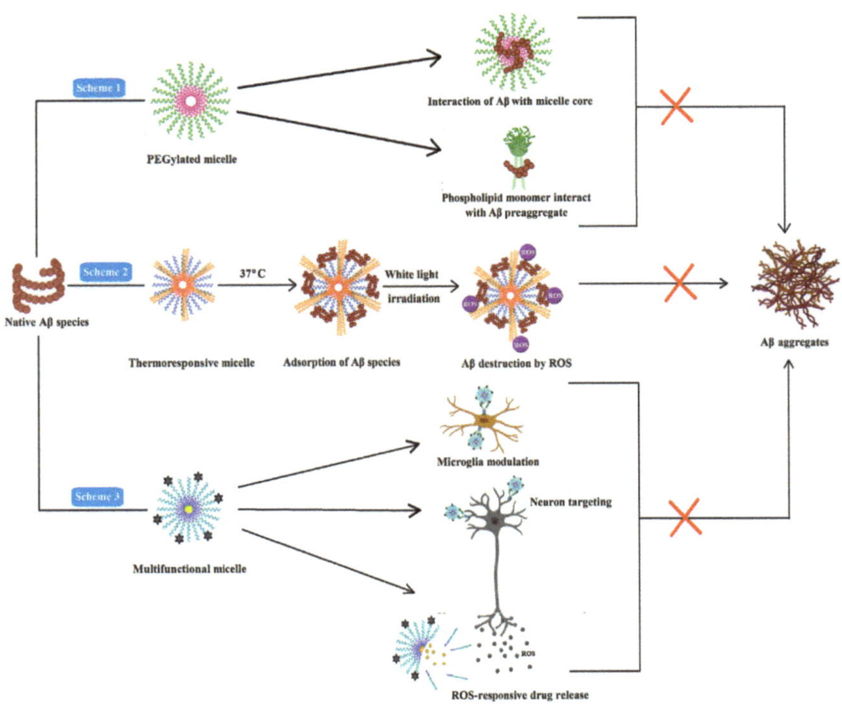

FIG. 8.1 The different possible mechanisms by which micelles interact with native Aβ species to prevent their aggregation.

which led to the proposal of a different mechanism. Thermoresponsive micelles were constructed using poly-2-(2-methoxy ethoxy)-ethyl methacrylate-*co*-oligo(ethylene glycol) methacrylate (PMO) and polyoligo(ethylene glycol) methacrylates (POEG) [21]. PMO is known to exhibit unique properties of changing conformation at physiological temperature and thus instantaneously transform from hydrophilic to hydrophobic nature. This hydrophobic domain, thereafter, forms the core of the micelles. Consequently, the hydrophobic Aβ preaggregates interact with this hydrophobic core and get adsorbed on the surface of the micelles. As a result, the process of Aβ fibrillation, as well as neurotoxic aggregate formation, is averted. On contrary, POEG limits excess capturing of Aβ monomers and also prevents self-aggregation of the micelles. Due to its hydrophilic character, POEG increases the overall hydrophilicity of the system and increases the biocompatibility of the micelles. Additionally, these micelles also produce ROS in presence of white light irradiation which in turn oxidizes the Aβ species (Fig. 8.1; Scheme 2) [22]. These oxidized species are incapable of forming aggregates and thus the process of Aβ fibrillation is prevented. However, a simultaneous phenomenon of Aβ disaggregation can also occur due to the destruction in aggregate conformation by ROS. Therefore, these micelles were capable of alleviating Aβ-induced cytotoxicity by both capturing the Aβ species as well as oxidizing their aggregates.

In AD conditions, a continuous process of neuronal loss exists which makes the microglia highly sensitive to immune responses. This leads to hyperactivity as well as the uncontrolled inflammatory response of microglia, thereby exaggerating AD further [23]. Additionally, a high level of ROS generation occurs from these microglia as well as mitochondria of the affected neurons which is a very substantial feature of AD brains. At later stages, Aβ amyloids also participate in ROS generation [24]. The damage caused due to ROS-generated oxidative stress further directs the development of pathological symptoms of the disease [25]. Accordingly, micelles have also been investigated for their ability to alleviate microglia overactivation and parallelly control other microenvironment changes responsible for AD. A multifunctional micelle was established using a receptor for advanced glycation end-products (RAGE) targeting peptide and poly(ethylene glycol) (PEG)-LysB polymer loaded with curcumin [26]. This peptide is derived from Aβ protein which makes it easy for the micelles to aggregate in AD region by mimicking the abnormal Aβ transport. Moreover, RAGE is responsible for the plasma Aβ influx into the brain. The micelles bind to the RAGE receptors expressed on the surface of microglia and neurons, subsequently preventing Aβ influx and thus averting AD progression [27]. Furthermore, PEG-LysB is a ROS-responsive polymer possessing the ability to scavenge ROS and thus reduce oxidative stress in the AD microenvironment. The payload, curcumin, is known for its targeting ability to Aβ aggregates which helps in producing a synergistic mechanism in the whole process of normalizing AD (Fig. 8.1; Scheme 3) [28]. However, the microglia modulation of this micelle was further confirmed by observing the mRNA expression of specific proteins associated with Aβ metabolism. The brains of AD-induced mice had high levels of glycogen synthase kinase-3β (GSK-3β) expression which increased APP/presenilin-1 (PS1) expression and finally Aβ production. After treatment with curcumin-loaded micelles, the expression of these proteins was found to decline significantly [26]. Overall, this multifunctional micelle could simultaneously mimic Aβ transportation to the brain, scavenge ROS, destroy Aβ aggregates, and modulate hyperactive microglia and damaged neurons.

8.3 Different routes for micelles delivery in dementia

Micelles are flexible enough to be administered via different routes. However, each route has its own advantages and drawbacks. There are a certain set of points that should be kept in mind before choosing the delivery route in case of neurological diseases. By far, micelles have been found suitable to be delivered via oral, intranasal, and intravenous routes in neurodegenerative conditions like dementia.

8.3.1 Oral route

The oral route offers a number of benefits especially when patient compliance is concerned. During chronic therapy, it becomes convenient for the patients to carry out effortless self-medication. Nonetheless, formulating a drug for oral administration remains very critical since a number of factors should be considered that influence drug bioavailability. The physiological barriers of the gastrointestinal tract provide significant hindrance in the absorption of the drug [29]. However, polymeric micelles have the potential to overcome these drawbacks due to their unique structure. The hydrophilic corona provides sufficient stability to the system which is surrounded by aqueous fluids, whereas the hydrophobic core solubilizes the poorly water-soluble drugs which would otherwise precipitate in the aqueous environment [30].

Mixed polymeric micelles have shown overwhelming results following oral administration in animal model. The micelles were prepared using Pluronics (P123&F127)/phosphatidylcholine/polysorbate 80 and nimodipine was chosen as the model drug. A greater drug bioavailability (208%) was observed in the brains of rats administered with micelles than those with the drug solution. Also, a higher circulation time was observed in the case of the drug-loaded micelles. Therefore, this study ensured that the micelles could pass through the nanopores of the intestinal membrane and reach the systemic circulation [31]. In a similar study, lactoferrin was attached to conjugated linoleic acid (CLA) to develop self-assembled micelles. Here, CLA served as a dual-purpose molecule as it formed the hydrophobic core of the micelle as well as possessed a therapeutic effect. The micelles exhibited a sustained CLA release behavior in intestinal pH after 4 hours. A reduction in ROS levels and Aβ aggregation in AD-induced rats ensured a better brain targeting by these micelles [32]. To conclude, oral administration of drugs could provide better brain targeting in neurodegenerative disease conditions.

8.3.2 Intranasal route

Among the various approaches used in brain targeting, the nasal route has exceptional advantages of delivering the drugs directly to the brain from the nasal cavity by surpassing the BBB noninvasively. It provides benefits of avoiding the various drawbacks of the invasive methods of administration such as safety, cost, and especially convenience. The intranasal route allows rapid absorption of the drug from the nasal cavity via trigeminal and olfactory nerves directly to the central nervous system (CNS) [33]. As a result, gastric degradation, hepatic metabolism, and systemic side effects of the drug can be avoided by this route.

Due to their exceptional intrinsic properties, the polymeric micelles have shown better brain targeting ability and easy permeation through nasal barriers. A thermosensitive gel was formed from rotigotine-loaded polymeric (Pluronic 407&188) micelles for nose-to-brain delivery of the drug. It was observed that the drug distribution in the cerebrum, cerebellum, olfactory bulb, and striatum was greater when administered through nasal route than those with i.v. administration [34]. In another study, the brain distribution of baicalein was improved by formulating it into poly (ethylene glycol)-block-poly (D, L-lactide) micelles. These micelles proved to be nontoxic and possessed antioxidant and anti-inflammatory properties. The brain distribution of baicalein was significantly higher in the nasal inhalation groups than the orally treated ones [35]. Therefore, the above-mentioned studies indicate that nasal drug delivery could be a better option in the management of dementia.

8.3.3 Intravenous route

This is the most common route for administering drugs straightaway to the systemic circulation. It has a number of advantages such as the rapid onset of action, avoiding first-pass metabolism and tissue irritation, and so on [36]. Accordingly, micelles have also shown improved action when administered i.v. in animal models. A significant reduction in Aβ deposition and tau hyperphosphorylation was caused by TPP-linked resveratrol micelles. Moreover, the cognitive performance of mice was restored following micelle treatment [37]. Furthermore, rapamycin-loaded ROS-responsive micellar systems were also developed for AD management. Higher drug delivery was found to the central neurons as well as an intracellular drug release was observed due to the ROS-mediated disaggregation of the micelles. As a result, these micelles were successful in restoring the autophagic flux which delayed the progression of AD [38].

8.4 Preparation methods of different micelles

In general, there are a number of methods used for the preparation of micelles. The selection of a particular method solely depends on the physicochemical properties of the polymers involved in the formation of the micelle [39]. Out of the several methods, this section elaborates on the dialysis method, direct dissolution method, and solvent evaporation method. These three methods have been frequently employed for the development of micelles that are intended for AD, PD, and other dementias.

8.4.1 Dialysis method

This is one of the most common methods of micelle preparation especially for amphiphilic copolymers having low aqueous solubility. Here, the drug and copolymer are mixed in an organic solvent [acetonitrile, dimethylsulfoxide (DMSO), N,N-dimethylformamide (DMF), tetrahydrofuran, etc.] and poured in a dialysis bag. The bag is kept in a water-containing beaker, where the water stimulates micelle formation. The dialysis is carried out for an extended period of time to remove the organic solvent and properly load the drug into the micelles [40]. Lactoferrin–CLA copolymer micelles were prepared by this method. Initially, lactoferrin and CLA were coupled by carbodiimide coupling reaction which was followed by dialysis against 40% DMSO for 24 hours and then against pure distilled water for the next 48 hours [32]. Similarly, Nano^{DOPA} micelles were prepared by dissolving PEG-*b*-P(L-DOPA$(OAc)_2$) copolymer in DMF followed by dialysis for 24 hours against water [41].

8.4.2 Direct dissolution method

This method is generally used for copolymers with high aqueous solubility. It involves the dissolving of drug and copolymer separately in aqueous media with increased temperature or stirring. Once dissolved, both the solutions are mixed together to obtain drug-loaded polymeric micelles [40]. Curcumin cocrystal micelles were fabricated by using this method. At the preliminary stage, the curcumin cocrystal, stabilizers, and surfactants were mixed by vigorous stirring to form a preconcentrate. Next, water was added to this preconcentrate with simultaneous stirring and self-assembled micelles were formed [42].

8.4.3 Solvent evaporation method

This method is also known as the thin-film hydration method. Here, the drug and copolymer are dissolved in a common organic solvent; however, a mixture of two miscible solvents may also be used to dissolve them. Next, the solvent is removed by evaporation which leads to the formation of a thin film of drug and copolymer. Further addition of water to the film leads to the spontaneous formation of drug-loaded micelles [43]. Morin hydrate-loaded micellar nanocarriers were developed by this method. Firstly, Pluronic P123 and Pluronic F127 as well as the drug were dissolved in methanol and the solvent was removed in Rota evaporator. After 24 hours, the film was hydrated with distilled water to obtain the dug-loaded micelles [44]. In a similar study, hydroxytyrosol-loaded micelles were formed from Pluronic F68 and dequalinium by dissolving the three components in methanol followed by hydration with distilled water [45].

8.5 Modified micelles for cellular targeting

8.5.1 Microglial targeting

Microglia originates from myeloid cells and covers nearly 12% of the brain. It remains in its resting state in normal conditions but undergoes activation during neuroinflammation and neurotoxicity [46]. Microglial can be categorized into amoeboid microglia, ramified microglia, and activated microglia [47]. In a resting state, it possesses a ramified shape that transforms into an amoeboid structure under certain conditions such as stress, trauma, and neurological problems. This causes disturbance in brain homeostasis, as well as genetic and functional alterations. Microglial activation elevates the levels of cytotoxic substances such as peroxynitrite and nitrite. However, a series of events take place following microglial activation such as neuronal death, higher levels of COX-2, interleukins (IL-1B, IL-6), and TNF-α. Additionally, the expressions of immune and recruitment molecules are also observed [47,48]. A modification in the brain's endothelial tight junction, surface protein, and microglia-induced neuroinflammation impacts the BBB permeability that results in a reduction in Aβ clearance, which leads to the development of different neurodegenerative disorders. RAGE and lipoprotein receptor-related protein transporters, involved in the Aβ clearance, are also downregulated due to the microglial-activated neurotoxicity that worsens the disease conditions [47]. Therefore, polymeric micelles were fabricated to modulate the activated microglia under a stress environment. These micelles are comprised of RAGE (microglial targeting) and curcumin along with ROS-sensitive polymers. Synergistic action of the micelle constituents led to the destruction of ROS species as well as normalizing the activated microglia in AD conditions [26]. In another study, researchers developed rosuvastatin-loaded polyethylene glycol-poly(ε-caprolactone) nanomicelles by the cosolvent evaporation method. The micelles possessed a particle size of about 23.37 nm. The microglia can exist either in M1 or M2 phenotypes depending on the surrounding environment. While the M1 type causes the upregulation of the proinflammatory cytokines, damage to BBB, and oxidative stress, the M2 type releases anti-inflammatory cytokines and promotes tissue recovery [49]. The regulatory effect of these micelles on microglia polarization was estimated by staining with M1-and M2-like markers. A significant increase in the levels of M2 type microglia and a decrease in M1 type microglia were observed over time post-treatment with micelles as compared to the vehicle group. Therefore, the drug-loaded micelles were capable of downregulating the pro-inflammatory cytokines like tumor necrosis factor (TNF)- α, interleukin (IL)-1β, IL-6, and IL-23 [50]. Apart from microglial targeting, efforts have been to target different cell organelles such as mitochondria, nucleus, etc. for specific and effective delivery of drugs in brain-localized disorders like dementia.

8.5.2 Mitochondrial targeting

Among the various cell organelles, mitochondria are a very unique subcellular structure present in a cell. It is known to be the energy factory of the cells that contain remarkable features and play a pivotal role in various cellular processes such as generating ATP through oxidative phosphorylation, maintaining calcium (Ca^{+2}) homeostasis, etc. Neurons are dependent on the mitochondria existing at the neuronal synapse since they are frequently involved in ATP production and Ca^{+2} homeostasis followed by neurotransmission and mitochondrial membrane potential maintenance [51]. Mitochondria in healthy neurons help to execute neuronal and cellular activities. Neuronal crisis leads to mitochondrial dysfunction that may alter several mitochondrial functions. This ultimately worsens the neuronal performance, consequently leading to the development of AD, PD, and several other neurodegenerative disorders. Mitochondrial malfunction results in the following changes:

1. Neuronal activities such as neurotransmitter release, membrane potential homeostasis, and neurotransmitter receptor affinity necessitate sufficient energy production that can be fulfilled by the brain or mitochondria. In the case of energy deprivation, activating mitochondrial ATP synthesis may help to mitigate the harmful effects in the brain. However, mitochondrial malfunction puts the brain's functioning and morphology under stress [52].
2. Although Ca^{+2} regulates neurotransmitter release at the synapse, mitochondria can buffer and maintain the Ca^{+2} concentration. As a result, mitochondrial impairment may result in the imbalance of the natural functioning of the brain, contributing to aging and AD [51].
3. There is a marked decrease in the levels of several metabolic enzymes (namely, α-ketoglutarate dehydrogenase, cyclooxygenase (COX), isocitrate dehydrogenase, pyruvate dehydrogenase) when higher levels of succinic and malate dehydrogenases disturb the mitochondrial membrane potential and its energy generation ability [53].
4. Mitochondrial biogenesis entails the fusion and fission processes that are required for metabolite and mitochondrial DNA mixing, mitochondrial growth and distribution, and cellular adaptability to the environment. Overexpression of APP in the neurons facilitates alterations in the mitochondrial fusion and fission proteins such as DrP1, Mfm1/2, Opa1, and Mfp1 that are ultimately responsible for the mitochondrial fragmentation [54].

Micelles boast an indispensable role in the cellular targeting of the drugs. Keeping this point in mind, Yang et al. [37] observed fabricated poly (ethylene glycol)-b-poly (Lactide) micelles modified with peptide C3 and triphenylphosphonium (TPP) utilizing the solvent diffusion method. The TPPs particular targeting affinity encourages mitochondrial targeting through the cell. The researchers investigated that resveratrol-loaded micelles (CTNM) decorated with 50% of TPP exhibited better brain targeting, accumulation, and BBB penetration than micelles with 10%–40% TPP decorated. Intravenous administration of CTNM has depicted higher drug concentration in the brain, with 1.89- and 105-fold increment in AUC values in comparison to micelles with TPP and drug alone, respectively. Further, it was observed that the oxidative stress marker, total antioxidant capacity, glutathione peroxidase, and superoxide dismutase levels reduced after i.v. treatment of APP/PS1 mice with CTNM. Interestingly, the prevention of neuronal synaptic degeneration by reversal of mitochondrial dysfunction was also observed [37]. In a similar study, the role of curcumin in protecting mitochondrial functioning was also interpreted. Due to its ROS scavenging potential, curcumin can maintain the integrity of mitochondria and fission–fusion mitochondrial protein. Hence DSPE-PE2000 micelles were synthesized to overcome the drug's hydrophobicity constraint and to boost protective activity in neuronal mitochondria [55]. Curcumin's intrinsic fluorescence property aided in estimating cellular uptake activity. The mitochondrial integrity was estimated via observing the mitochondrial membrane potential and morphology determination by using a mitochondria-specific probe (TPE-Ph-In). TPE-ph-In coupled to micelles could intensely stain inside the mitochondrial region of the selected cell lines indicating the mitochondrial targeting ability of these micelles. Also, a pretreatment with curcumin-loaded micelles resulted in the protection of HT22 cells from Aβ-induced cytotoxicity as well as prevented mitochondrial structure and distribution damage [55]. Mitochondrial swelling is another phenomenon that results from the opening of the mitochondrial permeability transition pore and is strongly correlated with mitochondrial function and neuronal cell death in progressive neurodegenerative diseases, such as AD and PD. Another study suggested that curcumin-loaded micelles had the potential to prevent mitochondrial swelling in the brains of aged NMRI mice. Drug-loaded micelles had a significant impact on nitrosative stress protection and brain accumulation than native drug micelles [56].

8.5.3 Nucleus targeting

Recently various genetic strategies have been employed for cellular targeting to the nucleus in different neurological disease conditions. For instance, ApoE is an apolipoprotein that originates from the astrocytes of which the ApoE2 component is mainly involved in the clearance of the Aβ plaque, hence impeding the accumulation of Aβ in the brain. Therefore, the delivery of a plasmid coded ApoE2 could be a promising avenue in the management of the disease [57]. However, the application is restricted because the gene or nucleic acid has to overcome different hurdles before reaching or targeting the nucleus. Several extracellular and intracellular barriers, that is, poor penetration, less transfection, endosomal, and lysosomal degradation limits gene delivery which necessitated an urge for a promising and suitable vector to overcome these obstacles [58]. In that consideration polymeric micelle is an excellent delivery vehicle/vector that provides better DNA condensation ability, good transfection, and promotes the proton buffering activity, allowing genes to safely enter the nucleus. Polymeric micelles fabricated via atom transfer radical polymerization were electrostatically attached to the negatively charged pDNA following maleimide-mediated covalent binding to conjugate TGN peptide (brain-specific ligand) [59]. This process ameliorated the targeting ability and facilitated better BBB permeability of the micelles. Fluorescent dyes were utilized to estimate the cellular uptake and translocation of the gene to the nucleus. The confocal microscopy observations demonstrated that the micelles initially localized in both the endosome and nucleus of BCE cells but after some time it got fully localized in the nucleus. It was assumed that the pDNA entered the nucleus via diffusion after getting released from the late endolysosomes. They significantly improved the biocompatibility, cellular uptake, and gene expression in BCEs cell lines and in vivo model. However, distribution studies displayed major distribution in the brain rather than the liver and kidney. The expression of green fluoresce protein was observed in all the seven regions of the mouse brain (i.e., cortical layer, hippocampus, hypothalamus, lateral ventricle, substantia nigra, third ventricle, and triangular nucleus) when treated with targeted micelles, which was not in the case of untargeted micelles [59]. This study demonstrated that such micelles could be exploited in future investigations as a promising vehicle for gene delivery.

8.6 Therapeutics-loaded micellar systems for different types of dementia

8.6.1 Drug-loaded systems

Reports from the past few years depict several clinical approaches for cognitive deficits and dementia; however, no specific medication therapy for the FTD and DLB has been reported. However, extensive research on cholinesterase inhibitors has suggested that the drugs rivastigmine, galantamine, and donepezil could be beneficial in the management of dementia, and that protein oxidation induces oxidative stress, which ultimately leads to neurodegeneration and dementia [60]. Several studies have suggested that oxidative stress may be a possible marker for AD. Overexpression of Aβ-protein in the retina, which is analogous to the brain, has been a progressive hallmark in the diagnosis of AD. Excessive lipid and protein oxidation have long been known to increase oxidative stress, culminating in neurodegeneration and dementia. Curcumin and hydroxytyrosol (HT), the two natural polyphenolic substances with high antioxidant activity, possess intriguing possibilities for dementia treatment. Curcumin, derived from the *Curcuma longa* plant, possesses an excellent binding affinity for Aβ plaque as well as inherent fluorescence characteristics. However, its use is limited due to its hydrophobic nature. Therefore, taking advantage of the excellent properties of micelles as nanocarriers, curcumin-encapsulated DSPE-PEG2000 micelles were developed as a tool to diagnose AD [61]. These micelles have been demonstrated to penetrate and stain Aβ plaque overexpressed in the retina of APPswe/PS1E9 mouse model, indicating that they could be used to detect AD via an intravitreal method. Apart from curcumin, the HTs also exhibit oxidative stress-reducing properties due to the arrangement of catechol in their structure. Hence, the HTs are capable of preventing fibrillation of α-synuclein in PD conditions [62]. Scientists have found that micelles prepared from Pluronic F68 (P68) and dequalinium (DQA) show exceptional features of liberating antioxidants in the mitochondria both in vitro and in vivo [63]. This nanoformulation displayed excellent antioxidant activity, biocompatibility, and dramatically enhanced BBB penetration than the free drug. BBB penetration study in hCMEC/D3 cell line demonstrated that a higher concentration of HT was present in the basolateral compartment, thereby validating the successful delivery of drug to the brain by these micelles. Over the last few decades, nose-to-brain delivery has been garnering prominent attention for AD management. Desai et al. [64] devised a nanomicellar carrier to stabilize curcumin cocrystal for AD. The micellar assembly of curcumin cocrystal exhibited 100% drug release and produced significant antioxidant activity in the U87MG cell line. However, in vivo studies demonstrated a 1.7-fold increment in absolute bioavailability of the cocrystal micelles. Also, a higher brain distribution and delayed clearance were observed for the micelles. This assured superior therapeutic effect of these micelles in AD treatment. The structural composition of the brain consists of a highly enriched tight junction of endothelial cells on the brain capillary wall which restricts drug penetration [65]. Poor BBB penetration of drugs is a major concern in the treatment of dementia. This issue can be easily resolved by successive modification of nanocarrier through ligands. For instance, α-lactoferrin CLA self-assembled micelles were successful in efficient brain targeting for AD management. The nanoassembly exhibited excellent biocompatibility along with improved cognitive abilities. Around 1.7-fold and 3-fold reduction in ROS and acetylcholinesterase activity were observed in the brains of micelle-treated rats, respectively. Moreover, a decrease in inflammatory and caspase-3 activities was demonstrated which led to the prevention of neuronal death [32]. Therefore, the micelles were successful in targeting CNS and proved to be of great use in the future.

Apart from AD and PD, micelles have also been developed for VaD management. Self-assembled nanomicelles were prepared by conjugating polysialic acid with octadecylamine (PSA-ODC) followed by loading with a calmodulin antagonist, DY9836. The particle size of the micelles was around 107.4 nm. In vitro cytotoxicity study showed that around 65% of cells were alive even after treatment with high concentration (1000 μg/mL). In vivo animal studies assured a 1.3-fold enhancement in C_{max} of the micelles than that of the plain drug. The micelles had excellent BBB penetrating ability. Also, the number of mature neurons was increased in hippocampus as well as the dephosphorylation of CaMKII and synapsin I was inhibited in micelle-treated mice [66]. Thus, these micelles were efficient in VaD management and may also be explored for other related diseases. A summary of several other micelles developed for different types of dementia has been enlisted in Table 8.1 mentioning their outcomes.

TABLE 8.1 Summary of micelles developed for different types of dementia.

Micelles	Drug	Particle size (nm)	Disease	Cell line	Outcome	References
Inulin-d-alfa-tocopherol succinate micelles	Curcumin	7.8 ± 2.1	Amyotrophic lateral sclerosis	Mesenchymal Stromal Cells (MSC)	The micelles showed no cytotoxicity in MSC, while significant cytotoxicity was observed in plain curcumin. Also, the micelles reached maximum loading in the cells within a few minutes.	[67]
PHEA-EDA-Sq17-PS80 copolymer micelles	Rivastigmine	34.1	AD	Neuro2a	Drug-loaded micelles exhibited concentration-dependent cellular uptake with good biocompatibility in neuroblastoma cells. Also, the micelles showed good stability in human plasma.	[68]
Phospatidyl ethanolamine-distearoyl methoxypoly-ethylene glycol micelles	Curcumin	21	AD	–	It has been observed that nanomicelles loaded with curcumin diminish protein fibrillation and β-sheet formation. The glycation process fascinated the release of curcumin in AD conditions.	[69]
Pluronic P127 & Pluronic F123 based micelles	Morin hydrate	52.8 ± 0.21 nm	AD	–	Micelles were prepared through the thin-film hydration method. They exhibited 17.63 ± 0.12 % drug release in pH 6.8 followed by 92.12± 0.50 % in gastric pH. The drug-loaded micellar assembly was capable of improving the locomotor activity, object reorganization activity and showed a significant effect in the Morris water maze test. However, the acetylcholinesterase level was attenuated after treatment. It was also observed that glutathione concentration was also enhanced after treatment with micelles.	[70]

Micelles	Drug	Particle size (nm)	Disease	Cell line	Outcome	References
Poly (ethylene glycol)-block-poly (O, O′-diacetyl-l-DOPA) micelles	Levodopa	52.2 nm	PD	BAEC cells	Amphiphilic micelles demonstrated stability at different gastrointestinal pH and were less cytotoxic in BAEC cells. A reversal of the behavioral activity and improvement in PD symptoms were observed after the intraperitoneal administration of the drug-loaded micelle.	[71]
Methoxy-poly-ethylene glycol-polycaprolactone micelle	Rapamycin	41.05 ± 1.20 nm	AD	HT22 cells	Micelles were fabricated by solvent diffusion method followed by modification with TPP. The micelles promoted significant enhancement in the cellular internalization in HT 22 cells and bEnd cells. Also, autophagy flux was observed that aided in Aβ plaque and p-tau clearance. Moreover, a reversal of neuronal and hippocampal damage was demonstrated in vivo post-treatment with the micelles.	[38]
RAGE peptide functionalized poly(ethylene glycol)-polylysine micelles	Curcumin	65 nm	AD	Brain capillary endothelium & SH-SY5Y cells	The curcumin encapsulated micelles internalized through micropinocytosis and clathrin-dependent pathway had the potential to downregulate free radical generation. They potentially improved the BBB penetration and cellular uptake. Additionally, endosome and lysosome degradation were prevented as well as Aβ plaque clearance was also demonstrated in the mice model. The micelles provided neuroprotection and microglial deactivation which is an important criterion for AD management.	[26]

(Continued)

Table 8.1 Cont'd

Micelles	Drug	Particle size (nm)	Disease	Cell line	Outcome	References
PEG-PLGA micelles thermosensitive gel	Rotigotine	88.62 ± 1.47	PD	–	Drug-loaded micellar gel exhibited approximately 93.5 ± 0.79 % encapsulation efficiency and 93.5 ± 0.79 % loading efficiency. Hydrogel with a gelation temperature of 32.3°C promoted the sustained release of the drug (52.9 % with 48 hours). At first, the drug reached the olfactory bulb followed by distribution to different regions of the brain. A higher brain distribution was observed in the gel-treated animals.	[34]
C3 peptide and triphosphonium modified poly (ethylene glycol)-b-poly (Lactide) micelles	Resveratrol	42.6 ± 0.53	AD	HT22 cells	Micelles were attached to TPP which provided better drug targeting in the brain. They were able to cross the BBB and efficiently reach the target site. Moreover, downregulated tau hyperphosphorylation, alleviated neuronal toxicity, and improved microgliosis was observed. Also, a reduction in the proinflammatory cytokines, that is, TNF-α and ILs further improved the cognitive functions.	[37]

8.6.2 Genetic material-loaded systems

Over the years, gene therapy (gene-editing technology) has been at par with drug-based therapy when disease recovery is concerned. Effective gene therapy leads to either restoring function or preventing the decline of the disease condition. RNA interference is one such gene-mediated approach carried out by small interfering RNA (siRNA) and microRNA (miRNA). It involves the manipulation of natural cellular mechanisms that leads to altered gene expression [72]. While the siRNA works by binding to a target mRNA and preventing its translation, the miRNA acts by regulating the expression of multiple functionally related genes [73]. The risk of miRNA misregulation and the ease of siRNA designing/working makes it convenient for scientists to choose siRNA for their research [74]. The gene therapy for dementia includes the transportation of nucleic acids/genetic materials to the affected areas of the brain. However, the presence of BBB limits the delivery of these genes to the CNS and makes the disease curing process difficult. The direct incorporation of drug into the CNS by intracerebral or intraventricular routes encompass the invasive method of drug delivery. But this method of treatment is greatly incompatible for patients and involves huge risk [75]. Thus, there lies the requirement of an appropriate carrier for delivering these genes to the target site. Recently, nanocarriers have been an effective approach for delivering therapeutic agents to CNS noninvasively. Further, receptor-mediated targeting of these nanocarriers aid in easy bypassing of BBB.

An attempt was made by Kanazawa et al. [76] to deliver siRNA to the brain by encapsulating it in nanomicelles. The nanomicelle was developed from a conjugate obtained from Tat (a cell-penetrating peptide) and polyethylene glycol-polycaprolactone (PEG-PCL). The efficacy of these micelles (MPEG-PCL-Tat) was compared post intravenous (i.v.) and intranasal (i.n.) treatments in rats. It was evident from the dynamics study that high distribution was found in brainstem, caudal brain tissue, olfactory bulb, and rostral brain tissue after i.n. administration (as depicted in Fig. 8.2). Moreover, the distribution of Tat peptide-modified micelles was higher than the nonmodified/naked ones, which proved that surface modification improved the targeting ability of the nanomicelles. To date, the majority of the studies carried out with micelles aimed for a single interference in gene expression by siRNA. It was just a few years back that advancement was made by Li and his coworkers [77] where they developed a double-interfering nano-magnesium oxide (MgO) micelles using plasmid DNA (pDNA) and α-synuclein-targeted mRNA. Initially, pDNA was adsorbed on the surface of MgO. This Mg(pDNA) was then encapsulated in a complex formed from polysaccharide pullulan (obtained from maize) and insulin protein. The mRNA was bound to the surface of Mg(pDNA) which further grafted nerve growth factor on it. The tissue distribution study revealed that the micelles reached the brain within a very short period and the Mg contents were notably higher in the micelle-treated groups when compared to the control groups. Also, these micelles proved to be safe as there were no visible pathological lesions

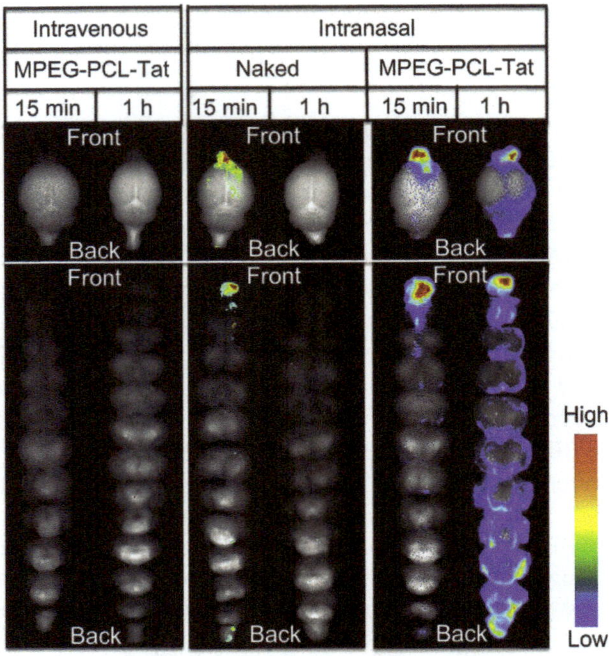

FIG. 8.2 Dynamics of distribution of MPEG-PCL-Tat complex in rat brain tissue following i.n. or i.v. administration (reproduced with permission from [76] copyright 2013, Elsevier).

observed in nontargeted organs (heart, liver, kidney, lung, and spleen). Overall, these micelles were successful in releasing pDNA and mRNA at the target site and inhibiting the expression of α-synuclein [77]. This study made a way for multifunctional nanocarriers to effectively deliver more than one RNA interfering molecule at a specific site of the brain. Although the above-mentioned investigations were successful in treating AD and PD, respectively, still there lies a need to explore this field in near future as the number of researches available presently are only handful.

8.7 Conclusion

In the past few years, the application of nanotechnology has shown a surge in the treatment of several neurodegenerative diseases. Simultaneously, a greater improvement has also been seen in understanding the disease pathology and progression. The major obstacle faced by conventional formulations is crossing BBB. Different nanocarriers take up unique pathways of bypassing the BBB and thus prevent the advancement of the disease. Dementia is a recently focused neurodegenerative disease when nanocarrier-mediated therapy is concerned. Micelles, in particular, have exhibited fruitful results in targeting the brain due to their lipophilic nature. Further advancements can be made by attaching ligands on the surface of the micelles which will enhance the targeting ability of these nanocarriers. Additionally, synergistic activity can be obtained by coloading these micelles with different drug-drug, drug-antibody, or drug-siRNA combinations. So far, there have been no stability and safety issues found related to the in vitro and in vivo studies of these micelles. However, certain harmful effects may be observed in their succeeding clinical studies. Therefore, robust studies should be carried out to validate these nanocarriers in order to make their way through clinical trials.

References

[1] Livingston G, Sommerlad A, Orgeta V, et al. Dementia prevention, intervention, and care. Lancet North Am Ed 2017;390(10113):2673–734.

[2] Lang L, Clifford A, Wei L, et al. Prevalence and determinants of undetected dementia in the community: a systematic literature review and a meta-analysis. BMJ open 2017;7(2):1–8.

[3] Barker W, Luis C, Kashuba A, et al. Relative frequencies of Alzheimer disease, Lewy body, vascular and frontotemporal dementia, and hippocampal sclerosis in the State of Florida Brain Bank. Alzheimer Dis Assoc Disord 2002;16(4):203–12.

[4] Emre M. Dementia associated with Parkinson's disease. The Lancet Neurology 2003;2(4):229–37.

[5] Langa KM, Foster NL, Larson EB. Mixed dementia: emerging concepts and therapeutic implications. JAMA 2004;292(23):2901–8.

[6] Atlanta GA. American Cancer Society. Cancer Facts and Figures 2013. Georgia, United States: American Cancer Society; 2013:7.

[7] Di Martino P, Censi R, Rosa Gigliobianco M, et al. Nano-medicine improving the bioavailability of small molecules for the prevention of neurodegenerative diseases. Curr Pharm Des 2017;23(13):1897–908.

[8] Hanafy NAN, El-Kemary M, Leporatti S. Micelles structure development as a strategy to improve smart cancer therapy. Cancers 2018;10(7):238.

[9] Xu W, Ling P, Zhang T. Polymeric micelles, a promising drug delivery system to enhance bioavailability of poorly water-soluble drugs. Journal of Drug Delivery 2013;2013:1–15.

[10] Wakaskar RR. General overview of lipid-polymer hybrid nanoparticles, dendrimers, micelles, liposomes, spongosomes and cubosomes. J Drug Targeting 2018;26(4):311–8.

[11] Kataoka K, Harada A, Nagasaki Y. Block copolymer micelles for drug delivery: design, characterization and biological significance. Adv Drug Deliv Rev 2001;47:113–31.

[12] Sezgin-bayindir Z, Ergin AD, Parmaksiz M, et al. Evaluation of various block copolymers for micelle formation and brain drug delivery: in vitro characterization and cellular uptake studies. J Drug Delivery Sci Technol 2016;36:120–9.

[13] Joseph M, Trinh HM, Mitra AK. Peptide and protein-based therapeutic agents. In: Emerging Nanotechnologies for Diagnostics, Drug Delivery and Medical Devices. Cambridge, United States: Elsevier; 2017;145–67.

[14] Sydow K, Nikolenko H, Lorenz D, et al. Lipopeptide-based micellar and liposomal carriers: influence of surface charge and particle size on cellular uptake into blood brain barrier cells. Eur J Pharm Biopharm 2016;109:130–9.

[15] Cabral H, Miyata K, Osada K, et al. Block copolymer micelles in nanomedicine applications. Chem Rev 2018;118:6844–92.

[16] Nel AE, Mädler L, Velegol D, et al. Understanding biophysicochemical interactions at the nano-bio interface. Nat Mater 2009;8:543–57.

[17] Alam P, Siddiqi MK, Chaturvedi SK, et al. Vitamin B12 offers neuronal cell protection by inhibiting Aβ-42 amyloid fibrillation. Int J Biol Macromol 2017;99:477–82.

[18] Lee SJC, Nam E, Lee HJ, et al. Towards an understanding of amyloid-β oligomers: characterization, toxicity mechanisms, and inhibitors. Chem Soc Rev 2017;46(2):310–23.

[19] Serpell LC. Alzheimer's amyloid fibrils: structure and assembly. Biochimica et Biophysica Acta (BBA) Molecular Basis of Disease 2000;1502(1):16–30.

[20] Pai AS, Rubinstein I, Önyüksel H. PEGylated phospholipid nanomicelles interact with β-amyloid(1-42) and mitigate its β-sheet formation, aggregation and neurotoxicity in vitro. Peptides 2006;27(11):2858–66.

[21] Geng H, Yuan H, Qiu L, et al. Inhibition and disaggregation of amyloid β protein fibrils through conjugated polymer-core thermoresponsive micelles. Journal of Materials Chemistry B 2020;8(44):10126–35.

[22] Yan Y, McCallum SA, Wang C. M35 oxidation induces Aβ40-like structural and dynamical changes in Aβ42. J Am Chem Soc 2008;130(16):5394–5.

[23] Niraula A, Sheridan JF, Godbout JP. Microglia priming with aging and stress. Neuropsychopharmacology 2017;42(1):318–33.

[24] Gackowski D, Rozalski R, Siomek A, et al. Oxidative stress and oxidative DNA damage is characteristic for mixed Alzheimer disease/vascular dementia. J Neurol Sci 2008;266(1-2): 57–62.

[25] Bonda DJ, Wang X, Perry G, et al. Oxidative stress in Alzheimer disease: a possibility for prevention. Neuropharmacology 2010;59(4-5):290–4.

[26] Lu Y, Guo Z, Zhang Y, et al. Microenvironment remodeling micelles for Alzheimer's disease therapy by early modulation of activated microglia. Advanced Science 2019;6(4).

[27] Deane R, Du Yan S, Submamaryan RK, et al. RAGE mediates amyloid-beta peptide transport across the blood-brain barrier and accumulation in brain. Nat Med 2003;9(7):907–13.

[28] Mehanny M, Hathout RM, Geneidi AS, et al. Exploring the use of nanocarrier systems to deliver the magical molecule; curcumin and its derivatives. Journal of Controlled Release: Official Journal of the Controlled Release Society 2016;225:1–30.

[29] Ensign LM, Cone R, Hanes J. Oral drug delivery with polymeric nanoparticles: the gastrointestinal mucus barriers. Adv Drug Deliv Rev 2012;64:557.

[30] Gaucher G, Satturwar P, Jones MC, et al. Polymeric micelles for oral drug delivery. Eur J Pharm Biopharm 2010;76:147–58.

[31] Basalious EB, Shamma RN. Novel self-assembled nano-tubular mixed micelles of Pluronics P123, Pluronic F127 and phosphatidylcholine for oral delivery of nimodipine: in vitro characterization, ex vivo transport and in vivo pharmacokinetic studies. Int J Pharm 2015;493(1-2):347–56.

[32] Agwa MM, Abdelmonsif DA, Khattab SN. Self- assembled lactoferrin-conjugated linoleic acid micelles as an orally active targeted nanoplatform for Alzheimer's disease Mona. Int J Biol Macromol 2020;162:246–61.

[33] Mistry A, Stolnik S, Illum L. Nanoparticles for direct nose-to-brain delivery of drugs. Int J Pharm 2009;379(1):146–57.

[34] Wang F, Yang Z, Liu M, et al. Facile nose-to-brain delivery of rotigotine-loaded polymer micelles thermosensitive hydrogels: in vitro characterization and in vivo behavior study. Int J Pharm 2020;577:119046.

[35] Zhang L, Yang S, Huang L, et al. Poly (ethylene glycol)-block-poly (D, L-lactide) (PEG-PLA) micelles for brain delivery of baicalein through nasal route for potential treatment of

neurodegenerative diseases due to oxidative stress and inflammation: an in vitro and in vivo study. Int J Pharm 2020;591:119981.

[36] Kwon GS. Polymeric micelles for delivery of poorly water-soluble compounds. Critical Reviews Therapeutic Drug Carrier Systems 2003;20:357–403.

[37] Yang P, Sheng D, Guo Q, et al. Biomaterials neuronal mitochondria-targeted micelles relieving oxidative stress for delayed progression of Alzheimer's disease. Biomaterials 2020;238:119844.

[38] Xu S, Yang P, Qian K, et al. Modulating autophagic flux via ROS-responsive targeted micelles to restore neuronal proteostasis in Alzheimer's disease. Bioactive Materials 2021.

[39] Torchilin VP. Structure and design of polymeric surfactant-based drug delivery systems. Journal of Controlled Release : Official Journal of the Controlled Release Society 2001;73:137–72.

[40] Cholkar K, Patel A, Dutt Vadlapudi A, et al. Novel nanomicellar formulation approaches for anterior and posterior segment ocular drug delivery. Recent Patents on Nanomedicine 2012;2:82–95.

[41] Vong LB, Sato Y, Chonpathompikunlert P, et al. Self-assembled polydopamine nanoparticles improve treatment in Parkinson's disease model mice and suppress dopamine-induced dyskinesia. Acta Biomater 2020;109:220–8.

[42] Desai PP, Patravale VB. Curcumin cocrystal micelles-multifunctional nanocomposites for management of neurodegenerative ailments. J Pharm Sci 2017;107(4):1–14.

[43] Letchford K, Zastre J, Liggins R, et al. Synthesis and micellar characterization of short block length methoxy poly(ethylene glycol)-block-poly(caprolactone) diblock copolymers. Colloids and Surfaces B, Biointerfaces 2004;35:81–91.

[44] Singh M, Thakur V, Deshmukh R, et al. Development and characterization of morin hydrate-loaded micellar nanocarriers for the effective management of Alzheimer's disease. 2018;35:137–48.

[45] System DC, Mursaleen L, Noble B, Somavarapu S, Zariwala MG. Micellar nanocarriers of hydroxytyrosol are protective against Parkinson's related oxidative stress in an in vitro. Antioxidants 2021;10:887–905.

[46] Block ML, Zecca L, Hong JS. Microglia-mediated neurotoxicity: uncovering the molecular mechanisms. Nat Rev Neurosci 2007;8(1):57–69.

[47] Cai Z, Hussain MD, Yan LJ. Microglia, neuroinflammation, and beta-amyloid protein in Alzheimer's disease. Int J Neurosci 2014;124(5):307–21.

[48] Bazan NG, Halabi A, Ertel M, et al. Neuroinflammation. Basic Neurochemistry 2012:610–20.

[49] Lan X, Han X, Li Q, et al. Modulators of microglial activation and polarization after intracerebral haemorrhage. Nat Rev Neurol 2017;13(7):420.

[50] Zi L, Zhou W, Xu J, et al. Rosuvastatin nanomicelles target neuroinflammation and improve neurological deficit in a mouse model of intracerebral hemorrhage. 2021;16:2933.

[51] Bhatia V, Sharma S. Role of mitochondrial dysfunction, oxidative stress and autophagy in progression of Alzheimer's disease. J Neurol Sci 2021;421:117253.

[52] Kumar V, Gurjeet T, Mehta V. Mitochondrion stressed mitochondria: a target to intrude Alzheimer's disease. Mitochondrion 2021;59:48–57.

[53] Ke J, Tian Q, Xu Q, et al. Mitochondrial dysfunction: a potential target for Alzheimer's disease intervention and treatment. Drug Discovery Today 2021;26(8):1–12.

[54] Pradeepkiran JA, Hemachandra Reddy P. Defective mitophagy in Alzheimer's disease. Ageing Res Rev 2020;64:101191.

[55] Jia F, Chibhabha F, Yang Y, et al. Detection and monitoring of the neuroprotective behavior of curcumin micelles based on an AIEgen probe. Journal of Materials Chemistry B 2021;9(3):731–45.

[56] Hagl S, Kocher A, Schiborr C, et al. Curcumin micelles improve mitochondrial function in neuronal PC12 cells and brains of NMRI mice Impact on bioavailability. Neurochem Int 2015;89:234–42.

[57] Kanekiyo T, Xu H, Bu G. ApoE and Aβ in Alzheimer's disease: accidental encounters or partners?. Neuron 2014;81:740.

[58] Arora S, Layek B, Singh J. Design and validation of liposomal ApoE2 gene delivery system to evade blood-brain barrier for effective treatment of Alzheimer's disease. Mol Pharmaceutics 2021;18(2):714–25.

[59] Qian Y, Zha Y, Feng B, et al. PEGylated poly(2-(dimethylamino) ethyl methacrylate)/DNA polyplex micelles decorated with phage-displayed TGN peptide for brain-targeted gene delivery. Biomaterials 2013;34(8):2117–29.

[60] Nussbaum ES. Diagnosis and management of carotid stenosis: a review. Minn Med 2000;83(1):45–9.

[61] Chibhabha F, Yang Y, Kuang Y, et al. Non-invasive optical imaging of retinal Aβ plaques using curcumin loaded polymeric micelles in APPswe/PS1ΔE9 transgenic mice for the diagnosis of Alzheimer's disease. Journal of Materials Chemistry B 2020;**8**:7438–52.

[62] Pathania A, Kumar R, Sandhir R. Hydroxytyrosol as anti-parkinsonian molecule: assessment using in-silico and MPTP-induced Parkinson's disease model. Biomed Pharmacother 2021;139:111525.

[63] Mursaleen L, Noble B, Somavarapu S, et al. Micellar nanocarriers of hydroxytyrosol are protective against Parkinson's related oxidative stress in an in vitro. Antioxidants 2021;10:887–905.

[64] Desai PP, Patravale VB. Curcumin cocrystal micelles-multifunctional nanocomposites for management of neurodegenerative ailments. J Pharm Sci 2018;107(4):1143–56.

[65] Oller-Salvia B, Sánchez-Navarro M, Giralt E, et al. Blood–brain barrier shuttle peptides: an emerging paradigm for brain delivery. Chem Soc Rev 2016;45(17):4690–707.

[66] Juan WX, Ping GY, Nan LN, et al. Endogenous polysialic acid based micelles for calmodulin antagonist delivery against vascular dementia. Applied Materials & Interfaces 2016;8(51):35045–58.

[67] Giuseppe A, Theodora T, Sara C, et al. Mesenchymal stromal cells loading curcumin-INVITE-micelles: a drug delivery system for neurodegenerative diseases. Colloids Surf B 2015;125:300–8.

[68] Scialabba C, Rocco F, Licciardi M, et al. Amphiphilic polyaspartamide copolymer-based micelles for rivastigmine delivery to neuronal cells. Informa Healthcare 2012;19(6):307–16.

[69] Mirzaie Z, Kordestani SS, Rezaei MH. Preparation and characterization of curcumin-loaded polymeric nanomicelles to interference with amyloidogenesis through glycation method. Biotechnol Appl Biochem 2019;66(4):537–44.

[70] Singh M, Thakur V, Deshmukh R, et al. Development and characterization of morin hydrate-loaded micellar nanocarriers for the effective management of Alzheimer's disease. 2018;35(2):137-148.

[71] Vong LB, Sato Y, Chonpathompikunlert P, et al. Self-assembled polydopamine nanoparticles improve treatment in Parkinson's disease model mice and suppress dopamine-induced dyskinesia. Acta Biomater 2020;109:220–8.

[72] Pappas TC, Bader AG, Andruss BF, et al. Applying small RNA molecules to the directed treatment of human diseases: realizing the potential. Expert Opin Ther Targets 2008;12(1):115–27.

[73] Shivdasani RA. MicroRNAs: regulators of gene expression and cell differentiation. Blood 2006;108(12):3646–53.

[74] Esquela-Kerscher A, Slack FJ. Oncomirs microRNAs with a role in cancer. Nat Rev Cancer 2006;6(4):259–69.

[75] Dhuria S, Hanson LR, Frey WH. Intranasal delivery to the central nervous system: Mechanisms and experimental considerations. J Pharm Sci 2010;99(4):1654–73.

[76] Kanazawa T, Akiyama F, Kakizaki S, et al. Delivery of siRNA to the brain using a combination of nose-to-brain delivery and cell-penetrating peptide-modified nano-micelles. Biomaterials 2013;34(36):9220–6.

[77] Li M, Hu K, Lin D, et al. Synthesis of Double Interfering Biodegradable Nano-MgO Micelle Composites and Their Effect on Parkinson's Disease. ACS Biomaterials Science & Engineering 2021;7(3):1216–29.

Chapter 9

Biologics for the management of dementia

Akash Chaurasiya, Sumeet Katke, Kanan Panchal, Jayabalan Nirmal
Translational Pharmaceutics Research Laboratory, Department of Pharmacy, Birla Institute of Technology and Science, Pilani, Hyderabad, India

9.1 Introduction

Dementia has become a common public health problem. The number of patients suffering from dementia is about 47 million worldwide, and the figures are expected to increase to 131 million by 2050 [11]. Dementia is a neuropathological syndrome of a chronic and progressive nature. The disease is represented by disturbances in the higher cortical functions such as memory, orientation, thinking, calculations, judgment, language, and comprehension. A typical characteristic of dementia is the impairment in the cognitive function along with deterioration in the emotional well-being and social behavior. Alzheimer's disease is the most common cause of dementia while other reasons include cerebrovascular diseases and dementia with Lewy bodies (DLB) [70].

Alzheimer's disease occurs in the elderly and the incidence increases with the advancing age. The known etiology for the Alzheimer's disease includes genetic factors and deposition of Aβ amyloid derived from amyloid precursor protein (APP) leading to formation of neuritic senile plaques and neurofibrillary tangles (Fig. 9.1). Neuritic senile plaques are the lesions consisting of a focal area with a central core containing Aβ amyloid and neurofibrillary tangle is a collection of neurofilaments and neurotubules within the cytoplasm of the neurons [68]. After Alzheimer's disease, cerebrovascular disease is a major contributor for the later-life dementia. Vascular dementia (VaD) arises as a loss of cognitive function due to cerebrovascular or cardiovascular disease. Atherosclerotic or arteriosclerotic mechanisms are most commonly involved in the pathogenesis of VaD. Most commonly, VaD is caused by small-vessel occlusions with multiple lacunas and by hypoperfusive lesions as a result of stenosis of medullary arterioles. Also, macrovascular diseases in the form of large vessel infarcts have also been reported as a cause of VaD [104]. DLB is a result of abnormal proteolytic processing and accumulation of the alpha-synuclein protein in the brain. Alpha-synuclein aggregation induces an inflammatory

Nanomedicine-Based Approaches for the Treatment of Dementia. https://doi.org/10.1016/B978-0-12-824331-2.00001-7
Copyright © 2023 Elsevier Inc. All rights reserved.

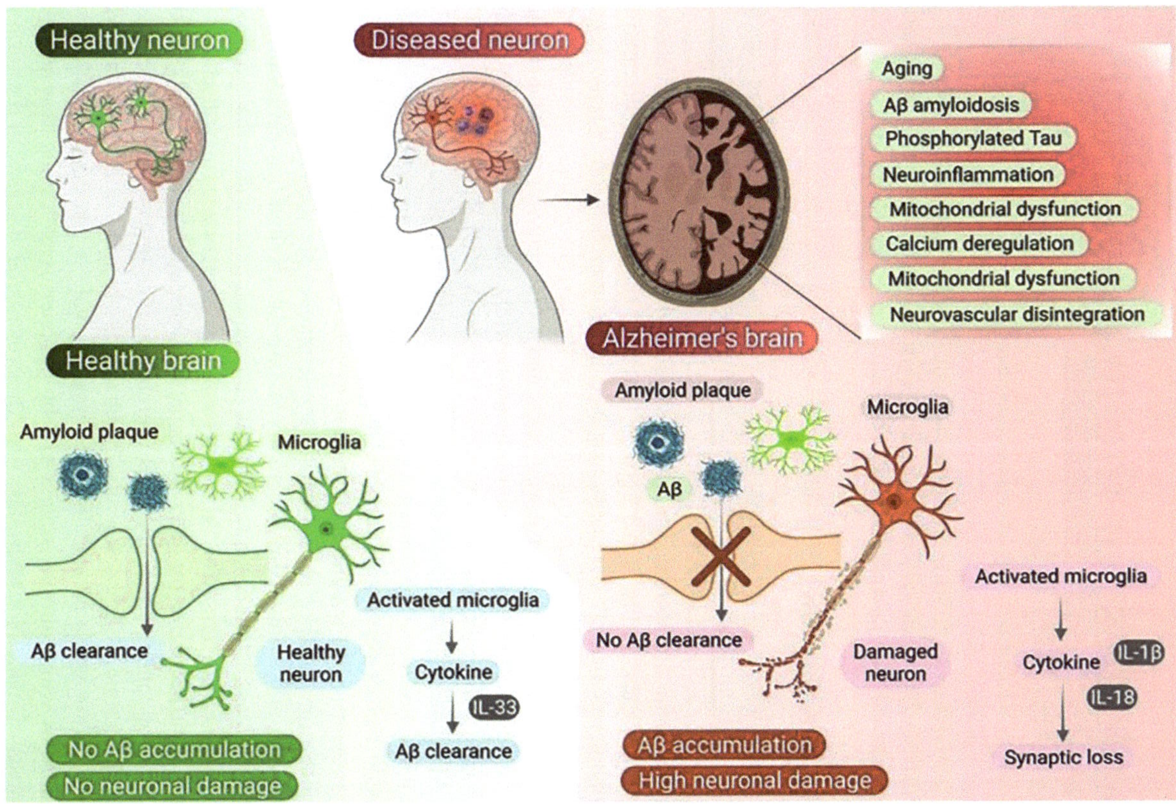

FIG. 9.1 Pathophysiology of Alzheimer's Disease. Image adopted from: Prasanna, P., Rathee, S., Rahul, V., Mandal, D., Chandra Goud, M. S., Yadav, P., Hawthorne, S., et al. (2021). Microfluidic platforms to unravel mysteries of Alzheimer's disease: how far have we come? Life, 11(10), 1022. MDPI AG. Retrieved from http://dx.doi.org/10.3390/life11101022 [184].

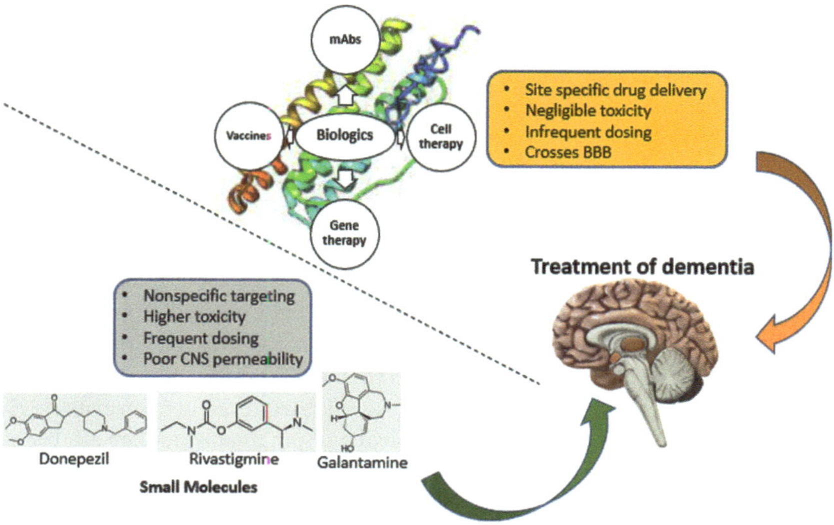

FIG. 9.2 Various approaches for dementia treatment.

response that promotes oxidative damage. This results in the dysregulation of ubiquitin-proteasome system responsible for the protein catabolism leading to neurodegeneration through apoptosis [66]. Recently, additional risk factors such as excessive consumption of alcohol, traumatic brain injury, and air pollution have been reported that may cause dementia. Since the risk of dementia increases with the increasing age, the number of people suffering from dementia is projected to rise because of the improving life expectancy of the population in both developed and developing countries due to betterment in medical treatments and nutrition [143].

Biological therapeutics or biologicals in simple term refers to those medicines which are derived from large-scale cell-cultures of bacteria, yeast, and cells from plant or animal origin. Biologicals are distinguished from the other medicines because these are usually proteins purified from blood or living culture systems whereas other medicines are considered small molecules usually manufactured synthetically or purified from plants [177]. Over the past few years, advancements have been made in understanding the disease pathogenesis and the underlying immune system. This has led to the development of biologic therapies consisting of monoclonal antibodies and fusion proteins. Diseases involving an underlying immune pathogenesis can be treated when the monoclonal antibodies or the fusion proteins are used to target the specific immune components, thus reducing the complications and improving the effectiveness compared to the conventional treatments [97]. Currently, with the progress in the field of biotechnology and advent of modern hybridoma technology, biologics are the fastest growing class of therapeutic class of drugs and surpassing the growth of small molecules. As drugs, biologics serve several advantages over the small molecules. Biological molecules are target-specific and unlike small molecules do not induce nontarget harmful side effects (Fig. 9.2). The biological drug products include a range of compounds from biological origin such as cytokines, peptides, nucleic acids, monoclonal antibodies, and recombinant proteins. Each of these biological moieties serve a specific purpose and are utilized accordingly. Biological products represent the highly advanced biomedical research and may offer effective means for the treatment of diseases that presently have no other treatments available [171]. These drug products have already proven their potential in critical disease areas such as cancer and have continued to fulfill unmet medical needs of the patients. Several biological drug products have been approved by USFDA like Bevencio, Imfinizi, Hemlibra, and Siliq along with cell therapies, such as Kymriah and Yescarta [93].

In recent years, the potential of biologics is also explored in neuropathological conditions like dementia. Several clinical and preclinical studies are being carried out to investigate the efficacy and safety of biologics for the treatment of dementia, Alzheimer's disease, etc. Aducanumab, a biological drug product has been successfully commercialized and is marketed as Aduhelm, showing the potential of biologics in the treatment of neuropathological conditions [169]. This chapter highlights the application of biologics for dementia treatment, their mechanism of action, and the key advantages of nanotechnology-based biological products for the management of these neuropathological conditions.

9.2 Existing treatments

There exists to be no drug in particular that is used for the complete mitigation of dementia. However, its causative indications like Alzheimer's, Parkinson's, and other diseases are being treated with some commonly prescribed drugs of both synthetic and natural origin [69]. **Memantine** is an N-Methyl-D-aspartate (NMDA) receptor antagonist used for the symptomatic treatment of Alzheimer's disease and for mitigating the symptoms of dementia [96]. On the other hand, **Tacrine** and its derivative **Velnacrine** are centrally acting cholinesterase inhibitors and are used to treat Alzheimer's disease. They act against monoamines and ion channels and also inhibit histamine N-methyltransferase [159]. Of these small molecules, **Donepezil**, an acetylcholinesterase inhibitor, is the leading medication used for the treatment of Alzheimer's disease. It is a piperidine derivative that reversibly binds to acetylcholinesterase and inhibits the hydrolysis of acetylcholine, thereby increasing the availability of acetylcholine at the synapses and thus enhancing cholinergic transmission [105]. For the treatment of dementia associated with Parkinson's disease, **Rivastigmine** is used. It is a semisynthetic derivative of the toxic alkaloid physostigmine which acts by covalently binding to active sites of both acetylcholinesterase and butyrylcholinesterase and thus inhibiting these enzymes and blocking their function [99,123]. There also exist several compounds of natural origin, described in Table 9.1, used for the treatment of dementia. Of many natural products, terpenoids are

TABLE 9.1 Natural compounds used for the treatment of dementia (Ref are cited in section 2).

Class	Source	Activity	References
Natural alkaloids			
Huperzine A	*Huperzia serrata, H. elmeri, H. carinata, H. aqualupian*	Acetylcholinesterase inhibitor	[111,115]
Galantamine	*Galanthus woronowii, Galanthus nivalis var. gracilis*	Anti- AD and dementia treatment	[106,124]
Physostigmine	Calabar beans	Cholinesterase inhibitor	[69]
Oxoassoamine	Leaves of *Narcissus assoanus, Sansevieria liberica, Talinum triangulare*	Anti- AD and dementia treatment, cholinesterase inhibitor	[17,90,91,122]
Assoanine		Cholinesterase inhibition in sensile dementia	
Voacangine, Rupicoline	Stalk of *Tabernaemontana australis*	Cholinesterase inhibitor	[8]
Hericerin, Erinacerin A, Hericenone B, Erinacene D	*Hericium erinaceum*	Dementia treatment	[69]
Moenjodaramine	Leaves of *Buxus papillosa*	Anti- AD and dementia treatment	[14]
Buxamine B	*Buxus macowanii*		
Natural terpenoids			
Ursolic acid pentacyclic (triterpenoids)	Leaves of *Bouvardia ternifolia, Cestrum diurnum, Funtumia latifolia, Mirabilis jalapa, Retanilla ephedra, Thymus vulgaris, Verbena stricta, Vinca minor, Nerium oleander, Salvia officinalis,* and seeds of *Cornus officinalis*	Anti- AD and dementia treatment	[31]

(Continued)

TABLE 9.1 Cont'd

Class	Source	Activity	References
Celastrol pentacyclic (triterpenoids)	Roots of *Tripterygium wilfordii, Celastrus regelii, C. hypoleucus,* Maytenus chuchuhuasca		[5]
α-onocerin	*Lycopodium clavatum, L. clavatum, L. selago, L. annotinum, L. alpinum, and L. complanatum ssp. chamaecyparissus*	Acetylcholinesterase inhibitor	[129]
Withaferin A (steroidal lactone)	Leaves and roots of *Acnistus arborescens, Withania somnifera*	Dementia treatment	[19]
Sitoindosidest IX	Leaves of *Withania somnifera*	Anti- AD and dementia treatment	
Carnosic acid (diterpene)	*Rosmarinus officinalis, Salvia officinalis*	Anti- AD and dementia treatment, cholinesterase inhibitor	[118]
Cryptotanshinone (diterpenoid)	Leaves and roots of *Salvia miltiorrhiza*	Anti- AD and dementia treatment	[142]
Dihydrotanshinone I	*Salvia miltiorrhiza*		[182]

AD, Alzheimer's disease.

the largest and most diverse group of organic compounds used to treat dementia. **Galantamine** is a tertiary alkaloid that is used to treat patients with VaD or Alzheimer's disease with cerebrovascular disease. This drug demonstrates a broad-spectrum and long-term efficacy in AD by competitively inhibiting acetylcholinesterase. Galantamine is a moderate and reversible inhibitor that allosterically modulates nicotinic acetylcholine receptors (nAChR) [84]. Of these, only five drugs have been approved by the USFDA for treating dementia of the mild-moderate stage of Alzheimer's disease symptomatically. Four of these are cholinesterase inhibitors, namely, tacrine, donepezil, rivastigmine, and galantamine, whereas memantine is an NMDA receptor antagonist [27].

Despite the drugs being clinically approved for this indication, there are several setbacks to this therapeutic scheme questioning their holistic effectiveness. These setbacks are either because of the chemical nature of the compound or the inherent physiology of the target tissue or due to the limitations of the drug formulation. As cholinesterase inhibitors increase the overall activity of acetylcholine in the peripheral nervous system, it contributes to several side effects. The common side effects include GIT upset, nausea, and diarrhea, whereas the lesser common ones are syncope, muscular weakness, and drastic weight loss [9,21]. Peripheral cholinergic side effects are more evident in patients receiving rivastigmine therapy [95]. A specific side effect associated with tacrine is the significant liver toxicity caused by it. Because of this very reason tacrine is now not being prescribed [138]. Besides the limitations associated with the drug molecules, drawbacks are also associated with the drug formulation. As these drugs are administered as oral tablets and capsules, their systemic delivery to the brain in therapeutic concentrations due to poor delivery remains a significant problem. Also, extensive first-pass metabolism reduces their half-life and overall effectiveness, and access to nontarget peripheral tissues poses additional side effects [163]. Even if the drug concentration crosses the therapeutic threshold within the systemic circulation, its absorption in the brain tissue is challenging. This is due to the blood–brain barrier (BBB), which impedes the drug influx inside the brain via the lipid cell membranes, tight junctions, and efflux systems such as the ABC efflux transporters [151].

As physiology cannot be altered, a shift from the conventional therapeutic compounds and drug delivery systems becomes extremely important in managing dementia. Various types of biologics like proteins, peptides, and antibodies are gaining importance for the treatment of dementia due to their increased efficacy and fewer side effects [63]. Aducanumab (Aduhelm), a human monoclonal antibody, is the first novel therapy approved by the USFDA in 2021 for the treatment of Alzheimer's disease [126,172]. Few other biologics like gantenerumab (human anti-amyloid β antibody), lecanemab (anti-amyloid β protofibril antibody), bapineuzumab (humanized monoclonal antibody), donanemab (humanized IgG1 monoclonal antibody), crenezumab (anti-amyloid β monoclonal antibody), and solanezumab (anti-amyloid monoclonal antibody) are being investigated under the phase 3 clinical trials [25,38,41,46,51,62,79,157]. Certain immunoglobulins like gammagard, gamunex, flebogamma have also proven their worth against cognitive impairment [103]. Additionally, proteins like cerebroprotein hydrolysate and multimodal neuropeptides like cerebrolysin are in the pipeline and are upcoming biologics to treat dementia and cognitive disorders [6,28]. These agents are shown to have better benefits over the risks of the current therapy because of their biological nature and direct action on the amyloid plaques.

Moreover, a nanotherapeutic approach to deliver these drugs is proving to be revolutionary for the treatment of cognitive impairments. Nanosystems prove to be promising as they can be chemically modified for selective targeting to bring about brain-specific activity and also help overcome the BBB. Furthermore, their property confers a desirable drug release pattern and protects the active agent from any enzymatic degradation, thus increasing its overall bioavailability and reducing the therapeutic dosage regimen. The carrier-based systems also minimize the off-target side-effects of the active molecules and thereby improve the patient's quality of life [100]. Thus, the gradual shift of the spectrum of medications from small molecules to biologics, from its conventional dosing to a finer nanosystemic dosing, is valuable and dynamic for the treatment and mitigation of dementia.

9.3 Biological drug product-based approaches

Biological drug products are also known as immunomodulators because they stimulate the body's immune system to act against certain targets in the body, hence treatment with biologics is also termed as immunotherapy. Depending on the manner in which these biological drug products interact in-vivo, they are classified into active and passive immunization. Active immunization involves the stimulation of body's immune system to produce specific antibodies by administration of antigens. Whereas in the case of passive immunization, antibodies are directly administered into the host that eliminates the need for production of own antibodies by the host [139]. In recent years, biologics-based drug products like antibodies, gene therapy, vaccines, etc., gained considerable importance for treating dementia due to their increased efficacy and fewer side effects. Various biological drug products have been explored preclinically and clinically to identify their potential in dementia treatment (Table 9.2). In this section, various types of biological products as investigated and approved for these neuropathological conditions are discussed.

9.3.1 Monoclonal antibodies

B cells produce the monoclonal antibodies (mAbs) and they specifically target the antigen. Initially, hybridoma technique as developed by Köhler and Milstein was used to obtain mouse mAbs in large amounts [114]. In recent time due to the technological advancements, the production of mAbs has transitioned from mouse, through chimeric, and humanized to fully humanized mAbs with a significant reduction in the immunogenic reaction of mouse components, which thereby also accelerated the basic research and clinical use of mAbs. These protein therapeutics serve advantages like high specificity, longer half-lives, precise action, and reduced frequency of dosing over the conventional small molecules [85]. They are structurally similar to immunoglobulin G (IgG) and mimic the function of a natural IgG in the body. They bind to the pathogens, extraceullular targets cells, or foreign bodies to effectively neutralize and clear them from the circulation [160].

The mAbs that have been designed to treat Alzheimer's disease or dementia are either "humanized mAbs" or "fully humanized mAbs." Passive immunization with mAbs clears the toxic amyloid-β species directly or through microglia or compliment activation. The microglial activation causes the phagocytosis of the deposited plaque. This clearance halts the amyloid cascade thus preventing the neurodegeneration and cognitive and functional decline. In this section, we shall discuss the mAbs that are available commercially or under clinical evaluation for the treatment of neurodegeneration and cognitive decline [147].

TABLE 9.2 Biologics drug product for dementia treatment.

Sr. No.	Novel drug	Innovator	Mechanism of action	Development status	References
Monoclonal antibody					
1.	JNJ-63733657	Janssen Research & Development, LLC	Humanized mAb, binds to phosphorylated tau, increases its clearance and slows AD progression.	Clinical Phase 2	[55]
2.	Gantenerumab	Hoffmann-La Roche	Humanized mAb, binds to aggregated Aβ and removes aggregated plaque by FCγ receptor mediated phagocytosis	Clinical Phase 3	[53]
3.	Solanezumab	Eli Lilly & Co.	Humanized mAb, binds to mid domain of the Aβ peptide, increases clearance of Aβ and slows AD progression.	Clinical Phase 3	[45]
4.	Pepinemab	Vaccinex Inc.	Humanized IgG4 mAb, inhibits semaphorin 4D (SEMA4D), blocks the neuroinflammation and slows neurodegeneration.	Clinical Phase 2	[54,136]
5.	Gosuranemab (BIIB092)	Biogen	Humanized anti-tau mAb, targets N-terminal tau, helps its clearance from the brain and slows neurological taupathies.	Clinical Phase 2	[49]
6.	TB006	TrueBinding, Inc.	A protein called Galectin-3 (Gal3) is abnormally present in higher levels in the brains of Alzheimer's patients. Gal3 binds to Aβ and acts as a glue to form toxic plaques. TB006, a humanized mAb, binds to Gal3 and prevents it from acting as a glue thus inhibiting the disease progression.	Clinical Phase 1	[58,165]
7.	Bapineuzumab	Pfizer Inc.	Humanized mAb, binds to N-terminal residues of Aβ peptides thus decreases the neurotoxicity caused by these peptides and further fibrillogenesis.	Clinical Phase 3	[40,101]

(Continued)

TABLE 9.2 Cont'd

Sr. No.	Novel drug	Innovator	Mechanism of action	Development status	References
8.	Ponezumab (PF-04360365)	Pfizer Inc.	Humanized IgG2Δa mAb, binds to soluble peptides of Aβ by targeting specific amino acids (30-40) in the C-terminus of the Aβ sequence.	Clinical Phase 1	[37,107]
9.	MEDI1814	AstraZeneca & Eli Lilly	Humanized mAb, selectively binds to Aβ-42, a form of Aβ responsible for neurodegeneration and helps its clearance from the brain.	Clinical Phase 1	[13,44]
10.	Crenezumab	Genentech Inc.	Humanized mAb with an IgG4 backbone. Higher affinity of binding toward oligomeric and fibrillar form of Aβ than monomeric Aβ. Stimulates Aβ phagocytosis and limits the release of cytokines thus preventing neurological inflammation and progression of disease.	Clinical Phase 3	[47,65]
11.	Donanemab	Eli Lilly & Co.	Humanized IgG1 mAb, recognizes and binds to pyroglutamate form of Aβ, Aβ(p3-42), that is aggregated in plaques. Helps in clearing the deposited Aβ plaques from the brain.	Clinical Phase 3	[59,74]
12.	Canakinumab	Novartis	Interleukin-1β (IL-1β) blocker, approved by USFDA for the treatment of autoimmune disorders such as Cryopyrin-Associated Periodic Syndromes (CAPS) and Familial Mediterranean Fever (FMF). It has been reported that treatment with anti-IL-1β biologics relieves proinflammatory action of amyloidosis and tau phosphorylation.	Clinical Phase 2	[16,60]
13.	Aducanumab (Aduhelm)	Biogen	Humanized IgG1 mAb, binds preferentially to aggregated parenchymal forms of Aβ in the brain.	Commercially available as Aduhelm	[2,169]

Sr. No.	Novel drug	Innovator	Mechanism of action	Development status	References
Gene therapy					
14.	PBFT02	Passage Bio Inc.	Patients with GRN mutations show reduced levels of progranulin, a protein essential for normal neuronal survival. PBFT01 is an adeno-associated viral vector serotype 1 carrying the gene encoding for human progranulin, helping in elevation of progranulin.	Clinical Phase 2	[56,87]
15	AAV-hTERT	Libella Gene Therapeutics	It has been reported that human gene, human telomerase reverse transcriptase improves neuronal health. Adeno associated virus (AAV) mediated gene therapy of human telomerase reverse transcriptase (hTERT) is hypothesized to affect the tau pathologies in the human hippocampus tissue thus supporting good neuronal health.	Clinical Phase 1	[52,127]
16	AAV2-BDNF	Mark Tuszynski, University of California, San Diego	AAV2- vector directed gene to express Brain Derived Neurotrophic Factor (BDNF) is expected to prevent the loss of neurons of the brain and activate the cells that have not yet deteriorated.	Clinical Phase 1	[61]
17	LX1001	Lexeo Therapeutics	The agent utilizes AAVrh.10hAPOE2, serotype rh.10 adeno-associated virus (AAV) gene transfer vector expressing the cDNA that codes for the human apolipoprotein E2 (APOE2) gene and is targeted toward APOE4 homozygotes in the CNS. The gene therapy is meant to convert APOE4 homozygotes to dual APOE2-APOE4 alleles on chromosome 19.	Clinical Phase 1	[48]

(Continued)

TABLE 9.2 Cont'd

Sr. No.	Novel drug	Innovator	Mechanism of action	Development status	References
18	Human Nerve Growth Factor (NGF)	The Shiley Family Trust	NGF potentially stimulates cell function and prevents neuronal death and further neurodegeneration. In this study, patients were screened for mild cognitive impairment, and skin biopsies would be obtained to produce cultures of primary, autologous fibroblasts. These fibroblasts were genetically modified to produce and secrete NGF molecules and injected into the patients through intracerebral route.	Clinical Phase 1	[35]
19	Intraparenchymal rAAV1 - (mi)RNA HTT	Voyager Therapeutics	Huntington's disease is an inherited disorder resulting in progressive neurodegeneration leading to cognitive dysfunction. The agent, VY-HTT01 is a gene therapy for designed to reduce the expression of huntingtin gene (HTT) thus altering the disease progression by knocking down the levels of HTT mRNA.	Clinical Phase 1	[57,173]
20	CERE-110	Ceregene	The agent is an adeno-associated virus-based delivery of gene expressing for NGF to treat the symptoms of Alzheimer's disease and progressive dementia.	Clinical Phase 1	[36]
Vaccine					
21	AFFITOPE AD02	Affiris AG	The agent is a synthetic peptide of 6 amino acids mimicking the N-terminus of Aβ. The innovator hypothesizes that the fragment will enable the recognition of Aβ and allow the production of anti-Aβ antibodies while minimizing the proinflammatory response by the host.	Clinical Phase 2	[3,42]

Sr. No.	Novel drug	Innovator	Mechanism of action	Development status	References
22	AADvac1	Axon Neuroscience SE	The agent is a synthetic peptide derived from tau sequences that are directed against tau proteins involved in pathological conditions of Alzheimer's disease. The agent is expected to produce the antibodies that reduce the neurofibrillary tangles, clear the phosphorylated tau protein and reduce the insoluble and oligomerized tau from the brain.	Clinical Phase 1	[43]
23	UB 311	United Biomedical	The agent consists of two synthetic $A\beta_{1-14}$ targeting peptides (B-cell isotope) linked to helper T-cell epitopes (UBITh) and formulated as Th2 delivery system. The agent induces strong immune response against the Aβ oligomers and reduces the plaque load from the CNS	Clinical Phase 2	[39]
24	Lu AF20513	H. Lundbeck A/S	The agent has been designed to overcome the weak immune system of geriatric population while avoiding the autoimmune responses of the host. Lu AF20513 is a mixed-peptide engineered agent where the epitope is the three repeats of first 12 amino acids of the Aβ peptide followed with the sequence of tetanus vaccine. This stimulates nonself-memory T-cells of the elderly patients to activate a B-cell response to produce polyclonal antibodies against Aβ.	Clinical Phase 1	[50,113]

9.3.1.1 *Bapineuzumab*

Bapineuzumab is a humanized prototypical mAb against the Aβ N-terminus. Bapineuzumab is an IgG1 antibody and by binding to the fibrillar and soluble Aβ results in its elimination through activation of microglial phagocytosis and cytokine production [15]. In the animal studies, the murine form of the antibody (3D6) was demonstrated to bind to fibrillar, monomeric, and oligomeric forms of Aβ, which lower the amount of Aβ in the brain and thereby improve the memory in transgenic mice. In clinical evaluation conducted by Janssen/Pfizer, the results from Phase 2 studies demonstrated a greater reduction in the amyloid on positron-emission tomographic amyloid imaging and reduced cerebrospinal fluid phosphorylated tau (phospho-tau), suggesting target engagement and attenuated neurodegeneration. In the subsequent clinical Phase 3 studies, discouraging results were obtained as no benefit in terms of clinical outcomes was observed though the biomarker results demonstrated that bapineuzumab could modify Aβ accumulation and phospho-tau, a downstream biomarker [148].

9.3.1.2 *Solanezumab*

Another mAb that has been evaluated under a clinical setting is Solanezumab developed by Eli Lilly. Solanezumab is a humanized mAb that binds to the mid domain of the Aβ peptide and slows down the neurodegeneration by increasing the clearance of soluble Aβ from the brain. In preclinical studies, formation of high-affinity antibody-Aβ peptide complexes was demonstrated resulting in a "peripheral sink" or in simple words, the efflux of Aβ from the brain to plasma, thus subsequently improved the cognitive performance in transgenic mouse models of neurodegenerative Alzheimer's disease [175]. A clinical study was carried out to evaluate the safety and tolerability along with the pharmacokinetic behavior of a single dose of solanezumab in subjects with mild to moderate Alzheimer's disease. The findings demonstrated that solanezumab is very well tolerated. In addition, robust plasma and dose-dependent CSF Aβ responses were obtained, suggesting a reduced pace of clinical progression of the disease [156].

9.3.1.3 *Gantenerumab*

Gantenerumab is a humanized anti-Aβ mAb that binds to both, an N-terminal and a mid-region epitope, on Aβ folded into a fibrillar conformation. The mechanism of action of gantenerumab is through glial recruitment and phagocytosis of the plaque resulting in its final burden into the brain. In preclinical studies carried onto the transgenic mice, the results demonstrated the binding of mAb to the cerebral Aβ and significant reduction in the cerebral plaques. Microglial phagocytosis of the fibrillar plaque from the brain was confirmed since the lysosomes showed internalized Aβ [64]. A clinical study was conducted to find out the mechanism of amyloid removal in the patients suffering from neurodegeneration related to Alzheimer's disease. The findings demonstrated that gantenerumab resulted in dose-dependent reduction in the brain amyloid level through an effector-cell mediated mechanism of action. Also, the drug was found to be very well tolerated in patients with very minor incidences of inflammation and vasogenic edema in category of subjects with highest dose. A phase 3 clinical study was carried out on subjects with prodromal Alzheimer's disease, that is, subjects with an early finding of biomarkers indicating disease burden and cognitive symptoms before reaching a clinical stage of dementia. The results were discouraging as there was a lack of efficacy of the treatment compared to the placebo, though the reduction in amyloid levels was observed. These results suggest that despite reduction in the amyloid levels at the minimum concentration of the drug, higher clinical dosing with gantenerumab is necessary to achieve clinical efficacy [131].

9.3.1.4 Crenezumab

Crenezumab is a fully humanized anti-Aβ mAb licensed by AC immune and genentech has a unique ability to bind to the multiple forms of Aβ such as soluble, fibrillar, and oligomeric. Unlike any other anti-Aβ developed for the Aβ immunotherapy, this mAb belongs to the IgG4 class. This novel approach of imparting IgG4 backbone to the molecule results in reduced activation of FcγRs in comparison to the IgG1. The reduced activation of FcγRs minimizes the inflammation of microglia caused by FcγRs mediated pathway, along with preserved microglial phagocytosis of the Aβ oligomers. Along with reduced toxicity, this isoform of IgG binds to multiple forms of Aβ like soluble, fibrillar, and oligomeric. Results from the in-vitro studies suggested that crenezumab has the ability to induce disaggregation of Aβ oligomers and reduce the oligomer-induced neurotoxicity. This novel mechanism of action and broad binding affinity of the mAb to Aβ suggested it to be a potential candidate for clinical evaluation [168]. The Phase 1 clinical studies demonstrated a good safety and tolerability profile for the drug, leading to further clinical Phase 2 studies [34]. The results from Phase 2 clinical trials showed failure to meet the coprimary end points of reduction in cognitive decline and functional global decline. Further Phase 3 clinical trials that used doses four times higher than that studied in the Phase 2 trials showed discouraging results again. This drug is also studied in individuals with an autosomal dominant mutation who are at risk to develop familial Alzheimer's disease [145].

9.3.1.5 Aducanumab

Aducanumab is a humanized Aβ directed mAb approved through accelerated approval pathway by USFDA for the treatment of Alzheimer's disease or mild dementia, originally developed by neurimmune and is marketed as Aduhelm by Biogen Inc. So far, aducanumab is the first-of-its-kind treatment approved by USFDA for the treatment of Alzheimer's disease [169]. This commercially successful mAb was developed using an antibody-based therapeutic approach by selecting human B-cell clones which get activated by the neo-epitopes present on the pathological Aβ aggregates (Fig. 9.3). The human memory B-cells were screened for their reactivity for aggregated Aβ including soluble oligomers and insoluble fibrils. In the preclinical studies, it was observed that the aducanumab could penetrate the (BBB), targeting the amyloid plaques and clearing it from the transgenic mouse brains. These results encouraged the investigators to proceed for clinical evaluation of the drug molecule [154]. The clinical studies were conducted on 3482 patients with Alzheimer's disease in three separate studies consisting of double-blind, placebo-controlled, randomized, and dose-ranging manner. The results from clinical evaluations suggested that patients receiving the treatment had significant reduction in the Aβ-amyloid in dose and time-dependent manner whereas the control group of patients had no reduction in the Aβ-amyloid plaque. Based on the surrogate endpoint of reduction of Aβ-plaque from the brain, the data from clinical trials supported the FDA's decision of accelerated approval of Aduhelm.

9.3.1.6 Donanemab

Donanemab, also known as N3pG, is a humanized IgG1 mAb derived from the mouse mE8-IgG2a. The biological drug molecule binds to pyroglutamate form of Aβ, which is the aggregated form of the Aβ amyloid plaque by recognizing the Aβ(p3-42). As we have already discussed, most of the mAbs currently under development or the approved one, aducanumab acting on Aβ amyloid bind to the soluble or insoluble components but have a very low affinity toward the deposited plaques, resulting in only partial removal of the Aβ amyloid from the CNS and limited therapeutic benefit. The rationale behind the development of donanemab was targeting the deposited plaque rather than merely removing the existing amyloid load from the brain. Previously studied, mAbs studied for the removal of amyloid bodies caused microhemorrhages in the brain and therefore were abandoned during development stating the safety reasons. Unlike other drug molecules, donanemab was reported to clear plaques in the mice without causing the microhemorrhages and encouraged the investigator, Lilly, to proceed for clinical studies. A clinical Phase 1 study was carried out on 100 people to study the safety, tolerability, and pharmacodynamics with mild cognitive impairment, followed by a clinical Phase 1 with a larger population of 150 patients with prodromal Alzheimer's disease. Results from both these clinical trials suggested that the amyloid burden from these patients reduced significantly [75]. Later, in Phase 2 studies conducted on 257 patients, significant reductions in the amyloid plaque level and the global tau load compared to the placebo was observed in the cohort receiving donanemab [119]. The investigator, Lilly announced the USFDA has granted breakthrough therapy designation for donanemab in June 2021 on the basis of results from the Phase 2 studies.

9.3.1.7 Canakinumab

Canakinumab is a human anti-Interleukin-1β (anti-IL-1β) mAb of the IgG1/κ isotype developed by Novartis [72]. Its works by neutralization of IL-1β signaling

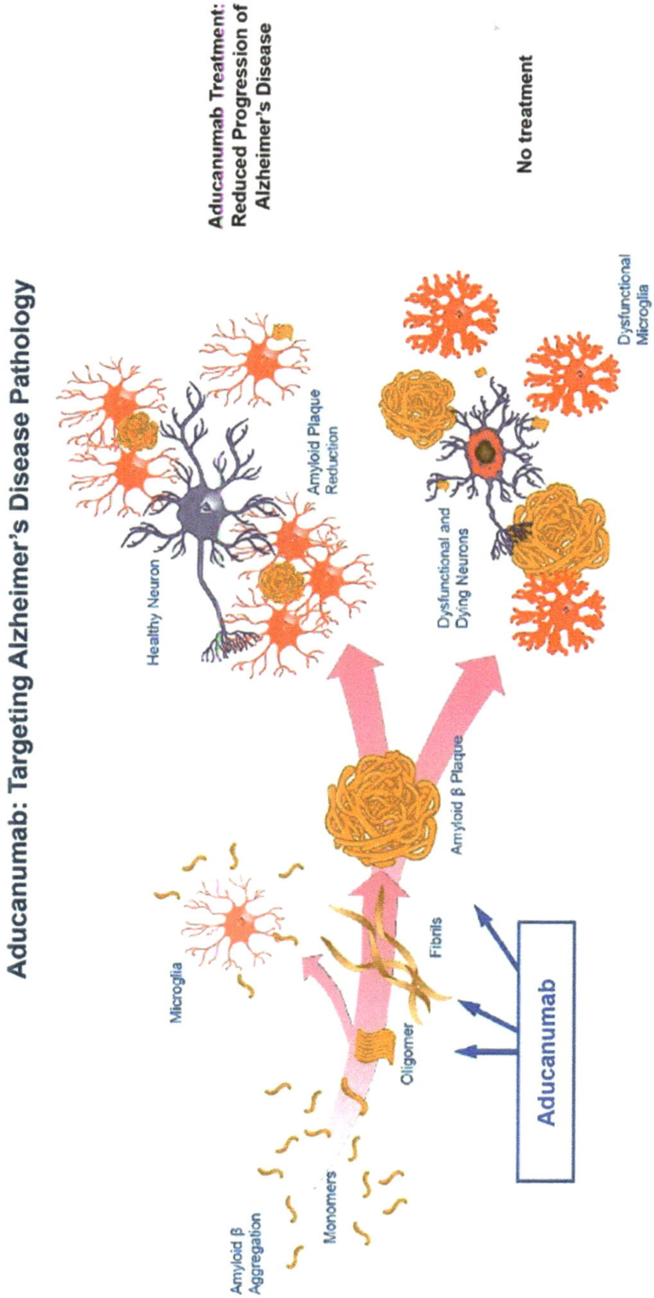

FIG. 9.3 Mechanism of action of Aducanumab. Image adopted from: Esang M, Gupta M (August 31, 2021) Aducanumab as a novel treatment for Alzheimer's disease: a decade of hope, controversies, and the future. Cureus 13(8): e17591. doi:10.7759/cureus.17591 [185].

which decreases inflammation in patients with autoimmune disorders. It was approved by USFDA in 2009 for the treatment of cryopyrin-associated periodic syndromes, tumor necrosis factor receptor-associated periodic syndrome, hyperimmunoglobulin D syndrome/mevalonate kinase deficiency and familial Mediterranean fever [170]. It has been reported that autoimmune diseases such as psoriasis, rheumatoid arthritis, and inflammatory bowel disease heighten the risk of Alzheimer's disease. TNF blocking agents are approved for the treatment of such autoimmune disorders. Studies have demonstrated that patients treated for autoimmune disorders with TNF blocking agents have a decreased risk of Alzheimer's disease compared to the general population [164]. In a study, patients treated with adalimumab demonstrated a reduced risk of neurodegeneration-related cognitive disorder [183]. On the basis of this supporting data, clinical study is being carried out by Novartis to evaluate the effect of anti-inflammatory agent such as canakinumab on cognition in early Alzheimer's disease [32].

9.3.2 Gene therapy

Gene therapy has various advantages as it is a delivery system and makes it an ideal strategy for treating the neurological disorders. Larger molecules like proteins and antibodies face the hurdle of BBB. However, in case of gene therapy, we can administer the gene through a delivery carrier such as a virus, and directly target the brain cells to modify the genetic defects via gene transduction and reduce the manifestation of the neurological disease. Another advantage of the gene therapy is the persistence of expression of proteins, so the therapy is needed to be administered only once making it very safe and effective [141]. Researchers have identified some specific genes, responsible for developing these cognitive disorders. Therefore, these targets have been evaluated as potential gene therapy-based strategies for the management of dementia.

9.3.2.1 Apolipoprotein E

Apolipoprotein E (APOE) is a protein that regulates metabolism and transport of lipids like cholesterol and triglycerides. Inside the brain, APOE is majorly expressed in the astrocytes and microglia and plays an important function of the delivery of lipoproteins to the neurons. APOE gene has been identified as one of the risk factors for developing the disease. Three different alleles of the APOE gene have been identified and the risk of developing the disease depends on which one is inherited.

1. APOE2: rarest of the alleles, reduces the risk of developing Alzheimer's disease by up to 40%.
2. APOE3: most common allele, does not affect the risk of developing Alzheimer's disease.
3. APOE4: reported to increase the risk of developing Alzheimer's disease along with lowering the age of onset of the disease.

The APOE4 protein increases the risk of developing neurodegenerative disorder like Alzheimer's disease because it prevents the clearance of Aβ plaques from the CNS and promotes it aggregation [89]. APOE4 induces the Aβ fibrillization to a greater extent compared to the other two isoforms which lead to high incidence of neuronal dysfunction and neurodegeneration.

It has been reported that cholesterol levels in the brain in Alzheimer's disease is lower compared to normal, therefore, it can be hypothesized that gene therapy directed toward APOE will help to manifest the APOE-related pathologies [125]. A gene delivery study was conducted on PDAPP transgenic mice, in which the three isoforms of APOE were gene-transferred using a lentiviral vector. The results demonstrated that the transgenic mice lacking in murine APOE showed increased Aβ burden after gene delivery of human APOE4 gene, while the other two isoforms, APOE2 and APOE3 did not affect the in-vivo Aβ levels. Also, it was reported that direct intracerebral gene-transfer of APOE2 through lentiviral vector dramatically reduced the hippocampal Aβ burden when compared with mice administered with other two lentiviral vector constructs. Thus, the data clearly suggest that gene delivery of human APOE2 may prevent and reduce the burden of Aβ in the brain followed by formation of plaques leading to dementia related to the Alzheimer's disease [73]. On the similar grounds, in one of the studies, transferrin and penetratin tagged liposomes were formulated for APOE2 targeted gene therapy. The in-vitro studies to evaluate the ability of the liposomes to cross BBB and transfect neuronal cells were carried out on triple coculture BBB model and the results showed enhanced transfection efficiency and penetration of BBB by the dual surface-modified liposomes. Also, in-vivo studies demonstrated enhanced APOE2 levels in the brain after intravenous administration of these dual surface-modified liposomes encapsulating the APOE2 [76].

9.3.2.2 *Endothelin-converting enzyme*

Endothelin-converting enzyme (ECE) is a membrane-integrated metalloproteinase that has an extracellular zinc-binding active site. As the name suggests, ECEs are characterized by their potential to hydrolyze big endothelins and biologically inactive intermediates. In the CNS, ECE is present in the cortex and hippocampus region along with other areas such as substantia nigra and Purkinje cells in the cerebellum. Three isoforms of ECE have been identified so far, ECE-1, ECE-2, and ECE-3. Unlike the other two isoforms, ECE-3 is not present in the CNS and is mostly found in the erythroid tissue [132]. In one of the studies, it has been identified that ECE-1 can degrade Aβ in both in-vitro and in-vivo conditions. In the in-vitro study, treatment of endogenous ECE-expressing cell lines with the ECE metalloprotease inhibitor, phosphoramidon, caused 2–3 times elevation in the extracellular Aβ levels due to reduction in the intracellular Aβ degradation. Further, in the in-vivo study, overexpression of ECE-1 in the Chinese Hamster Ovary cells lacking endogenous ECE activity, significantly reduced the extracellular Aβ concentration and this effect was completely reversed by treatment of the cells with phosphoramidon [78]. These results suggest that ECE-1 is capable of hydrolyzing Aβ and reducing its concentration, which may help to ameliorate the in-vivo neurodegeneration. In another study, potential of ECE gene transfer for the treatment of Alzheimer's disease and related neurodegeneration was studied. Here, the effects of an intracranial administration of ECE-1 synthetic gene loaded into the serotype 5 recombinant adeno-associated viral vector (rAAV) on Aβ deposition in APP plus PSEN1 transgenic mice were evaluated. The results demonstrated that the Aβ levels decreased in the CNS of the mice receiving the treatment when compared to the control. Thus, these promising results indicate that increasing the expression of Aβ degrading enzymes through gene therapy could be a novel approach for the treatment of Alzheimer's disease which a primary cause of dementia [26].

9.3.2.3 Cathepsin B

Cathepsin is a lysosomal cysteine protease involved in neuropathological and neurodegenerative diseases such as dementia, Alzheimer's disease, and traumatic brain injury. Formation of α-synuclein (α-Syn) aggregates is one of the key steps in progression of neuropathological condition such as DLB and Parkinson's disease (PD) [88]. In a study, expression of cathepsin B in formation of α-Syn was studied and the results suggested that lysosomal protease cathepsin B is involved in stimulation of intracellular aggregate formation of α-Syn fibrils, leading to neurological disorders like PD and DLB [166].

9.3.2.4 BACE1 proteins

BACE1 (β-site APP cleaving enzyme 1) is an aspartyl protease involved in the abnormal production of the Aβ plaques, which is a hallmark of Alzheimer's disease and related dementia. Various reports have suggested a strong link between expression of BACE1 proteins in the CNS and neuropathological conditions like Alzheimer's disease and dementia. The production of Aβ is enhanced in the presence of BACE1 because it initiates the proteolysis of APP, thus BACE1 is supposed to be one of the prime targets for the prevention of Aβ production in the Alzheimer's disease [150]. In a study, BACE1 targeted siRNA delivery into the hippocampus region of APP transgenic mice was carried out using lentivirus mediated gene therapy. The results demonstrated that siRNA targeting the BACE1 reduced the Aβ production and subsequently the Alzheimer's disease-related dementia. From these findings, it can be suggested that the approach of siRNA loaded into lentiviral vectors could have potential therapeutic value for the treatment of neuropathological diseases [158].

9.3.2.5 Nerve growth factor

Nerve growth factor (NGF) is a protein that is useful in reversing or stopping the progression of neurodegenerative diseases related to the cholinergic basal forebrain. There are various reports suggesting that improved levels of NGF could be useful in treating the disorders such as Alzheimer's disease related dementia. On the basis of these findings, approaches such as gene therapy have been adopted for the improvement of NGF levels in the CNS for the treatment of neuropathological disorders [153]. It has also been proposed that basal forebrain cholinergic degeneration in Alzheimer's disease can be treated with NGF. In a study, CERE-110, a genetically modified, replication defective adeno-associated virus serotype 2 (AAV2) vector containing the complete human β-NGF cDNA was developed for the delivery of NGF for the Alzheimer's disease treatment. Findings from these studies described sustained and stable transgene expression over prolonged period of time, also the efficacy studies carried out in the rodents showed promising results. These findings from preclinical studies encouraged the investigators to proceed for Phase 1 clinical trials [22]. Further, results from the clinical Phase 1 studies carried out in small group of eight individuals showed no long-term adverse effects with the therapy. Also, decline in the cholinergic neurodegeneration and cognitive improvement was reported. The investigators further suggest additional extensive clinical trials to establish safety and efficacy of the delivery system in larger population to support the data for commercialization of drug product [167].

9.3.3 Stem cell-based therapeutics

As discussed earlier, Alzheimer's disease is a leading cause of dementia and occurs due to neurodegeneration. Restoring the lost cells through differentiation, stimulation of neurogenesis and effectively delivering the therapeutic agents to the brain is a possibility through the revolutionary discovery of stem cells for the treatment of such conditions. There are several reports suggesting promising results of treatment of Alzheimer's disease using cell therapy which were followed by clinical evaluations of these novel formulations [112]. Most commonly used stem cells in the treatment of Alzheimer's disease are mesenchymal stem cells (MSCs), embryonic stem cells (ESCs) and neural stem cells (NSCs) originated from brain. In the following section we have discussed the application of these stem cells using in-vitro and in-vivo tools for the treatment of neuropathological conditions.

9.3.3.1 Embryonic stem cell

ESCs are derivatives of pluripotent blastocysts and possess the ability to generate cell types from ectoderm, mesoderm, and endoderm. A study was carried out to investigate the production of cholinergic neurons from mouse ESCs and the potential of utilizing ESC-derived neuronal precursor cells (NPCs) and primed NPCs (PNPCs) in rodent model of Alzheimer's disease. The results of immunohistochemical analysis from the study demonstrated that there was no tumor formation upon administration indicating safety of the transplantation of the cells in-vivo. Also, improvement in the cholinergic neurology of the rodent model of Alzheimer's disease was reported [121].

9.3.3.2 Mesenchymal stem cell

MSCs are obtained from tissues of umbilical cord blood (ucb-MSCs), Wharton jelly, and bone marrow and adipose tissue of adults. The ucb-MSCs have demonstrated a great potential in the treatment of neurological disorders. In a study, ucb-MSC transplantation into APP and PSEN1 double transgenic mice was carried out. The results from this study demonstrated significantly improved decline in the memory and learning in the rodent species. Also, evidence of reversal of the disease was shown on the basis of decreased microglia-induced proinflammatory cytokines and neuroinflammation. These findings suggest that ucb-MSC could be a potential advantageous approach for ameliorating the cognitive decline [108]. On the similar grounds, Medipost Co. Ltd. has developed a product called NEUROSTEM (ucb-MSCs) to treat patients with Alzheimer's disease. The administration is done using a medical device tube (Ommaya Reservoir) inserted into the patient's head to deliver the product directly into the ventricles in the brain. Currently, Phases 1 and 2 studies have been carried out to investigate the safety, dose-limiting toxicity and efficacy of the repeated intra-ventricular administration of NEUROSTEM in patients with Alzheimer's disease [33,116].

9.3.3.3 Neural stem cell

NSCs have a unique potential of self-renewal and differentiation into one of the three neuroectodermal specifications. Depending on the factors such as the location within the CNS and development phase, NSCs may be differentiated into astrocytes, oligodendrocytes or neurons. There are various reports suggesting neurogenesis and repair of the damaged CNS is stimulated through the differentiation of NSCs. Therefore, external administration of NSCs to support the neurogenesis and repair the damage could be an effective strategy to combat Alzheimer's disease [24]. In a study carried out on Alzheimer's disease mouse model demonstrated that the implanted human NSCs differentiated into neuronal and glial cells resulting in improved spatial memory in these mice along with reduction in tau phosphorylation and Aβ levels. Thus, this study provides a substantial preclinical evidence that human NSCs transplantation could be a safe and advantageous option for the treatment of Alzheimer's disease and related neuropathological conditions [109].

9.3.4 Vaccines

From the previous reports related to the advancements in the treatment of neuropathological disorders like Alzheimer's disease and related dementia, it has been established that the anti-Aβ antibodies are capable of binding to the Aβ peptides and preventing their fibrillization, promoting breakdown of the preformed fibrils, and combating the fibril dependent neurotoxicity. The process of stimulating the immune system of the host through agents like preformed antigen to produce antibodies is known as active immunization. Unlike active immunization, passive immunization serves problems such as hemorrhagic risks, difficulty in identification of correct antigen targets, higher cost of development, frequent administration in case of chronic disorders, and stimulation of immune response by the host for the externally administered antibodies [176]. We have already discussed the various antibodies belonging to the passive immunization currently in the commercial and development phase in the previous section of the book chapter.

A novel anti-Aβ synthetic peptide vaccine UB-311 has been developed for the treatment of mild to moderate Alzheimer's disease. UB-311 is designed with two synthetic Aβ targeting peptides linked to different helper T-cell epitopes (UBITh) and formulated in a Th-2-based delivery system. Th-2 cells are involved in mediating immune responses. Preclinical studies were conducted on transgenic mice model of Alzheimer's disease, hAPP751, and baboons and macaques were utilized as nonrodent species. The results from the preclinical studies demonstrated the drug product to be safe, effective, well-tolerated, and showed a potential cognitive improvement on the basis of Alzheimer's disease assessment scale-cognitive (ADAS-cog) [174]. Clinical studies of UB-311 have been carried out. In Phase 1 study carried out in the year 2010–2011, safety, immunogenicity, and tolerability of UB-311 were evaluated with three doses in 19 patients with mild to moderate Alzheimer's disease. The results were reported to have shown that the vaccine is safe and effective with only mild inflammation at the site of action. In 2015, Phase 2 study was conducted in 43 patients diagnosed with mild Alzheimer's disease. Besides evaluation of primary outcomes such as safety, tolerability, and safety of the multiple doses, assessment of cognitive, functional, and neuropsychiatric outcomes was also carried out. Promising results were reported in the study and therefore the clinical evaluation progressed to Phase 3 studies. The Phase 3 study was commenced in the year 2020 that consisted of two identical, placebo-controlled, double-blind studies to be carried out for 73 weeks. The data related to this clinical trial have not appeared in the clinical registries yet [162].

9.4 Biological products-based combination therapy

Neurodegenerative disease like dementia is usually multifaceted and thus require a multimodal therapeutic approach. This could employ addressing various molecular targets of the disease synergistically. It has been proven that combination therapy is clinically more efficacious to monotherapy. It is a known fact that a single agent is usually effective at high concentrations as a result of dose-dependent action, which could lead to more severe side effects and could also cause drug resistance. So as monotherapy has multiple limitations of safety, efficacy, and disease modification, utilizing combination therapy of drugs having varied mechanism of action is more beneficial in this framework. Combination therapy would not only help overcome these deficiencies but could also increase the overall efficacy of the treatment by synergistic or additive actions. As it is not dependent on a single therapeutic agent, such therapy proves to be efficacious at lower doses thus improving the safety and tolerability of the therapy. Additionally, combination therapy also provides neuroprotective actions, extending the symptomatic benefits, and eventually delays the progression of the disease. Combination therapy has been shown to have more effectiveness if initiated in the early phases at the slowing rate of cognitive impairment [98].

The clinical trial of a biologics product combination therapy is carried out by testing the two drugs independently, and in combination and along with placebo in a 2 × 2 trial design. However, in the case of drugs to be used for dementia add-on trials are conducted in which the new chemical entity (NCE) is compared with placebo in patients who are receiving some background treatment [67]. Thus, there exist some limitations with the clinical testing of these drugs. Inspite of this Aduhelm (Aducanumab), a human monoclonal antibody has been approved by the FDA in 2021 [169]. Besides certain other biologics of the monoclonal antibody class such as gantenerumab, lecanemab, solanezumab, and donanemab are currently being investigated in placebo controlled phase III clinical trials, whereas bapineuzumab has successfully completed its phase III trials. These large molecules are being evaluated as an add-on therapy to existing treatment in patients with prodromal or mild Alzheimer's disease [38,41,46,51,62]. Additionally, solanezumab is being investigated parallel to gantenerumab in a phase III trial in the dominantly inherited Alzheimer network trials unit (DIAN-TU) trials [18]. These add-on combinations are speculated to target the amyloid cascade to bind and cause an immunological response against β-amyloid peptide which thereby increases the amyloid clearance and improving the overall cognitive function [152].

Also, certain immunoglobulins are being explored for their synergistic effect with other molecules or therapy to combat dementia. Gamunex is a potential combination therapy currently being investigated in phase III clinical trials. This therapy utilizes human albumin in combination with an intravenous immunoglobulin which helps in the eradication of β-amyloid. Plasma exchange with albumin effectively sequesters β-amyloid which crosses the BBB, and clears it out of the central nervous system. An infusion with this works in a continuous fashion, depleting its reserves. Moreover, intravenous infusion with immunoglobulins further enhances this clearance from the brain. Additionally, albumin also possesses antioxidant property which further helps in improving the therapeutic activity of this regimen [23,144]. Thus, a combination therapy involving serum protein and immunoglobulins prove to be synergistically effective.

Attributing to the complexities involved in this neurodegenerative disease, there exists a lack of effective FDA-approved monotherapy regimen. Thus, there is a constant urge for designing and developing a combination therapy which would holistically help in the efficient treatment of dementia. As it would be difficult to develop a single moiety having properties of various pharmacophores, employing a combination approach using biologics could simplify the therapeutic regimen. This would not only have a multitargeted action but it would further ameliorate patient compliance. Clinical trials for various biologic combinations as an add-on therapy are being explored to treat moderate-to-severe dementia. Clinical trials also exhibited better clinical efficacy in comparison to monotherapy with reasonable or similar tolerability and safety. However, stand-alone 2 × 2 trial design is required to explore the efficiency of biologics as a combination therapy. Besides, factors like neuroprotective effects, potential benefit to the patients and overall cost-effectiveness of the regimen need to be assessed in clinical studies to further reinforce usefulness of combination therapy in the treatment of dementia.

9.5 Nanotechnology-based biological drug products

It is understood that biologics have a great potential to not only reduce the symptoms but also mitigate the disease. However, making it available at the site of action in therapeutic concentrations remains a challenge. This is attributed to the BBB, which only allows the passage of smaller molecules having a molecular weight within 400 Da and forming fewer than eight hydrogen bonds [133]. Although biologics can pass through this barrier in the case of lesions, its distribution within the neural tissue is not extensive and uniform [1,20]. Because of the unfavorable pharmacokinetic and pharmacodynamic properties of the actives, there is a failure in the therapy [10]. This is because of unsuitable physicochemical properties of the drug, undesirable absorption, distribution, and metabolism, and the off-target toxicity it causes. Additionally, the instability of the drug, such as hydrolysis, oxidation or photolysis, further decreases its effectiveness [155,161].

Nanotherapeutics are now proving to be a promising approach for the treatment of neurodegenerative diseases. This is because it helps overcome several hurdles and challenges which a conventional formulation face. Nanotechnology helps by enhancing the active agent's pharmacokinetic and pharmacodynamic profile and exhibit minimal toxicity [130]. The carrier system protects the drug residing within from enzymatic degradation and the first-pass metabolism effect. These nanoparticles additionally provide targeting action to the brain and possess long-acting properties and controlled release at the site of action. This further helps in increasing the therapeutic concentrations, namely, the biodistribution of the biologics in the brain. Nanotechnology also helps minimize several adverse effects as well as motor complications [100]. Therefore, nanosystems like liposomes, microemulsions, solid lipid nanoparticles, polymeric nanoparticles, liquid crystals, and hydrogels are being developed to carry the drugs across the BBB [80] (Fig. 9.4). The surface of these nanoparticles can be chemically modified for selective targeting and cell-specific action, which has shown promising results in targeting the brain tissue [100]. Hence, the nanoparticles are functionalized with surfactants like polysorbate 80 or ligands, enabling them to bind to the brain receptors, thereby promoting their transport through the BBB.

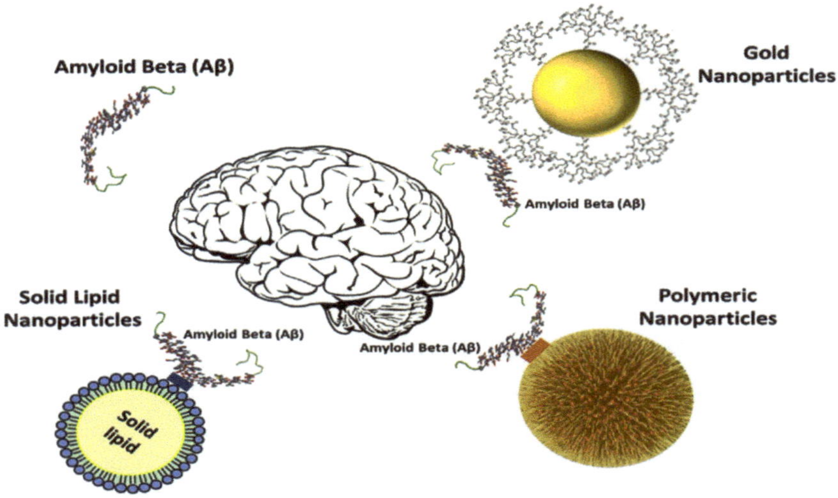

FIG. 9.4 Nanotherapeutics in treating the accumulation of Amyloid-Beta peptide in Alzheimer's patients. Image adopted from: Abbas M. Potential role of nanoparticles in treating the accumulation of amyloid-beta peptide in Alzheimer's patients. Polymers. 2021; 13(7):1051. https://doi.org/10.3390/polym13071051 [186].

Moreover, nanosystems are also being utilized as theranostic agents employed to detect amyloid β (Aβ) aggregates and thereby predict dementia [110]. The administration of these formulations is not only restricted to the oral route for intestinal absorption but also comprises noninvasive routes like intranasal and intravitreal delivery. Notable improvement has been made in delivering biologics through nanoparticulate systems using the nose-to-brain route. The encapsulated drug is protected from biological and chemical degradation and also surpasses the efflux by the P-gp proteins [120]. Among various colloidal carrier systems, lipid-based nanoparticles such as liposomes, niosomes, cubosomes, nanoemulsions, and solid lipid nanoparticles are promising for nasal delivery [4]. There also exist specific invasive techniques for the local delivery of drugs, such as injecting implants and hydrogels intracranially [163]. However, these are explored at very late stages of the diseases and are rarely used.

9.5.1 Polymeric nanoparticles

Polymeric nanoparticles like the ones composed of PLGA (poly(D,L-lactide-co-glycolide)) and PBCA (poly(butyl cyanoacrylate)) are being explored for sustained and targeted delivery of a range of biologics, owning to their biocompatibility and GRAS status [86,135]. These polymers have been successfully employed to encapsulate enzymes like superoxide dismutase (SOD), polypeptides like erythropoietin (EPO), and other proteins; and deliver them to the brain in therapeutic concentrations [30,140]. Additionally, coating the nanoparticles with nonionic surfactants or modifying its surface with glycoproteins like

Tween 80 (polysorbate 80) and g7, respectively, helps facilitate the delivery of macromolecules to the brain tissues [83,149]. A study utilized PLGA nanoparticles coated with Tween 80 to load tissue inhibitor of matrix metalloproteinases 1 (TIMP-1) and exhibited desirable protein penetration inside the brain on intravenous administration [29]. Another nanoparticulate drug delivery system was developed to carry a β-sheet breaker peptide H102 having dual functionality. In this, the surface of the pegylated PLA nanoparticle was conjugated into two peptides, namely TGN and QSH. TGN helped transport the carrier across the BBB, whereas QSH brought about Aβ42 targeting, resulting in the therapeutic action. Due to this dual function, there was an effective increase in the H102 accumulation at the desired site in the brain and thus provided better neuroprotective action [181]. To further retain the therapeutic activity, enzymes are cross-linked as aggregates and then encapsulated into PLGA nanoparticles. On validation with specific enzyme aggregates, these carriers could efficiently deliver the biologics at the target site in a sustained manner for a period of 48 hours [81]. Macromolecule-loaded nanoparticles were also formulated using pegylated poly(ε-caprolactone) (PEG-PCL) to target the fibrin in the CNS [71]. In addition to the conventional polymers used as nanocarriers, other types of materials, like the pH-sensitive polymersome, poly (oligo (ethylene glycol) methylmethacrylate)-co-poly(2-(diisopropylamino)ethyl methacrylate) (POEGMA-PDPA), is used in the encapsulation of certain proteins. On testing IgG-loaded angiopep-2 modification of this polymersome in mice intravenously, it was found to show an increased accumulation inside the brain [180]. Another study utilized Lys-Leu-Val-Phe-Phe (KLVFF) and Fmoc-KLVFF fluorescent peptide nanoparticles to detect Aβ aggregation and which thereby helps diagnose dementia due to Alzheimer's disease [110].

9.5.2 Liposomes

The use of liposomes in enhancing protein accumulation within the brain on intravenous administration is a well-established method. Formulation of liposomes utilizes neutral, cationic, and anionic lipids; however, cationic and neutral lipids exhibit better uptake than the anionic ones [137]. β-GAL and SOD1 were successfully encapsulated in anionic and cationic liposomes, respectively. They could cross the BBB to effectively deliver the enzymes in therapeutic concentrations than the free enzyme [92,128]. PEGylation of these liposomes further improved their pharmacokinetic profile and tissue uptake. Using this, NGF was efficiently carried to the brain intravenously by PEGylated liposomes. These liposomes were further conjugated to RMP-7, a ligand to the B2 receptor on the brain endothelial cells [178]. Moreover, doubly conjugated lipids were developed to exhibit a chemo-responsive behavior across the brain. In this, peptides targeting the brain were conjugated at the N-terminus to matrix metalloproteinase-9 (MMP-9) responsive peptides, and this was further conjugated at the N-terminus to the lipid. The resulting nanoparticle composed showed higher transport across the BBB when MMP-9 levels were increased, attributed to the responsive nature of the ligand [94]. Similarly, glutathione, a tripeptide, was conjugated to PEGylated liposomes for delivering β-amyloid targeting antibody fragments to the brain [146].

9.5.3 Micelles

Studies have explored the use of polymeric micelles to deliver therapeutic proteins to the brain. Pluronics are highly investigated among various poloxamers due to their efficiency in carrying macromolecules. Pluronics are a triblock polymer comprising of the PEO-PPO-PEO structure, where PEO stands forpoly(ethylene oxide), and PPO stands for poly(propylene oxide) [180]. Conjugating pluronic F127 with chitosan and further functionalizing it with a brain-targeting peptide-like (rabies virus glycoprotein (RVG29)) resulted in desirable CNS accumulation. It was found to be significantly better than the carrier conjugated only to (RVG29) [102]. A comparative study of free β-GAL and β-GAL loaded in a mixed micelle composed of pluronic F127 and D-α-tocopheryl PEG succinate resulted in enhanced drug delivery of the latter. The former showed no detectable enzymatic activity in the brain [117]. An investigation is also being made to explore the functionality of polyion complex micelles. These micelles are formed by the coacervation of two hydrophilic block copolymers that are oppositely charged. These are a class of nanocarriers that would help deliver charged proteins. Also, the nanozymes would improve the loading efficiency of the protein as well as impart some preservation to the enzyme activity [82].

9.5.4 Inorganic nanoparticles

Surface-modified gold nanoparticles have also been explored to carry drugs to the brain. The gold particles were functionalized with mimosine, a plant-based amino acid, which helped in the passage through the BBB. Additionally, mimosine-gold nanoparticles were found to initiate the disassembly of matured Aβ fibers, reduce phosphorylation of tau proteins, and the production of oxy-radicals. This thus resulted in an increase in the neuronal viability, attenuated Aβ fibrillization, and overall neuronal toxicity [7].

9.6 Future direction in the management of dementia

Currently approved medications by FDA for the treatment of dementia and Alzheimer's disease are acetylcholinesterase inhibitors, such as galantamine, donepezil, rivastigmine, and the NMDA antagonist, memantine. However, these small molecules provide a symptomatic relief and due to their nonspecific mechanism of action cause potential adverse effects, such as bradycardia, syncope, sleep behavior disorder, and gastrointestinal side effects. Also, these approved drugs are contraindicated in conditions like cardiac arrythmias [179]. In the future, the management of dementia is predicted to include novel nanotechnology and biological drug product-based approaches to either reverse the brain damage or to effectively deliver the drug to the brain [12]. Biological therapeutics provide a disease-modifying therapy for the management of neurodegenerative disorders such as dementia and Alzheimer's disease. But these biological drug products have undergone multiple failures during the clinical evaluation and the major reasons could be too late starting of therapies in the disease development, erroneous main target for the treatment, or unsuitable drug doses. To overcome such issues during the clinical evaluation of the newer interventions, a guidance document has been drafted by USFDA. In the coming future, such guidance from the regulatory bodies would assist sponsors in the clinical development of drugs for the treatment of neurological disorders such as early onset of dementia or Alzheimer's disease [77]. Another major reason for failure of the biologics in the clinical studies is the hurdle posed by BBB to reach therapeutic levels in the brain. In the upcoming research, emphasis is being laid on re-engineering the biologic drugs as BBB penetrating agents [134].

Recent advancements in understanding the pathophysiology of dementia and the underlying pathways for Alzheimer's disease have resulted in creation of vast libraries of drug targets. The single largest encouraging factor for the growth of biologics in the treatment of neurological disorders is the safety and efficacy of these drugs. The novel approaches such as gene therapy, immunotherapy, antibody-drug conjugate, and cell therapy will offer greater promise for the development of regenerative medicine for the treatment of neurodegenerative disorder such as dementia. If all the efforts starting from the identification of correct targets to the development of BBB penetrating biological drugs and novel drug delivery systems come to fruition, the concept of precision medicine could be applied in every patient suffering from dementia in the near future for any risk-factor elimination and personalized care.

Considering the advantages and opportunities served by the biological drug products, various biotechnology firms are collaborating with pharmaceutical giants for marketing the new therapies, like AstraZeneca's agreement to buy the biotechnology major MedImmune at a premium cost. Rapid advances in the areas of neurobiology will create a demand for biologics. Through the research in genetics, gene expression, structural biology of neurons such as understanding of chemical skeleton of nerves, axons, receptors, and synapses and deeper understanding of neuro-regeneration and repair, new target pathways especially for biologics are likely to be revealed. The future of biologics in the treatment of neurological disorders appears to be bright and lucrative for industries because of its cutting-edge science, therapeutic and safety advantages and a huge commercial potential considering the positive long-term growth in the market value of biologics.

9.7 Concluding remark

The inadequacies of the small molecules proven to be overcome by biologics, thereby providing appropriate treatment for dementia. Application of nanotechnology to deliver the biologics could improve the overall safety, efficacy, and effectiveness of the product. However, there remains a constant requirement to develop new therapeutic agents, and discover new routes for further mitigating the limitations. Despite the expected future advancements, biologics remains to be a significant means of treating dementia.

References

[1] Abulrob A, Brunette E, Slinn J, Baumann E, Stanimirovic D. Dynamic analysis of the blood-brain barrier disruption in experimental stroke using time domain in vivo fluorescence imaging. Mol Imaging 2008;7(6). doi:10.2310/7290.2008.00025 7290.2008.00025.

[2] *Aduhelm.* https://www.alzforum.org/news/research-news/aducanumab-approved-treat-alzheime [Accessed 19 August 2022].

[3] In Surprise, Placebo, not Aβ Vaccine, Said to Slow Alzheimer's. https://www.alzforum.org/therapeutics/affitope-ad02 [Accessed 19 August 2022].

[4] Akel H, Ismail R, Csóka I. Progress and perspectives of brain-targeting lipid-based nanosystems via the nasal route in Alzheimer's disease. Eur J Pharm Biopharm 2020;148:38–53. https://doi.org/10.1016/j.ejpb.2019.12.014.

[5] Allison AC, Cacabelos R, Lombardi VR, Alvarez XA, Vigo C. Celastrol, a potent antioxidant and anti-inflammatory drug, as a possible treatment for Alzheimer's disease. Prog Neuropsychopharmacol Biol Psychiatry 2001;25(7):1341–57. https://doi.org/10.1016/s0278-5846(01)00192-0.

[6] An L, Han X, Li H, Ma Y, Shi L, Xu G, Yuan G, Sun J, Zhao N, Sheng Y, Wang M, Du P. Effects and mechanism of cerebroprotein hydrolysate on learning and memory ability in mice. Genetics and Molecular Research : GMR 2016;15(3). https://doi.org/10.4238/gmr.15038804.

[7] Anand BG, Wu Q, Karthivashan G, Shejale KP, Amidian S, Wille H, Kar S. Mimosine functionalized gold nanoparticles (Mimo-AuNPs) suppress β-amyloid aggregation and neuronal toxicity. Bioactive Materials 2021;6(12):4491–505. https://doi.org/10.1016/j.bioactmat.2021.04.029.

[8] Andrade MT, Lima JA, Pinto AC, Rezende CM, Carvalho MP, Epifanio RA. Indole alkaloids from Tabernaemontana australis (Muell. Arg) Miers that inhibit acetylcholinesterase enzyme. Bioorg Med Chem 2005;13(12):4092–5. https://doi.org/10.1016/j.bmc.2005.03.045.

[9] Areosa SA, Sherriff F, McShane R. Memantine for dementia. Cochrane Database Syst Rev 2005;2:CD003154, https://doi.org/10.1002/14651858.CD003154.pub3.

[10] Arias JLNanotechnology and Drug Delivery, Volume One: Nanoplatforms in Drug Delivery. Vol. 2. Boka Raton, FL: CRC Press; 2014.

[11] Arvanitakis Z, Shah RC, Bennett DA. Diagnosis and management of dementia: review. JAMA 2019;322(16):1589–99. https://doi.org/10.1001/jama.2019.4782.

[12] Astell AJ, Bouranis N, Hoey J, Lindauer A, Mihailidis A, Nugent C, Robillard JM. Technology and dementia: the future is now. Dement Geriatr Cogn Disord 2019;47(3):131–9. https://doi.org/10.1159/000497800.

[13] *AstraZeneca Press Release.* https://www.astrazeneca.com/media-centre/press-releases/2016/Astrazeneca-and-Lilly-to-develop-second-potentially-disease-modifying-treatment-for-alzheimers-disease-09122016.html#! [Accessed 19 August 2022].

[14] Ata A, Andersh BJ. Buxus steroidal alkaloids: chemistry and biology. Alkaloids Chem Biol 2008;66:191–213 https://doi.org/10.1016/s1099-4831(08)00203-4.

[15] Bapineuzumab-Overview. https://www.creativebiolabs.net/bapineuzumab-overview.htm [Accessed 19 August 2022].

[16] Bartfai T, Lees GV. Alzheimer drug trials: combination of safe and efficacious biologicals to break the amyloidosis-neuroinflammation vicious cycle. ASN Neuro 2020;12. 1759091420918557 https://doi.org/10.1177/1759091420918557.

[17] Bastida J, Viladomat F, Llabrés JM, Codina C, Rubiralta M. Alkaloids from narcissus jacetanus1. Planta Med 1988;54(04):362.

[18] Bateman RJ, Benzinger TL, Berry S, Clifford DB, Duggan C, Fagan AM, Fanning K, Farlow MR, Hassenstab J, McDade EM, Mills S, Paumier K, Quintana M, Salloway SP, Santacruz A, Schneider LS, Wang G, Xiong C. The DIAN-TU next generation Alzheimer's prevention trial: adaptive design and disease progression model. Alzheimer's & Dementia : The Journal of the Alzheimer's Association 2017;13(1):8–19. https://doi.org/10.1016/j.jalz.2016.07.005.

[19] Bhattacharya SK, Bhattacharya D, Sairam K, Ghosal S. Effect of Withania somnifera glycowithanolides on a rat model of tardive dyskinesia. (Letter to the Editor). Phytomedicine: International Journal of Phytotherapy & Phytopharmacology 2002;9:167+. https://link.gale.com/apps/doc/A92544757/AONE?u=anon~da038e49&sid=googleScholar&xid=55c009b7.

[20] Bien-Ly N, Boswell CA, Jeet S, Beach TG, Hoyte K, Luk W, Shihadeh V, Ulufatu S, Foreman O, Lu Y, DeVoss J, van der Brug M, Watts RJ. Lack of widespread BBB disruption in Alzheimer's disease models: focus on therapeutic antibodies. Neuron 2015;88(2):289–97. https://doi.org/10.1016/j.neuron.2015.09.036.

[21] Birks J. Cholinesterase inhibitors for Alzheimer's disease. Cochrane Database Syst Rev 2006;1:CD005593. https://doi.org/10.1002/14651858.CD005593.

[22] Bishop KM, Hofer EK, Mehta A, Ramirez A, Sun L, Tuszynski M, Bartus RT. Therapeutic potential of CERE-110 (AAV2-NGF): targeted, stable, and sustained NGF delivery and trophic activity on rodent basal forebrain cholinergic neurons. Exp Neurol 2008;211(2):574–84. https://doi.org/10.1016/j.expneurol.2008.03.004.

[23] Boada M, Ramos-Fernández E, Guivernau B, Muñoz FJ, Costa M, Ortiz AM, Jorquera JI, Núñez L, Torres M, Páez A. Treatment of Alzheimer disease using combination therapy with plasma exchange and haemapheresis with albumin and intravenous immunoglobulin: Rationale and treatment approach of the AMBAR (Alzheimer Management By Albumin Replacement) study. Neurologia (Barcelona, Spain) 2016;31(7):473–81. https://doi.org/10.1016/j.nrl.2014.02.003.

[24] Boese AC, Hamblin MH, Lee J-P. Neural stem cell therapy for neurovascular injury in Alzheimer's disease. Exp Neurol 2020;324:113112. https://doi.org/10.1016/j.expneurol.2019.113112.

[25] Bohrmann B, Baumann K, Benz J, Gerber F, Huber W, Knoflach F, Messer J, Oroszlan K, Rauchenberger R, Richter WF, Rothe C, Urban M, Bardroff M, Winter M, Nordstedt C, Loetscher H. Gantenerumab: a novel human anti-Aβ antibody demonstrates sustained cerebral amyloid-β binding and elicits cell-mediated removal of human amyloid-β. Journal of Alzheimer's Disease : JAD 2012;28(1):49–69. https://doi.org/10.3233/JAD-2011-110977.

[26] Carty NC, Nash K, Lee D, Mercer M, Gottschall PE, Meyers C, Muzyczka N, Gordon MN, Morgan D. Adeno-associated Viral (AAV) Serotype 5 vector mediated gene delivery of endothelin-converting enzyme reduces Aβ deposits in APP + PS1 transgenic mice. Mol Ther 2008;16(9):1580–6. https://doi.org/10.1038/mt.2008.148.

[27] Casey DA, Antimisiaris D, O'Brien J. Drugs for Alzheimer's disease: are they effective?. P & T : A Peer-Reviewed Journal for Formulary Management 2010;35(4):208–11. https://pubmed.ncbi.nlm.nih.gov/20498822.

[28] Cerebrolysin®. https://www.cerebrolysin.com/en/cerebrolysin/about-cerebrolysin/. [Accessed 19 August 2022].

[29] Chaturvedi M, Molino Y, Sreedhar B, Khrestchatisky M, Kaczmarek L. Tissue inhibitor of matrix metalloproteinases-1 loaded poly(lactic-co-glycolic acid) nanoparticles for delivery across the blood-brain barrier. Int J Nanomed 2014;9(1):575–88. https://doi.org/10.2147/IJN.S54750.

[30] Chen H, Spagnoli F, Burris M, Rolland WB, Fajilan A, Dou H, Tang J, Zhang JH. Nanoerythropoietin is 10-times more effective than regular erythropoietin in neuroprotection in a neonatal rat model of hypoxia and ischemia. Stroke 2012;43(3):884–7. https://doi.org/10.1161/STROKEAHA.111.637090.

[31] Chung YK, Heo HJ, Kim EK, Kim HK, Huh TL, Lim Y, Kim SK, Shin DH. Inhibitory effect of ursolic acid purified from Origanum majorana L on the acetylcholinesterase. Mol Cells 2001;11(2):137–43.

[32] Clinical trial. *NCT04795466*. https://clinicaltrials.gov/ct2/show/NCT04795466?term=canakinumab&cond=Alzheimer+Disease&draw=2&rank=1. [Accessed 19 August 2022].

[33] *Clinical trial.NCT02054208*. https://clinicaltrials.gov/ct2/show/NCT02054208?term=stem+cell&cond=Alzheimer+Disease&draw=2&rank=7. [Accessed 19 August 2022].

[34] *Clinical trial NCT no: NCT02427243*. https://clinicaltrials.gov/ct2/show/NCT02427243?term=crenezumab&phase=0&draw=2&rank=1. [Accessed 19 August 2022].

[35] *ClinicalTrials.gov Identifier: NCT00017940*. https://clinicaltrials.gov/ct2/show/NCT00017940?term=gene+therapy&cond=Dementia&draw=2&rank=6. [Accessed 19 August 2022].

[36] ClinicalTrials.gov Identifier: *NCT00087789*. https://clinicaltrials.gov/ct2/show/NCT00087789 [Accessed 19 August 2022].

[37] *ClinicalTrials.gov Identifier: NCT00455000*. https://clinicaltrials.gov/ct2/show/NCT00455000?term=monoclonal+antibody&cond=Dementia&draw=2&rank=15. [Accessed 19 August 2022].

[38] *ClinicalTrials.gov Identifier: NCT00574132*. https://clinicaltrials.gov/ct2/show/NCT00574132 [Accessed 19 August 2022].

[39] *ClinicalTrials.gov Identifier: NCT00965588*. https://clinicaltrials.gov/ct2/show/NCT00965588?term=vaccine&cond=Dementia&draw=2&rank=9 [Accessed 19 August 2022].

[40] *ClinicalTrials.gov Identifier: NCT00996918*. https://clinicaltrials.gov/ct2/show/NCT00996918?term=bapineuzumab&cond=Dementia&draw=2&rank=3 [Accessed 19 August 2022].

[41] *ClinicalTrials.gov Identifier: NCT02008357*, https://www.clinicaltrials.gov/ct2/show/NCT02008357 [Accessed 19 August 2022].

[42] *ClinicalTrials.gov Identifier: NCT02008513*. https://clinicaltrials.gov/ct2/show/NCT02008513?term=vaccine&cond=Dementia&draw=2&rank=7 [Accessed 19 August 2022].

[43] ClinicalTrials.gov Identifier: *NCT02031198*. https://clinicaltrials.gov/ct2/show/NCT02031198?term=vaccine&cond=Dementia&draw=2&rank=8 [Accessed 19 August 2022].

[44] ClinicalTrials.gov Identifier: *NCT02036645*. https://clinicaltrials.gov/ct2/show/NCT02036645?term=monoclonal+antibody&cond=Dementia&draw=2&rank=17 [Accessed 19 August 2022].

[45] *ClinicalTrials.gov Identifier: NCT02760602*. https://clinicaltrials.gov/ct2/show/NCT02760602?term=monoclonal+antibody&cond=Dementia&draw=2&rank=9 [Accessed 19 August 2022].

[46] *ClinicalTrials.gov Identifier: NCT03443973*. https://clinicaltrials.gov/ct2/show/NCT03443973 [Accessed 19 August 2022].

[47] *ClinicalTrials.gov Identifier: NCT03491150*. https://clinicaltrials.gov/ct2/show/NCT03491150?term=crenezumab&cond=Dementia&draw=2&rank=1 [Accessed 19 August 2022].

[48] ClinicalTrials.gov Identifier: NCT03634007. https://clinicaltrials.gov/ct2/show/NCT03634007?term=gene+therapy&cond=Dementia&draw=2&rank=5 [Accessed 19 August 2022].

[49] ClinicalTrials.gov Identifier: NCT03658135. https://clinicaltrials.gov/ct2/show/NCT03658135?term=monoclonal+antibody&cond=Dementia&draw=2&rank=7 [Accessed 19 August 2022].

[50] *ClinicalTrials.gov Identifier: NCT03668405*. https://clinicaltrials.gov/ct2/show/NCT03668405?term=vaccine&cond=Dementia&draw=2&rank=25 [Accessed 19 August 2022].

[51] *ClinicalTrials.gov Identifier: NCT03887455*. https://clinicaltrials.gov/ct2/show/NCT03887455 [Accessed 19 August 2022].

[52] *ClinicalTrials.gov Identifier: NCT04133454*. https://clinicaltrials.gov/ct2/show/NCT04133454?term=gene+therapy&cond=Dementia&draw=2&rank=3 [Accessed 19 August 2022].

[53] *ClinicalTrials.gov Identifier: NCT04339413*. https://clinicaltrials.gov/ct2/show/NCT04339413?term=gantenerumab&draw=2&rank=4 [Accessed 19 August 2022].

[54] ClinicalTrials.gov Identifier: *NCT04381468*. https://clinicaltrials.gov/ct2/show/NCT04381468?term=monoclonal+antibody&cond=Dementia&draw=2&rank=6 [Accessed 19 August 2022].

[55] *ClinicalTrials.gov Identifier: NCT04619420*. https://clinicaltrials.gov/ct2/show/NCT04619420?term=monoclonal+antibody&cond=Dementia&draw=2&rank=1 [Accessed 19 August 2022].

[56] *ClinicalTrials.gov Identifier: NCT04747431*. https://clinicaltrials.gov/ct2/show/NCT04747431?term=gene+therapy&cond=Dementia&draw=3&rank=1 [Accessed 19 August 2022].

[57] *ClinicalTrials.gov Identifier: NCT04885114*. https://clinicaltrials.gov/ct2/show/NCT04885114?term=gene+therapy&cond=Dementia&draw=2&rank=7 [Accessed 19 August 2022].

[58] *ClinicalTrials.gov Identifier: NCT04920786*. https://clinicaltrials.gov/ct2/show/NCT04920786?term=monoclonal+antibody&cond=Dementia&draw=2&rank=10 [Accessed 19 August 2022].

[59] *ClinicalTrials.gov Identifier: NCT05026866*. https://clinicaltrials.gov/ct2/show/NCT05026866?term=donanemab&cond=Dementia&draw=2&rank=4 [Accessed 19 August 2022].

[60] *ClinicalTrials.gov Identifier: NCT05026866*. https://clinicaltrials.gov/ct2/show/NCT04795466?term=canakinumab&cond=Dementia&draw=2&rank=1 [Accessed 19 August 2022].

[61] *ClinicalTrials.gov Identifier: NCT05040217*. https://clinicaltrials.gov/ct2/show/NCT05040217?term=gene+therapy&cond=Dementia&draw=2&rank=4 [Accessed 19 August 2022].

[62] *ClinicalTrials.gov Idneufier: NCT04437511*. https://clinicaltrials.gov/ct2/show/NCT04437511?term=donanemab&cond=Alzheimer+Disease&draw=2&rank=1 [Accessed 19 August 2022].

[63] Craik DJ, Fairlie DP, Liras S, Price D. The Future of Peptide-based Drugs. Chemical Biology & Drug Design 2013;81(1):136–47. https://doi.org/10.1111/cbdd.12055.

[64] Crehan H, Lemere CA. Chapter 7 - Anti-Amyloid-β Immunotherapy for Alzheimer's Disease. MA, United States: Academic Press; 2016. p. 193–226. M. S. B. T.-D. T. for A. D. Wolfe [Ed.] https://doi.org/10.1016/B978-0-12-802173-6.00007-1.

[65] *Crenezumab Overview*. https://www.creativebiolabs.net/crenezumab-overview.htm#:~:text=Mechanism%20of%20Action%20of%20Crenezumab&text=It%20was%20engineered%20to%20clear,effects%20such%20as%20vasogenic%20edema [Accessed 19 August 2022].

[66] Cummings JL. Dementia with Lewy bodies: molecular pathogenesis and implications for classification. J Geriatr Psychiatry Neurol 2004;17(3):112–9. https://doi.org/10.1177/0891988704267473.

[67] Cummings JL, Tong G, & Ballard C (2019). Treatment Combinations for Alzheimer's Disease: current and future pharmacotherapy options. Journal of Alzheimer's Disease : JAD, 67(3), 779–794. https://doi.org/10.3233/JAD-180766.

[68] Damjanov I, Mohan H. Textbook of Pathology, 7th ed. New Delhi, India: Jaypee Brothers Medical Publishers (P) Ltd; 2003.

[69] Dembitsky VM, Dzhemileva L, Gloriozova T, & D'yakonov V. Natural and synthetic drugs used for the treatment of the dementia. Biochem Biophys Res Commun 2020;524(3):772–83. https://doi.org/10.1016/j.bbrc.2020.01.123.

[70] *Dementia A NICE–SCIE*. Guideline on Supporting People with Dementia and Their Carers in Health and Social Care. Leicester (UK): The British Psychological Society and Gaskell; 2007.

[71] Deng J, Mei H, Shi W, Pang Z, Zhang B, Guo T, Wang H, Jiang X, Hu Y. Recombinant tissue plasminogen activator-conjugated nanoparticles effectively targets thrombolysis in a rat model of middle cerebral artery occlusion. Current Medical Science 2018;38(3):427–35. https://doi.org/10.1007/s11596-018-1896-z.

[72] Dhimolea E. Canakinumab. MAbs 2010;2(1):3–13. https://doi.org/10.4161/mabs.2.1.10328.

[73] Dodart J-C, Marr RA, Koistinaho M, Gregersen BM, Malkani S, Verma IM, Paul SM. Gene delivery of human apolipoprotein E alters brain Aβ burden in a mouse model of Alzheimer's disease. Proc Natl Acad Sci 2005;102(4):1211–6. https://doi.org/10.1073/pnas.0409072102.

[74] IUPHAR/ BPS Guide to Pharmacology. https://www.guidetopharmacology.org/GRAC/LigandDisplayForward?tab=clinical&ligandId=8357 [Accessed 19 August 2022].

[75] Lilly's donanemab receives U.S. FDA's Breakthrough Therapy designation for treatment of Alzheimer's disease. https://investor.lilly.com/news-releases/news-release-details/lillys-donanemab-receives-us-fdas-breakthrough-therapy [Accessed 19 August 2022].

[76] dos Santos Rodrigues B, Kanekiyo T, Singh J. ApoE-2 brain-targeted gene therapy through transferrin and penetratin tagged liposomal nanoparticles. Pharm Res 2019;36(11):161 https://doi.org/10.1007/s11095-019-2691-7.

[77] Early Alzheimer's disease: developing drugs for treatment guidance for industry. https://www.fda.gov/media/110903/download [Accessed 19 August 2022]

[78] Eckman EA, Reed DK, Eckman CB. Degradation of the Alzheimer's amyloid β peptide by endothelin-converting enzyme*. J Biol Chem 2001;276(27):24540–8. https://doi.org/10.1074/jbc.M007579200.

[79] Eisai. *Eisai initiates rolling submission to the U.S. FDA for biologics license application of lecanemab (BAN2401) for early alzheimer's disease under the accelerated approval pathway*. https://www.eisai.com/news/2021/news202177.html [Accessed 19 August 2022].

[80] Fonseca-Santos B, Gremião MPD, Chorilli M. Nanotechnology-based drug delivery systems for the treatment of Alzheimer's disease. Int J Nanomed 2015;10:4981–5003. https://doi.org/10.2147/IJN.S87148.

[81] Galliani M, Santi M, Del Grosso A, Cecchettini A, Santorelli FM, Hofmann SL, Lu J-Y, Angella L, Cecchini M, Signore G. Cross-linked enzyme aggregates as versatile tool for enzyme delivery: application to polymeric nanoparticles. Bioconjugate Chem 2018;29(7):2225–31. https://doi.org/10.1021/acs.bioconjchem.8b00206.

[82] Gaydess A, Duysen E, Li Y, Gilman V, Kabanov A, Lockridge O, Bronich T. Visualization of exogenous delivery of nanoformulated butyrylcholinesterase to the central nervous system. Chem Biol Interact 2010;187(1–3):295–8. https://doi.org/10.1016/j.cbi.2010.01.005.

[83] Gelperina S, Maksimenko O, Khalansky A, Vanchugova L, Shipulo E, Abbasova K, Berdiev R, Wohlfart S, Chepurnova N, Kreuter J. Drug delivery to the brain using surfactant-coated poly(lactide-co-glycolide) nanoparticles: Influence of the formulation parameters. Eur J Pharm Biopharm 2010;74(2):157–63. https://doi.org/10.1016/j.ejpb.2009.09.003.

[84] Grantham C, Geerts H. The rationale behind cholinergic drug treatment for dementia related to cerebrovascular disease. J Neurol Sci 2002;203–204:131–6. https://doi.org/10.1016/s0022-510x(02)00274-5.

[85] Hansel TT, Kropshofer H, Singer T, Mitchell JA, George AJT. The safety and side effects of monoclonal antibodies. Nat Rev Drug Discovery 2010;9(4):325–38. https://doi.org/10.1038/nrd3003.

[86] Hasadsri L, Kreuter J, Hattori H, Iwasaki T, George JM. Functional protein delivery into neurons using polymeric nanoparticles*. J Biol Chem 2009;284(11):6972–81. https://doi.org/10.1074/jbc.M805956200.

[87] Hinderer C, Miller R, Dyer C, Johansson J, Bell P, Buza E, Wilson JM. Adeno-associated virus serotype 1-based gene therapy for FTD caused by GRN mutations. Annals of Clinical and Translational Neurology 2020;7(10):1843–53. https://doi.org/10.1002/acn3.51165.

[88] Hook V, Yoon M, Mosier C, Ito G, Podvin S, Head BP, Rissman R, O'Donoghue AJ, Hook G. Cathepsin B in neurodegeneration of Alzheimer's disease, traumatic brain injury, and related brain disorders. Biochimica et Biophysica Acta Proteins and Proteomics 2020;1868(8):140428. https://doi.org/10.1016/j.bbapap.2020.140428.

[89] Horizny C*New gene therapy for the treatment of Alzheimer's disease*. https://www.taconic.com/taconic-insights/alzheimers-disease/ad-gene-therapy-trial.html [Accessed 19 August 2022].

[90] Ikewuchi C, Ayalogu E, Onyeike E, Ikewuchi J. Study on the alkaloid, allicin, glycoside and saponin composition of the leaves of sansevieria liberica Gérôme and Labroy by gas chromatography. Pacific Journal of Science and Technology 2011;12:367–73.

[91] Ikewuchi C, Ikewuchi J, Ifeanacho M. Bioactive phytochemicals in an aqueous extract of the leaves of Talinum triangulare. Food Science & Nutrition 2016;5. https://doi.org/10.1002/fsn3.449.

[92] Imaizumi S, Woolworth V, Fishman RA, Chan PH. Liposome-entrapped superoxide dismutase reduces cerebral infarction in cerebral ischemia in rats. Stroke 1990;21(9):1312–7. https://doi.org/10.1161/01.STR.21.9.1312.

[93] Industry news: key differences in small molecule, biologics drug development. https://pharmanewsintel.com/news/key-differences-in-small-molecule-biologics-drug-development [Accessed 19 August 2022].

[94] Islam Y, Ehtezazi P, Cashmore A, Marinsalda E, Leach AG, Coxon CR, Fatokun AA, Sexton DW, Khan I, Zouganelis G, Downing J, Pluchino S, Sivakumaran M, Teixido M, Ehtezazi T. The inclusion of a matrix metalloproteinase-9 responsive sequence in self-assembled peptide-based brain-targeting nanoparticles improves the efficiency of nanoparticles crossing the blood-brain barrier at elevated MMP-9 levels. J Pharm Sci 2021;110(3):1349–64. https://doi.org/10.1016/j.xphs.2020.12.004.

[95] Jackson S, Ham RJ, Wilkinson D. The safety and tolerability of donepezil in patients with Alzheimer's disease. Br J Clin Pharmacol 2004;58(*Suppl 1*):1–8. Suppl 1 https://doi.org/10.1111/j.1365-2125.2004.01848.x.

[96] Jarvis B, Figgitt DP. Memantine. Drugs Aging 2003;20(6):465–76. https://doi.org/10.2165/00002512-200320060-00005.

[97] Johnston SL. Biologic therapies: what and when?. J Clin Pathol 2007;60(1):8–17. https://doi.org/10.1136/jcp.2005.032300.

[98] Kabir MT, Uddin MS, Mamun AAl, Jeandet P, Aleya L, Mansouri RA, Ashraf GM, Mathew B, Bin-Jumah MN, Abdel-Daim MM. Combination drug therapy for the management of Alzheimer's disease. Int J Mol Sci 2020;21(9):3272. https://doi.org/10.3390/ijms21093272.

[99] Kandiah N, Pai M-C, Senanarong V, Looi I, Ampil E, Park KW, Karanam AK, Christopher S. Rivastigmine: the advantages of dual inhibition of acetylcholinesterase and butyrylcholinesterase and its role in subcortical vascular dementia and parkinson's disease dementia. Clinical Interventions in Aging 2017;12:697–707. https://doi.org/10.2147/CIA.S129145.

[100] Kassem LM, Ibrahim NA, Farhana SA. Nanoparticle therapy is a promising approach in the management and prevention of many diseases: does it help in curing Alzheimer disease?. Journal of Nanotechnology 2020;2020. 8147080 https://doi.org/10.1155/2020/8147080.

[101] Khorassani F, Hilas O. Bapineuzumab, an investigational agent for Alzheimer's disease. P & T : A Peer-Reviewed Journal for Formulary Management 2013;38(2):89–91. https://pubmed.ncbi.nlm.nih.gov/23599675.

[102] Kim J-Y, Choi WI, Kim YH, Tae G. Brain-targeted delivery of protein using chitosan- and RVG peptide-conjugated, pluronic-based nano-carrier. Biomaterials 2013;34(4):1170–8. https://doi.org/10.1016/j.biomaterials.2012.09.047.

[103] Klaver AC, Finke JM, Digambaranath J, Balasubramaniam M, Loeffler DA. Antibody concentrations to Aβ1–42 monomer and soluble oligomers in untreated and antibody–antigen-dissociated intravenous immunoglobulin preparations. Int Immunopharmacol 2010;10(1):115–9. https://doi.org/10.1016/j.intimp.2009.10.005.

[104] Knopman DS. Cerebrovascular disease and dementia. Br J Radiol 2007;80(SPEC. ISS. 2):1–10. https://doi.org/10.1259/bjr/75681080.

[105] Kumar A, Gupta V, S. S. Donepezil. In: StatPearls [Internet]. Treasure Island (FL): StatPearls Publishing; 2021, https://www.ncbi.nlm.nih.gov/books/NBK513257/.

[106] Bubeva-Ivanova L. Phytochemical investigation of Galanthus nivalis var. gracilis. Fr Polit 1957;7.

[107] Landen JW, Cohen S, Jr B, C. B, Cronenberger C, Styren S, Burstein AH, Sattler C, Lee J-H, Jr J, C. R, Kantarci K, Schwartz PF, Duggan WT, Zhao Q, Sprenger K, Bednar MM, Binneman B. Multiple-dose ponezumab for mild-to-moderate Alzheimer's disease: Safety and efficacy. Alzheimer's & Dementia (New York, N Y) 2017;3(3):339–47. https://doi.org/10.1016/j.trci.2017.04.003.

[108] Lee HJ, Lee JK, Lee H, Carter JE, Chang JW, Oh W, Yang YS, Suh J-G, Lee B-H, Jin HK, Bae J. Human umbilical cord blood-derived mesenchymal stem cells improve neuropathology and cognitive impairment in an Alzheimer's disease mouse model through modulation of neuroinflammation. Neurobiol Aging 2012;33(3):588–602. https://doi.org/10.1016/j.neurobiolaging.2010.03.024.

[109] Lee I-S, Jung K, Kim I-S, Lee H, Kim M, Yun S, Hwang K, Shin JE, Park KI. Human neural stem cells alleviate Alzheimer-like pathology in a mouse model. Molecular Neurodegeneration 2015;10:38. https://doi.org/10.1186/s13024-015-0035-6.

[110] Liu D, Fu D, Zhang L, Sun L. Detection of amyloid-beta by Fmoc-KLVFF self-assembled fluorescent nanoparticles for Alzheimer's disease diagnosis. Chin Chem Lett 2021;32(3):1066–70. https://doi.org/10.1016/j.cclet.2020.09.009.

[111] Liu J-S, Zhu Y-L, Yu C-M, Zhou Y-Z, Han Y-Y, Wu F-W, Qi B-F. The structures of huperzine A and B, two new alkaloids exhibiting marked anticholinesterase activity. Can J Chem 1986;64(4):837–9. https://doi.org/10.1139/v86-137.

[112] Liu X-Y, Yang L-P, Zhao L. Stem cell therapy for Alzheimer's disease. World Journal of Stem Cells 2020;12(8):787–802. https://doi.org/10.4252/wjsc.v12.i8.787.

[113] Alves RP, Yang MJ, Batista MT. Ferreira LC. Alzheimer's disease: is a vaccine possible? Braz J Med Biol Res 2014;47(6):438–44. doi:10.1590/1414-431x20143434.

[114] Lu R-M, Hwang Y-C, Liu I-J, Lee C-C, Tsai H-Z, Li H-J, Wu H-C. Development of therapeutic antibodies for the treatment of diseases. J Biomed Sci 2020;27(1):1. https://doi.org/10.1186/s12929-019-0592-z.

[115] Ma X, Tan C, Zhu D, Gang DR, Xiao P. Huperzine A from Huperzia species—an ethnopharmacolgical review. J Ethnopharmacol 2007;113(1):15–34. https://doi.org/10.1016/j.jep.2007.05.030.

[116] *MEDIPOSTCompletes Phase 2a clinical trial of NEUROSTEM for Alzheimer's Disease*. https://www.medi-post.com/stem-cell-therapeutic/2020/01/36435/ [Accessed 19 August 2022]

[117] Meng X, Liu J, Yu X, Li J, Lu X, Shen T. Pluronic F127 and D-α-Tocopheryl Polyethylene Glycol Succinate (TPGS) mixed micelles for targeting drug delivery across the blood brain barrier. Sci Rep 2017;7(1). doi:10.1038/s41598-017-03123-y.

[118] Merad M, Soufi W, Ghalem S, Boukli F, Baig MH, Ahmad K, Kamal MA. Molecular interaction of acetylcholinesterase with carnosic acid derivatives: a neuroinformatics study. CNS & Neurological Disorders Drug Targets 2014;13(3):440–6. https://doi.org/10.2174/18715273113126660157.

[119] Mintun MA, Lo AC, Duggan Evans C, Wessels AM, Ardayfio PA, Andersen SW, Shcherbinin S, Sparks J, Sims JR, Brys M, Apostolova LG, Salloway SP, Skovronsky DM. Donanemab in early Alzheimer's disease. N Engl J Med 2021;384(18):1691–704. https://doi.org/10.1056/NEJMoa2100708.

[120] Mistry A, Stolnik S, Illum L. Nanoparticles for direct nose-to-brain delivery of drugs. Int J Pharm 2009;379(1):146–57. https://doi.org/10.1016/j.ijpharm.2009.06.019.

[121] Moghadam FH, Alaie H, Karbalaie K, Tanhaei S, Nasr Esfahani MH, Baharvand H. Transplantation of primed or unprimed mouse embryonic stem cell-derived neural precursor cells improves cognitive function in Alzheimerian rats. Differentiation 2009;78(2):59–68. https://doi.org/10.1016/j.diff.2009.06.005.

[122] Mukherjee PK, Kumar V, Mal M, Houghton PJ. Acetylcholinesterase inhibitors from plants. Phytomedicine : International Journal of Phytotherapy and Phytopharmacology 2007;14(4):289–300. https://doi.org/10.1016/j.phymed.2007.02.002.

[123] Müller T. Rivastigmine in the treatment of patients with Alzheimer's disease. Neuropsychiatric Disease and Treatment 2007;3(2):211–8. https://doi.org/10.2147/nedt.2007.3.2.211.

[124] Proskurnina NF, L. YA. Alkaloids of Galanthus woronowi. I. Isolation of galanthamine. J Gen Chim Gen USSR 1947;17.

[125] Nilsson P, Iwata N, Muramatsu S, Tjernberg LO, Winblad B, Saido TC. Gene therapy in Alzheimer's disease – potential for disease modification. J Cell Mol Med 2010;14(4):741–57. https://doi.org/10.1111/j.1582-4934.2010.01038.x.

[126] Nisticò R, Borg JJ. Aducanumab for Alzheimer's disease: a regulatory perspective. Pharmacol Res 2021;171:105754. https://doi.org/10.1016/j.phrs.2021.105754.

[127] *No Title*. (n.d.).

[128] Onodera H, Takada G, Tada K, Desnick RJ. Microautoradiographic study on the tissue localization of liposome-entrapped or unentrapped ^{3}H-Labeled β-galactosidase injected into rats. Tohoku J Exp Med 1983;140(1):1–13. https://doi.org/10.1620/tjem.140.1.

[129] Orhan I, Terzioglu S, Sener B. Alpha-onocerin: an acetylcholinesterase inhibitor from Lycopodium clavatum. Planta Med 2003;69(3):265–7. https://doi.org/10.1055/s-2003-38489.

[130] Orive G, Hernández RM, Rodríguez Gascón A, Domínguez-Gil A, Pedraz JL. Drug delivery in biotechnology: present and future. Curr Opin Biotechnol 2003;14(6):659–64. https://doi.org/10.1016/j.copbio.2003.10.007.

[131] Ostrowitzki S, Lasser RA, Dorflinger E, Scheltens P, Barkhof F, Nikolcheva T, Ashford E, Retout S, Hofmann C, Delmar P, Klein G, Andjelkovic M, Dubois B, Boada M, Blennow K, Santarelli L, Fontoura PInvestigators, for the Sc. R. A phase III randomized trial of gantenerumab in prodromal Alzheimer's disease. Alzheimer's Research & Therapy 2017;9(1):95. https://doi.org/10.1186/s13195-017-0318-y.

[132] Pacheco-Quinto J, Herdt A, Eckman CB, Eckman EA. Endothelin-converting enzymes and related metalloproteases in Alzheimer's disease. Journal of Alzheimer's Disease : JAD 2013;33(*Suppl 1*):S101–10. 0 1. https://doi.org/10.3233/JAD-2012-129043.

[133] Pardridge WM. Delivery of biologics across the blood-brain barrier with molecular trojan horse technology. BioDrugs : Clinical Immunotherapeutics, Biopharmaceuticals and Gene Therapy 2017;31(6):503–19. https://doi.org/10.1007/s40259-017-0248-z.

[134] Pardridge WM. Alzheimer's disease: future drug development and the blood-brain barrier. Expert Opin Investig Drugs 2019;28(7):569–72. https://doi.org/10.1080/13543784.2019.1627325.

[135] Patel T, Zhou J, Piepmeier JM, Saltzman WM. Polymeric nanoparticles for drug delivery to the central nervous system. Adv Drug Deliv Rev 2012;64(7):701–5. https://doi.org/10.1016/j.addr.2011.12.006.

[136] VX15 Anti-Semaphorin 4D Antibody (pepinemab) Increases FDG-PET Signal and is a Potential Treatment for Alzheimer's Disease. https://ir.vaccinex.com/static-files/7b26635c-d97b-48b1-bcc0-bd77d8df5ce4 [Accessed 19 August 2022].

[137] Postmes THJ, Hukkelhoven M, van den Bogaard AEJM, Halders SG, Coenegracht J. Passage through the blood-brain barrier of thyrotropin-releasing hormone encapsulated in liposomes. J Pharm Pharmacol 1980;32(1):722–4. https://doi.org/10.1111/j.2042-7158.1980.tb13051.x.

[138] Qaseem A, Snow V, Cross JTJ, Forciea MA, Hopkins RJ, Shekelle P, Adelman A, Mehr D, Schellhase K, Campos-Outcalt D, Santaguida P, Owens DK. Current pharmacologic treatment of dementia: a clinical practice guideline from the American College of Physicians and the American Academy of Family Physicians. Ann Intern Med 2008;148(5):370–8. https://doi.org/10.7326/0003-4819-148-5-200803040-00008.

[139] Qosa H, Volpe DA. The development of biological therapies for neurological diseases: moving on from previous failures. Expert Opin Drug Discovery 2018;13(4):283–93. https://doi.org/10.1080/17460441.2018.1437142.

[140] Reddy MK, Labhasetwar V. Nanoparticle-mediated delivery of superoxide dismutase to the brain: an effective strategy to reduce ischemia-reperfusion injury. FASEB J 2009;23(5):1384–95. https://doi.org/10.1096/fj.08-116947.

[141] Rees V*Delivering gene therapies to the brain to treat Alzheimer's*. https://www.drugtargetreview.com/article/96311/delivering-gene-therapies-to-the-brain-to-treat-alzheimers/?__cf_chl_rt_tk=JQ_nVmL_99VDuhbSNlwD3Kp0AJc8q4_zxLYwCDbbW1Q-1639632887-0-gaNycGzNCKU [Accessed 19 August 2022].

[142] Ren Y, Houghton PJ, Hider RC, Howes M-JR. Novel diterpenoid acetylcholinesterase inhibitors from Salvia miltiorhiza. Planta Med 2004;70(3):201–4. https://doi.org/10.1055/s-2004-815535.

[143] Ringertz HG (1993). Radiology and the Swedish council on technology assessment in health care. In *Investigative Radiology* (Vol. 28, Issue June). 10.1097/00004424-199308003-00023

[144] Roche M, Rondeau P, Singh NR, Tarnus E, Bourdon E. The antioxidant properties of serum albumin. FEBS Lett 2008;582(13):1783–7. https://doi.org/10.1016/j.febslet.2008.04.057.

[145] Roche Media Release. https://www.roche.com/media/releases/med-cor-2019-01-30.htm [Accessed 19 August 2022].

[146] Rotman M, Welling MM, Bunschoten A, de Backer ME, Rip J, Nabuurs RJA, Gaillard PJ, van Buchem MA, van der Maarel SM, van der Weerd L. Enhanced glutathione PEGylated liposomal brain delivery of an anti-amyloid single domain antibody fragment in a mouse model for Alzheimer's disease. J Controlled Release 2015;203:40–50. https://doi.org/10.1016/j.jconrel.2015.02.012.

[147] Rygiel K. Novel strategies for Alzheimer's disease treatment: an overview of anti-amyloid beta monoclonal antibodies. Indian Journal of Pharmacology 2016;48(6):629–36. https://doi.org/10.4103/0253-7613.194867.

[148] Salloway S, Sperling R, Fox NC, Blennow K, Klunk W, Raskind M, Sabbagh M, Honig LS, Porsteinsson AP, Ferris S, Reichert M, Ketter N, Nejadnik B, Guenzler V, Miloslavsky M, Wang D, Lu Y, Lull J, Tudor IC…, Brashear HR. Two Phase 3 trials of bapineuzumab in mild-to-moderate Alzheimer's disease. N Engl J Med 2014;370(4):322–33. https://doi.org/10.1056/NEJMoa1304839.

[149] Salvalaio M, Rigon L, Belletti D, D'Avanzo F, Pederzoli F, Ruozi B, Marin O, Vandelli MA, Forni F, Scarpa M, Tomanin R, Tosi G. Targeted polymeric nanoparticles for brain delivery of high molecular weight molecules in lysosomal storage disorders. PLoS One 2016;11(5):e0156452. https://doi.org/10.1371/journal.pone.0156452.

[150] Sathya M, Premkumar P, Karthick C, Moorthi P, Jayachandran KS, Anusuyadevi M. BACE1 in Alzheimer's disease. Clin Chim Acta 2012;414:171–8. https://doi.org/10.1016/j.cca.2012.08.013.

[151] Saunders NR, Habgood MD, Møllgård K, Dziegielewska KM. The biological significance of brain barrier mechanisms: help or hindrance in drug delivery to the central nervous system?. F1000Research 2016;5. https://doi.org/10.12688/f1000research.7378.1.

[152] Schenk D, Basi GS, Pangalos MN. Treatment strategies targeting amyloid β-protein. Cold Spring Harb Perspect Med 2012;2(9):a006387. https://doi.org/10.1101/cshperspect.a006387.

[153] Scott SA, Crutcher KA. Nerve growth factor and Alzheimer's disease. Rev Neurosci 1994;5(3):179–211. https://doi.org/10.1515/revneuro.1994.5.3.179.

[154] Sevigny J, Chiao P, Bussière T, Weinreb PH, Williams L, Maier M, Dunstan R, Salloway S, Chen T, Ling Y, O'Gorman J, Qian F, Arastu M, Li M, Chollate S, Brennan MS, Quintero-Monzon O, Scannevin RH, Arnold HM…, Sandrock A. The antibody aducanumab reduces Aβ plaques in Alzheimer's disease. Nature 2016;537(7618):50–6. https://doi.org/10.1038/nature19323.

[155] Sharma S. Nanotechnology Based Targeted Drug Delivery: Current Status and Future Prospects for Drug Development. London: IntechOpen; 2011. A. S. E.-I. M. Kapetanovic [Ed.]; p. Ch. 19. https://doi.org/10.5772/28902.

[156] Siemers ER, Friedrich S, Dean RA, Gonzales CR, Farlow MR, Paul SM, DeMattos RB. Safety and changes in plasma and cerebrospinal fluid amyloid β after a single administration of an amyloid β monoclonal antibody in subjects with Alzheimer disease. Clin Neuropharmacol 2010;33(2). https://journals.lww.com/clinicalneuropharm/Fulltext/2010/03000/Safety_and_Changes_in_Plasma_and_Cerebrospinal.3.aspx [Accessed 19 August 2022.].

[157] Siemers ER, Sundell KL, Carlson C, Case M, Sethuraman G, Liu-Seifert H, Dowsett SA, Pontecorvo MJ, Dean RA, Demattos R. Phase 3 solanezumab trials: Secondary outcomes in mild Alzheimer's disease patients. Alzheimer's & Dementia : The Journal of the Alzheimer's Association 2016;12(2):110–20. https://doi.org/10.1016/j.jalz.2015.06.1893.

[158] Singer O, Marr RA, Rockenstein E, Crews L, Coufal NG, Gage FH, Verma IM, Masliah E. Targeting BACE1 with siRNAs ameliorates Alzheimer disease neuropathology in a transgenic model. Nat Neurosci 2005;8(10):1343–9. https://doi.org/10.1038/nn1531.

[159] Sinha K, Sun C, Kamari R, Bettermann K. Current status and future prospects of pathophysiology-based neuroprotective drugs for the treatment of vascular dementia. Drug Discovery Today 2020;25(4):793–9. https://doi.org/10.1016/j.drudis.2020.01.003.

[160] Strohl WR, Strohl LMBT-TAE. 1 - Introduction to biologics and monoclonal antibodies. In: Woodhead Publishing Series in Biomedicine Woodhead Publishing; 2012. p. 1–595. https://doi.org/10.1533/9781908818096.1.

[161] Suri K, Wolfram J, Shen H, Ferrari M. Advances in nanotechnology-based drug delivery platforms and novel drug delivery systems. In: Novel Approaches and Strategies for Biologics, Vaccines and Cancer Therapies. USA: Elsevier Inc.; 2015:41–58. https://doi.org/10.1016/B978-0-12-416603-5.00003-1.

[162] *ClinicalTrials.gov Identifier: NCT02760602*. https://clinicaltrials.gov/ct2/show/NCT02551809 [Accessed 19 August 2022].

[163] Tonda-Turo C, Origlia N, Mattu C, Accorroni A, Chiono V. Current limitations in the treatment Parkinson's and Alzheimer's diseases: state-of-the-art and future perspective of polymeric carriers. Curr Med Chem 2018;25. doi:10.2174/0929867325666180221125759.

[164] Torres-Acosta N, O'Keefe JH, O'Keefe EL, Isaacson R, Small G. Therapeutic potential of TNF-α inhibition for Alzheimer's disease prevention. Journal of Alzheimer's Disease : JAD 2020;78(2):619–26. https://doi.org/10.3233/JAD-200711.

[165] TrueBinding. https://www.truebinding.com/ourscience [Accessed 19 August 2022].

[166] Tsujimura A, Taguchi K, Watanabe Y, Tatebe H, Tokuda T, Mizuno T, Tanaka M. Lysosomal enzyme cathepsin B enhances the aggregate forming activity of exogenous α-synuclein fibrils. Neurobiol Dis 2015;73:244–53. https://doi.org/10.1016/j.nbd.2014.10.011.

[167] Tuszynski MH, Thal L, Pay M, Salmon DP, U HS, Bakay R, Patel P, Blesch A, Vahlsing HL, Ho G, Tong G, Potkin SG, Fallon J, Hansen L, Mufson EJ, Kordower JH, Gall C, Conner J. A phase 1 clinical trial of nerve growth factor gene therapy for Alzheimer disease. Nat Med 2005;11(5):551–5. https://doi.org/10.1038/nm1239.

[168] Ultsch M, Li B, Maurer T, Mathieu M, Adolfsson O, Muhs A, Pfeifer A, Pihlgren M, Bainbridge TW, Reichelt M, Ernst JA, Eigenbrot C, Fuh G, Atwal JK, Watts RJ, Wang W. Structure of Crenezumab complex with Aβ Shows Loss of β-Hairpin. Sci Rep 2016;6:39374. https://doi.org/10.1038/srep39374.

[169] USFDA. *AduhelmTM label*. https://www.accessdata.fda.gov/drugsatfda_docs/label/2021/761178s000lbl.pdf [Accessed 19 August 2022].

[170] USFDA. *ILARIS label*. https://www.accessdata.fda.gov/drugsatfda_docs/label/2020/125319s100lbl.pdf/ [Accessed 19 August 2022].

[171] USFDA. (a). www.fda.gov/about-fda/center-biologics-evaluation-and-research-cber/what-are-biologics-questions-and-answers [Accessed 19 August 2022].

[172] USFDA. (b). *FDA's Decision to Approve New Treatment for Alzheimer's Disease*. https://www.fda.gov/drugs/news-events-human-drugs/fdas-decision-approve-new-treatment-alzheimers-disease [Accessed 19 August 2022].

[173] Voyager Therapeutics Press Release. https://ir.voyagertherapeutics.com/news-releases/news-release-details/voyager-therapeutics-receives-fda-clearance-ind-application-gene [Accessed 19 August 2022].

[174] Wang CY, Wang P-N, Chiu M-J, Finstad CL, Lin F, Lynn S, Tai Y-H, De Fang X, Zhao K, Hung C-H, Tseng Y, Peng W-J, Wang J, Yu C-C, Kuo B-S, Frohna PA. UB-311, a novel UBITh(®) amyloid β peptide vaccine for mild Alzheimer's disease. Alzheimer's & Dementia (New York, N Y) 2017;3(2):262–72. https://doi.org/10.1016/j.trci.2017.03.005.

[175] Willis BA, Sundell K, Lachno DR, Ferguson-Sells LR, Case MG, Holdridge K, DeMattos RB, Raskin J, Siemers ER, Dean RA. Central pharmacodynamic activity of solanezumab

in mild Alzheimer's disease dementia. Alzheimer's & Dementia: Translational Research & Clinical Interventions 2018;4(1):652–60. https://doi.org/10.1016/j.trci.2018.10.001.

[176] Wisniewski T, Goñi F. Immunotherapeutic approaches for Alzheimer's disease. Neuron 2015;85(6):1162–76. https://doi.org/10.1016/j.neuron.2014.12.064.

[177] World Health Organization. https://www.who.int/health-topics/biologicals#tab=tab_1 [Accessed 19 August 2022].

[178] Xie Y, Ye L, Zhang X, Cui W, Lou J, Nagai T, Hou X. Transport of nerve growth factor encapsulated into liposomes across the blood-brain barrier: in vitro and in vivo studies. J Controlled Release 2005;105(1–2):106–19. https://doi.org/10.1016/j.jconrel.2005.03.005.

[179] Yiannopoulou KG, Papageorgiou SG. Current and future treatments in Alzheimer disease: an update. Journal of Central Nervous System Disease 2020;12. https://doi.org/10.1177/1179573520907397.

[180] Zaghmi A, Drouin-Ouellet J, Brambilla D, Gauthier MA. Treating brain diseases using systemic parenterally-administered protein therapeutics: dysfunction of the brain barriers and potential strategies. Biomaterials 2021;269:120461. https://doi.org/10.1016/j.biomaterials.2020.120461.

[181] Zhang C, Zheng X, Wan X, Shao X, Liu Q, Zhang Z, Zhang Q. The potential use of H102 peptide-loaded dual-functional nanoparticles in the treatment of Alzheimer's disease. J Controlled Release 2014;192:317–24. https://doi.org/10.1016/j.jconrel.2014.07.050.

[182] Zhang X-Z, Qian S-S, Zhang Y-J, Wang R-Q. Salvia miltiorrhiza: a source for anti-Alzheimer's disease drugs. Pharm Biol 2015;54:1–7. https://doi.org/10.3109/13880209.2015.1027408.

[183] Zhou M, Xu R, Kaelber DC, Gurney ME. Tumor Necrosis Factor (TNF) blocking agents are associated with lower risk for Alzheimer's disease in patients with rheumatoid arthritis and psoriasis. PLoS One 2020;15(3):e0229819. https://doi.org/10.1371/journal.pone.0229819..

[184] Prasanna P, Rathee S, Rahul V, Mandal D, Chandra Goud MS, Yadav P, et al. Microfluidic Platforms to Unravel Mysteries of Alzheimer's Disease: How Far Have We Come? Life 2021;11(10). doi:10.3390/life11101022.

[185] Esang M, Gupta M. Aducanumab as a novel treatment for alzheimer's disease: a decade of hope, controversies, and the future. Cureus 2021;13(8). doi:10.7759/cureus.17591.

[186] Abbas M. Potential role of nanoparticles in treating the accumulation of amyloid-beta peptide in alzheimer's patients. Polymers 2021;13(7). doi:10.3390/polym13071051.

Chapter 10

Nanocarriers-based noninvasive approaches for dementia

Priyanka Kumari, Rusham Das, Amit Kumar Goyal
Department of Pharmacy, School of Chemical Sciences, & Pharmacy, Central University of Rajasthan

10.1 Introduction

Dementia is a severe illness that causes patients, society, and their caregivers enormous physical, psychological, and pecuniary burdens. A clinical condition exhibits gradual cognitive deterioration that impairs an individual's capacity to operate independently [1]. Globally, the number of cases of dementia is expected to be rise from 57.4 (50.4–65.1 interval with 95% uncertainty) million in 2019 to 153 (130.8–175.9 interval) million in 2050 [2]. Dementia should be seen as an inherited trait with various plausible origins, rather than a disease in and of itself [3]. The information must be recorded, stored, and retrieved in memory. The most prevalent clinical manifestation of Alzheimer's disease (AD) is a gradual loss of memory, usually accompanied by a difficulty to learn new knowledge, especially introspective information such as recent events in one's life. This is due to the fact that AD primarily damages neural circuits involved in episodic memory [4]. Mild cognitive impairment is characterized as performance on objective neuropsychological cognition tests that are lower than expected but usual everyday functioning. Neurodegenerative diseases (such as early phases of Lewy body disease), cerebrovascular disease (e.g., sporadic small strokes), psychiatric conditions (e.g., depression, anxiety), etc., and medications that affect cognition (e.g., opioids), all-cause fluctuations during cognition and variability in cognitive test results [5]. Schwarz et al. concluded after focusing on its pathophysiology that only symptomatic cure is available to overcome dementia with limited therapy licensed for AD. The approved drug as a monotherapy were cholinesterase inhibitors and memantine, which in combination may provide advanced therapeutic activity [6,7]. The other conventional therapy given orally were galantamine, donepezil, and rivastigmine, whereas galantine was preferred mostly via transdermal route. There are various immediate drug delivery systems that are available via sublingual, pulmonary, or transdermal routes with low therapeutic index and high systemic side effects

Nanomedicine-Based Approaches for the Treatment of Dementia. https://doi.org/10.1016/B978-0-12-824331-2.00004-2
Copyright © 2023 Elsevier Inc. All rights reserved.

[8]. For specific and targeted drug delivery use of nanocarrier and nanotechnology has been found to be an effective and successive tool to deliver biologically active molecules through blood–brain barrier (BBB). It elevates the healing efficacy and curtails adverse effects confederated with typical drug. Encapsulation of traditional drug in the form of nanomedicine works on increasing its potency to the site of action and its bioavailability [9].

10.2 Approaches for the treatment of dementia

Approaches to the treatment of dementia have advanced rapidly and the treatment schemes range from noninvasive to invasive methods along with behavioural techniques for the betterment of the quality of life for the patients suffering from dementia [10,11].

10.2.1 Molecule-based approaches

The molecular-based approaches range from the application of medications or drug molecules and other methods that are still under development. These work on the mechanisms ranging from the removal of Amyloid β plaque to the prevention of plaque formation [12,13]. Details of the methods that are under the developmental stage are also furnished in the chapter.

10.2.1.1 Medication-based therapies

In the current scenario, no treatment for AD, available therapies only provide relief from the symptoms. It was observed many promising molecules could not make it through the clinical trials in the past decade, hence the introduction suggested by the British Association for Psychopharmacology that existing dementia diagnosing standards are accurate enough to be used in clinical management [14]. Brain scanning is done using a morphological approach like MRI and CT scan, and a functional approach like single-photon emission computerized tomography and positron emission tomography as these can enhance diagnosis performance in specific conditions [15]. Cholinesterase inhibitors like galantamine, rivastigmine, and donepezil were found to be useful to enhance perception for minor to intermediate AD, whereas memantine [16] is efficient in intermediate to extreme AD [17–19]. Combined treatment (cholinesterase inhibitors with memantine) can also prove advantageous. Drugs must not be interrupted simply because the magnitude of dementia worsens. Certain medications, such as statins, anti-inflammatory drugs, vitamin E, dietary nutraceuticals, and *Ginkgo biloba* [20], can never be advised to exhibit counteractive action and therapy of AD unless additional data is obtained. In people with modest cognitive deficits, both cholinesterase inhibitors and memantine are useful [21]. Cholinesterase inhibitors seem ineffective and might even increase irritation in people with front temporal dementia, however, serotonin reuptake inhibitors may aid with behavioural (and not perceptual) symptoms [22]. Cholinesterase inhibitors, including memantine, must be administered to cure persons having both Parkinson's disease (PD) dementia as well as dementia due to Lewy bodies [23]. In vascular dementia, no medicines are obviously useful, however cholinesterase inhibitors seem helpful in mixed dementia. Multifactorial therapies do have the ability to prohibit or postpone the symptoms of dementia, according to preliminary research. However, the general approach concentrates on medicine, both behavioural and noncognitive disorders can benefit from psychiatric therapies in combination with pharmacotherapy [24]. Numerous innovative pharmaceutical treatments for reducing amyloid and/or tau accumulation in persons having or under elevated danger of AD are now in the works. Although crucial study findings in the initial (prodromal/mild) AD remain pending, outcomes in further advanced (light to medium) AD show ambiguity, along with no disease-modifying drugs are presently approved nor suggested for clinical administration [10].

Atypical antipsychotic medication for behavioural and psychiatric abnormalities in individuals suffering from serious dementia has now been studied in multiple randomized regulated studies. Risperidone in a dose of roughly 1 mg/d as well as olanzapine at a level of 5–10 mg/d appears to be more highly beneficial than that of the placebo in trials. Regulatory agencies have published advisories in recent times that these two medications raise the chance of cerebrovascular episodes [25].

10.2.1.2 Methods that prevent formation of amyloid-β

To minimize or prevent the generation of Amyloid-β, the main rogue in AD, the accompanying treatments have been recommended.

10.2.1.2.1 α-secretase activation

Reversing APP conversion into nonamyloidogenic pathway via increasing α -secretase function results in a decrease in entire Aβ synthesis and, as a result, a significantly lower risk of AD. As a result, the development of α-secretase catalysts as well as α-secretase mimetics are being considered as a promising treatment strategy for treating cytotoxic A [26].

10.2.1.2.2 γ-secretase or β-secretase inhibition

Hazardous Aβ peptides are produced by the aberrant breakdown of amyloid progenitor protein with the help of β- as well as γ-secretase in AD [27]. Blocking action of the abovementioned proteolytic enzymes may help to prevent the progression of AD [28]. For inhibiting this type of proteases, a range of γ as well as β-secretase blockers were created [29].

10.2.1.3 Methods that promote blocking of Aβ self-assembly

Self-assembling Aβ components have the ability to create hazardous hydrophilic oligomers. The capacity of such improperly folded oligomers, also referred to as seeds, to catalyze a cascade of events driving the agglomeration of nontoxic, non agglomerated Aβ particles [30] to a hazardous oligomeric form has now been documented. One of the most widely used techniques toward finding possible treatments of AD has been used to prevent Aβ from self-assembling [31].

10.2.1.3.1 Modulators based on small molecules

Small molecule-based prospective treatment approaches work by segregating the monomeric state of amyloid-β, hindering subsequent self-assembly as well as preventing Aβ oligomerization, modifying the epitaxial development of dangerous Aβ oligomers, therefore controlling the advancement of the amyloidogenic mechanism [32]. Small molecule activators are organic molecules with a low molecular mass that can bind to the monomeric Aβ peptide. Numerous polyphenol-containing drugs prevent mental impairment by inhibiting Aβ oligomerization. Oleuropein, a polyphenol produced from olive oil was found possessing anti-inflammatory, antioxidant, and hypocholesterolemic properties [33].

10.2.1.3.2 Immunotherapy

Immunotherapy stimulates the development of antibodies that aim the elimination of Aβ oligomers or plaques in order to prevent plaque [34] buildup by activating the host defence mechanisms to recognize as well as stop Aβ. As a treatment strategy for inhibiting Aβ oligomerization, either active or passive Aβ immunization can be used [35]. Antibody-mediated immobilization of hydrophilic or oligomeric state of the peptide is possible because the markers of Aβ are uncovered and approachable. Anti-Aβ antibodies promote amyloid plaque removal by microglia that redirect the Aβ peptide through the brain to the circulatory system [36]. In recent years, a slew of anti-A immunotherapeutics was approved for clinical studies, some of which can bind to particular Aβ epitopes. The Phase III clinical studies for BAN-2401, aducanumab, gantenerumab, crenezumab, solanezumab, as well as IV immunoglobulin G (IVIG) are now underway [37]. In a rat model of AD, research indicates that cancer therapeutics on the basis of immunotherapy, which is also cleared by the FDA and is called programmed death-1 inhibitors were effective in eliminating Aβ plaques while improving cognition. Advancement in science & clinical research has positioned immunotherapy as a possible disease-modifying treatment for AD [38].

10.2.1.3.3 Modulators based on peptide

The utilization of peptides as Aβ agglomeration activators is a viable alternative that has significant benefits, including biological compatibility, low toxic effects, good selectivity, low tissue accumulation, chemically diversified design domain, and a higher likelihood of BBB permeability. The sensitivity of peptides toward proteolytic processing has limited their employment in perturbance.

Altered peptides with unnatural as well as D-amino acids, on the other hand, showed lower protease penetration [39].

A rising number of small peptides were seen to have antiamyloid agglomeration properties. These Aβ analogues relying on peptides can be divided into various types. The following are the two most frequent sequence-based strategies [40]:

i. **Peptides founded on Aβ's core detection pattern:** The brief peptide fragment "KLVFF" (Aβ 16–20) has been dubbed "core recognition motif" for creating effective antagonists of Aβ self-assembly by certain scientists. The peptide-dependent perturbants that bound to this area were similarly able to attach to entire Aβ as well as prevent it from fibrillating. Several peptides addressing the core Aβ section were produced ever since to restrict Aβ from aggregating into -sheet-rich fibrils; such peptides generally designated as the β-sheet destroyers [41].
ii. **N-methylated peptides:** N-methylation is thought to reduce hydrogen bonding amongst amyloidogenic proteins due to its steric impact. As a result, a large number of N-methylated peptides were successfully utilized to inhibit amyloid fibrillation [42].

10.2.1.3.4 Metal ion-based chelators

The metal ion theory proposes that metal ion (Cu^{2+}, Zn^{2+}, and Fe^{2+}) equilibrium plays an important part in brain function. Metal ion equilibrium disturbance is speculated to have a considerable part in the neuropathogenesis of AD [43], which has sparked immense curiosity about its treatment potential. As a result, a large number of metal ion chelating agents were being tested for potential effectiveness in the treatment of Aβ self-association [44,45].

10.2.1.3.5 Chaperone proteins

Molecular chaperones are a kind of protein that plays an important part in protein equilibrium, with one of its main tasks being to prevent improper folding of proteins as well as agglomeration. As a result, attempts to develop molecular chaperone duplicates with function as well as selectivity over amyloidogenic proteins, which might be used as therapeutic solutions to address amyloid disorders, have sparked [46]. Hsp70 chaperone subtypes with higher selectivity for Aβ42 over wild-type strain Hsp70 have been developed by a group of researchers. The produced fibrils were fragmented by these variations, which impeded A42 self-assembly [47]. Researchers have established the ability of artificial nanochaperones designed on mixed-shell polymeric micelles (MSPM) to strongly attach to Aβ monomers as well as oligomers, limit Aβ fibrillation, & reduce induced neurotoxicity in a remarkable investigation. Numerous groups have used the chaperone method to stop the agglomeration of additional amyloidosis-inducing proteins, suggesting that it might be a viable option in the implementation of novel amyloidosis therapeutics [48].

10.2.1.4 Therapies that target tau protein

Recent tau research suggests that tau impairment has a stronger link to dementia intensity than amyloid deposition. As a result, preventing tau accumulation or eliminating the accumulated varieties of tau will be much more therapeutically successful than eradicating Aβ agglomerates as a treatment method [49]. Treatments dependent on tau protein regulation are still in their early stages, with the sole possibility now in Phase III clinical research having phenothiazine methylene blue (a tau protein blocker). The tau-based treatment strategy has run across major roadblocks. Because tau pathophysiology is associated with over 30 neurological illnesses, designing an AD-specific tau antagonist is difficult [50]. The tau pathophysiology is even not replicated in the developmental mice models. No tau alteration has so far been linked to AD. The significance of tau hyper phosphorylation in Alzheimer's pathogenesis is still debated. However, a worldwide Phase 3 study is currently looking into the idea of utilizing a tau agglomeration antagonist to treat AD [51].

10.2.1.4.1 Immunotherapy

Because the configuration of the tau motif fluctuates during the disorder, immunotherapeutic treatments are solely reliant on the degree of the ailment. Antibodies can be directed against hyper phosphorylated tau, overall tau, exact tau, multimeric tau, as well as segments of tau [52].

10.2.1.4.2 Polyphenols

Polyphenols that work to suppress tau accumulation do so via stopping it from oligomerizing as well as fibrillating. Polyphenols such as "phenothiazines, porphyrins, benzothiazoles, cyanines, phenylthiazole-hydra-zides, N-phenylamines, thioxothiazolidinone, aminothienopyridazines, and anthraquinones" were demonstrated to possess anti-amyloid properties [53]. Natural polyphenols such as epigallocatechin gallate (found in green tea), oleocanthal, and oleuropein (from olive oil) are tau blockers that primarily attack tau monomers [54,55].

10.2.1.4.3 Peptides that target the core identifying pattern of tau

Two hexapeptide sequences found in tau's "repeat domain," VQIVYK and VQIINK, were found to be critical for tau accumulation to neurofibrillary tangles [56]. As a result, such fragments are thought to compose tau protein's fundamental identification pattern, making them an attractive template for designing structure-based blockers of tau self-assembly. There were previously been a number of peptide-based inducer described. They might act as a blueprint for creating new peptide-based therapies for AD [57,58].

10.2.2 Noninvasive approaches

Noninvasive approaches are more utilized for the therapy of AD in order to improve quality of life of the patient, improve cognitive ability, and bring

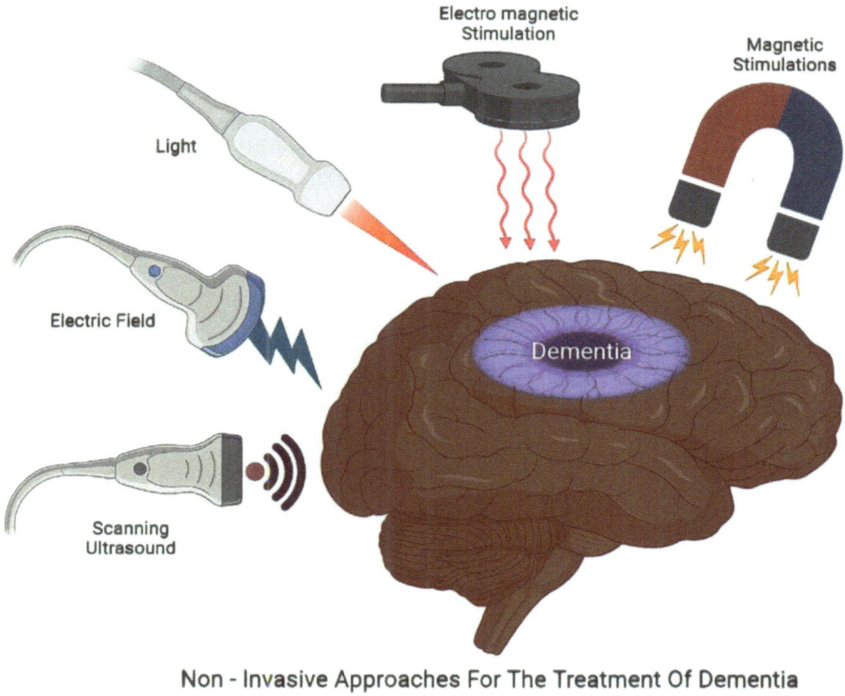

FIG. 10.1 Conventional noninvasive approaches for the treatment of dementia.

behavioral changes. The most popularly utilized approaches are explored thoroughly by scientists and have been found to be helping in the symptomatic relief. A graphical representation of the conventional noninvasive methods is shown in Fig. 10.1.

10.2.2.1 Light therapy

By interference of amyloid accumulation, light individually as well as in collaboration with chemical stimulators can stop neurodegeneration. Numerous research on-amyloid and tau hybrid animal designs indicate that therapy with near-infrared radiation has beneficial impacts [59]. Therapy utilizing near-infrared radiation reduces plaques and clumps in the brain, oxidative distress, and inflammatory processes. It also improves mitochondrial performance, leading to high ATP synthesis, from these researches [60]. Natural light in association with xanthene pigments inhibited A self-assembly via blocking the structural transformation of monomeric to sheet structure, according to research. The decrease of Aβ-imparted cytotoxic activity was mainly due to the suppression of self-assembly [61].

10.2.2.2 Scanning ultrasound therapy

Scanning ultrasound (SU) is a nonsurgical technique that has recently been found to decrease plaque burden as well as improve cognition inside an animal system of AD. SU lowers plaques via temporarily breaching the BBB thus promoting the internalization of amyloid plaques within microglial lysosomes by phagocytosis [62]. The capacity of SU that breaches the BBB could be used in medication administration as well. A nonthermal targeted ultrasound paired to an I.V. injection comprising microparticles was shown to possess the ability of unlocking the BBB for therapy purposes, as in combination with SU [63]. The short & long term consequences of SU were also studied, and thus the findings suggest that ultrasonic can also be utilized effectively to prevent the age-related degeneration of dendrites inside a neuron while not harming synaptic excitement [64].

10.2.2.3 Electric field

Several researches looking into the overall impact of an externally applied electrostatic current upon amyloidogenic peptides and proteins have found that the external electric field causes a permanent alteration in the shape. The administered external electric field generates a significantly stable or transitory dipole to develop alongside the supplied field's path, modifying the amyloid-sheet structure. Molecular dynamical predictions involving Aβ amyloid peptides as well as insulin there in the vicinity of an exogenous applied electric field have clearly anticipated the influence of such an outer electric field in altering protein structure [65]. Current research looked at utilizing an electrostatic force to decouple amyloid fibrils via promoting conformational changes together into the α-helical configuration, which reduced its β-sheet structure. A steady electric field, according to one speculative investigation, may affect a transition from just a β-sheet to a helical arrangement. Electric fields can cause molecules containing a polarity across the amide surfaces to rotate as well as orient the polarity in the field vector's path. A collaborative alteration within the organization of bacteriorhodopsin might be caused by introducing a relatively mild intensity (150 V/cm) electric field, according to a different investigation. The impact of intensity-based AC electromagnetic current produced vibration in detaching prefabricated amyloid fibrils was investigated in a laboratory investigation. A scientific team has established the potential therapeutic effectiveness of electric-induced self-assembly regulation in three distinct laboratory investigations. Researchers discovered that combined AC and DC fields may influence overall nanoarchitecture of diphenylalanine, as well as agglomeration along with lethality of amyloid-beta as well as tau's central peptide sections. On the exploratory aspects, the utilization of electromagnetic current as a treatment is still not fully studied. The findings of speculative investigations are incongruent. Low-amplitude electric fields have the ability to be a useful, noninvasive weapon in the fight against AD as well as related amyloid disfunctionalities. However, in order to be considered as a prospective treatment alternative, the area needs additional experimental investigation for effectiveness as well as toxicity [66–68].

10.2.2.4 Brain stimulation (noninvasive)

Noninvasive cerebral excitation, namely transcranial magnetic excitation as well as a transcranial directed electrical stimulus, seems to be a viable substitute for invasive pharmaceutical treatments for AD. Transcranial magnetic stimulations work by using Faraday's electromagnetic technique to electrical impulses in specified cerebral areas. Transcranial magnetic stimulation treatments had also been proven to improve the recollection and cognitive ability of dementia sufferers in numerous trials [69]. Transcranial magnetic stimulation therapy provides some symptomatic alleviation, despite inconsistent outcomes documented by several organizations using diverse methodologies. The transcranial direct current stimulation modifies cerebral responsiveness by delivering minimal DC voltage to the patient's skull using probes [70]. According to the latest studies, transcranial direct current stimulation can help Alzheimer's patients enhance their vision, phonemic awareness capacity, attentiveness control, executive function, and syllable retention. The success of preclinical noninvasive brain stimulation techniques necessitates regulated, multisite randomized clinical studies to establish their treatment possibilities for AD [71].

10.3 Nanocarrier-based invasive approaches

As the genetic carrier systems have the incapability of crossing the BBB in order to deliver the genetic materials to brain following administration intravenously, its potential as a carrier agent cannot be utilized in the treatments for the brain ailments including cancer, Parkinsonism, and AD. It was investigated whether a lactoferrin-bearing generation 3-diaminobutyric polypropylenimine (DAB) dendrimer will indeed permit transmission of plasmid DNA to the brain upon IV administration, based on the fact that lactoferrin could indeed successfully approach the brain through utilizing particular receptors for passing the BBB. *In vitro*, coupling of lactoferrin to dendrimer resulted in a 2.1-fold increase in DNA absorption in bEnd.3 murine brain capillary endothelial cells especially in comparison to unaltered dendrimer. *In vivo*, intravenous treatment of lactoferrin-bearing DAB dendriplex raised the expression of genes in the brain by over 6.4 times when matched to DAB dendriplex, although lowering gene expression of lung as well as kidneys [72]. The brain has much greater gene expression compared to any significant organ in the body. As a result, a DAB dendrimer represents a potential transport strategy for systemic gene transfer to the brain [73].

Inconsistencies in brain insulin signaling have been [74] linked with pathophysiology of AD. In this context, the neuroprotective benefit of metformin, which acts like a sensitizer for insulin, was already proven in previous research. Incorporating a genomic transceiver, romidepsin, with metformin in the current study will enhance neurotrophic factor as well as the expression of gene and minimize AD-associated molecular and physiological modifications through packing them primarily into a nanocarrier surface-modified [75] template for enhanced treatment efficacy & biocompatibility. The model's generated intracerebroventricular streptozocin (3 mg/kg) AD was packed using metformin as well as romidepsin into a poloxamer stabilized polymer nanoparticle (NP) drug delivery framework in the current study. In comparison to both free individual medication (romidepsin 50 mg/kg and metformin 10 mg/kg) and free combined medication treatment (romidepsin 25 mg/kg & metformin 5 mg/kg), decreased molecular as well as physiological changes across 21 days was observed. The nanomaterials (romidepsin 25 mg/kg & metformin 5 mg/kg) have also exhibited higher neurological efficacy than that of the unrestricted combo of medications, as evidenced by dramatically reduced anxiety and increased neurotrophic factors. The combinatorial neuroprotective activity of metformin plus romidepsin was subsequently boosted, thanks to the poloxamer sturdy polymeric nanocarrier platform [76].

The development of dementia is thought to be influenced by brain energy problems and oxidative stress caused by prolonged hypoperfusion. The goal of a research was to look at how brain creatine kinase (BB-CK) response as well as mitochondrial respiratory chain activity changed in male Wistar rats that were given prolonged cerebral hypoperfusion. The blockage of brachiocephalic trunk along with the left common carotid artery was achieved with no need for a thoracotomy utilizing a less operative method (CCA). At 2 as well as 10 weeks of persistent 3-VO, the advance rate for creatine kinase (kfor) had been determined *in vivo* using maximal transfer 31P magnetic resonance spectroscopy. At 10 weeks following 3-VO, the activity of mitochondrial respiratory cycle in vitro was evaluated polarographically [77]. The considerable 42% decreasing trend in kfor at 2 as well as 10 weeks particularly in comparison to controls implied brain energy metabolism dysfunction, that is consistent to the 12% decline in the oxidative phosphorylation coefficient (ADP:O) as well as the fourteen percent reduction in the oxidative phosphorylation rate assessed in separated mitochondria. Persistent 3-VO may therefore contribute to a vascular intellectual disability including neuronal degradation through oxidative alteration of creatine kinase mechanism (enzyme inactivation), but also metabolic problems [78].

AD is characterized by growing cognitive impairment including behavioral dysfunction (AD). We created an epigallocatechin-3-gallate (EGCG) as well as β-site amyloid antecedent protein (APP) cleaving enzyme 1 antisense (BACE1-AS) shRNA-encoded plasmid [79] as a therapeutic for AD. RVG29 peptide-targeted multipurpose NPs were packed with plasmid (REGS-PFlow cytometry, biological compatibility test, pharmacokinetic assessment, western blot assessment, as well as the Morris water maze evaluation were used to characterize the polymeric NPs. The variations in plasma along with brain NP buildup after IV treatment revealed that EGS-PN & REGS-PN had a considerably prolonged circulatory duration in the blood. Free EGCG, on the other hand, was quickly removed from circulation. The MWM experiment demonstrated that delivering a functional gene but also EGCG (REGS-PN) at the same time significantly enhanced the spatial memory but also recollection capacities of APP/PS1 as well as wild-type mice when matched to the free EGCG-treated collective. Based on the findings, argument took place about codelivery of a target genome (shRNA) plus EGCG in a multipurpose nanocarrier might reach greater remedial proportions in the brain, making it a promising technique for treating AD [80].

Inconsistencies in brain insulin signaling are said to have a role in AD pathogenesis. A research hypothesized that combining an epigenetic transceiver, Vorinostat, with rosiglitazone could enhance neurotrophic factor gene expression and reduce molecular and physiological changes linked with AD, primarily by packing these substances into a surface-modified nanocarrier framework for increased bioavailability and clinical performance. As a result, in this investigation, rosiglitazone & Vorinostat had been packed onto a poloxamer stabilized polymeric nanocarrier platform & delivered to mice in a streptozocin (3 mg/kg) caused Alzheimer's paradigm. When contrasted to either therapy alone (rosiglitazone 10 mg/kg, Vorinostat 50 mg/kg), therapy with free medication combo (rosiglitazone 5 mg/kg, Vorinostat 25 mg/kg) over 3 weeks reduced behavioral, biochemical, but also cellular changes. Furthermore, as shown by enhanced behavioral outcome, decreased oxidative stress, and higher concentrations of neurotrophic factors, the nanoformulation (rosiglitazone 5 mg/kg, Vorinostat 25 mg/kg) coencapsulated, showed superior neuroprotective activity compared to the medication combo. Finally, the poloxamer stabilized polymeric nanocarrier framework improved additive neuroprotective effectiveness exhibited by rosiglitazone as well as Vorinostat [81].

Some more nanocarrier-based invasive studies have been performed which show promising results but as we are focusing on the nanocarrier-based noninvasive approaches for the treatment of dementia so we are not exploring this invasive domain much more.

10.4 Nanocarrier-based noninvasive approaches

Encapsulating therapeutics, proteins, and peptides in nanocarriers can efficiently deliver them for the treatment of neurodegenerative illnesses like dementia, AD, and PD [82]. By addressing the difficulty of drug penetration via the BBB, nanocarriers enhance drug targeting, diminishes drug toxicity, and promotes therapeutic efficacy [83]. Any invasive technique that enables for direct drug delivery into the brain lesions is associated with a high neurosurgery cost and an elevated risk of infection because unwanted components may reach to the system when the BBB is breached. Because of the tangible nature of these approaches, the brain might be subjected to a variety of severe lesions, such as parent vessel thrombosis or brain herniation [84]. Nanocarriers are nanosized molecules (less than 200 nm) that may circulate across obstacles

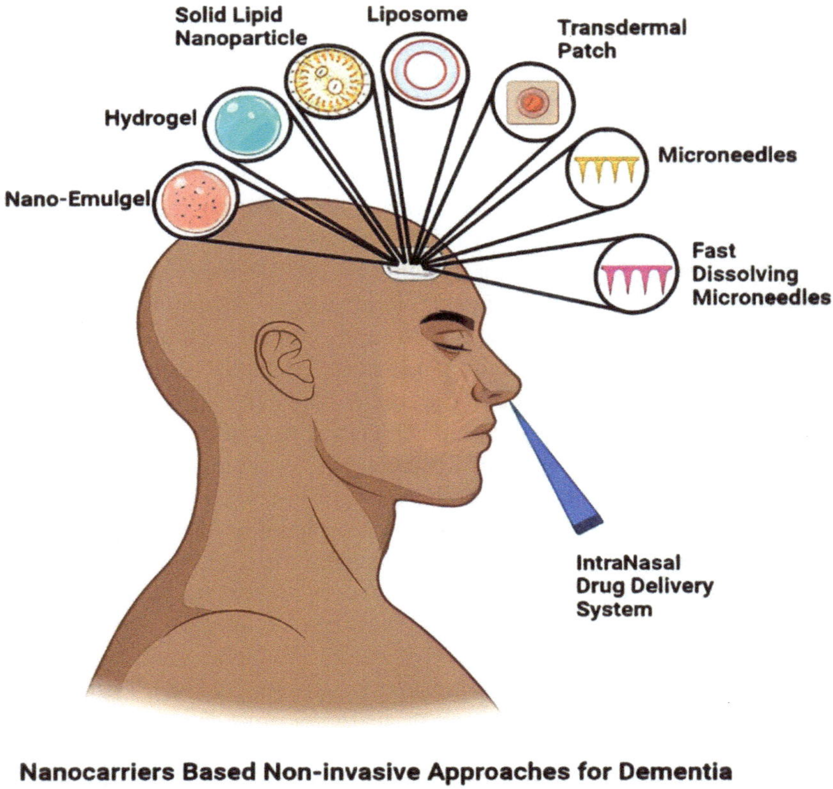

Fig. 10.2 Nanocarrier-based noninvasive approaches for the treatment of dementia.

while preserving the therapeutic effect of the active moieties. The nanocarriers relatively small size provides a large surface area that facilitates absorption, the potential to bind or absorb theranostics and cellular penetration when delivered through transdermally or intranasally via noninvasive techniques (Fig. 10.2) [85]. Lipid-based carrier systems in regards to noninvasive nanotechnology, emerged as the most preferable drug delivery system in terms of brain targeting. Being a lipid drug delivery system, its favors biocompatibility features, such as its high rate of crossing BBBs, regulated drug release, increased dissolution and solubilization within the intestinal milieu, and reduced stomach emptying rate with increased mucosal permeability; these techniques are also favored for adaption and improvement of poorly soluble drug bioavailability [86].

10.4.1 Nanocarriers approaches for dementia

Transdermal route is found to be an alternative to avoid drug first-pass metabolism in order to prevent drug degradation whereas the major hurdle is the permeation of drug though stratum corneum. The SC being a protective layer and barrier of foreign molecules can be invaded by ultradeformable liposomes as it has the capacity to deform itself through the pores of the skin. The property of squeezing out of liposomes is due to the presence of edge activator and fluidity of the bilayered membrane was achieved by lipids. The poor bioavailability (orally—10%) of drug Noopept (Npt), neuroprotective therapeutics demanded nanocarriers to increase its stability, retentivity, efficacy and safety in treating dementia. Ultradeformable liposomes (UDL) encapsulated Npt was delivered transdermally by embedding them into fast dissolvable microneedle patch. The lipid used to form the bilayer was Phospholipon 90G/90H, and the deforming agent was sodium deoxycholate. The UDL was prepared by ethanol injection method and optimized by QbD approach. The requirement of axial needle fracture force of microneedle was 0.688 N, sufficient to pierce the stratum corneum, and revealed drug dissolution within 2 minutes. More than 99% of Npt was found to be retentive when it was encapsulated with in the liposomal structure and in vitro cytotoxicity study on HaCaT cell descripted 94.27% viability. The increase in the pharmacological response in comparison to oral Npt suspension in Dawley rat concluded reduction of dose and its frequency as well as increases its effectiveness by recruiting patient compliance [87]. To solve the problem of bioavailability and short half-life, Srivastava and Thakkar developed an infusion-like distribution of vinpocetine (VPN) through transdermal channel using fast-dissolving microneedle as reservoir of drug. The length of the fast-dissolving microneedle was reduced by greater than 50% within 60 seconds, leading to 100% within 2 minutes, indicating a fast dissolution rate. The entrapment efficiency and particle size (PS) analyzed after the dissolution of microneedle exhibited 86.85 ± 1.57% and 76.24 ± 2.68 nm, respectively. In contrast to the value of flux produced by vinpocetine suspension, ex vivo permeation on pig's ear skin showed a constant flux of 11.091 g/cm^2 /h via drug-loaded UDL in microneedle patch (Fig. 10.3). In a nutshell, VPN's newly created fast-dissolving microneedle patch exhibited excellent results, with the possibility of reducing doses and dosing periodicity for better patient compliance while treating dementia [88]. Solid lipid nanoparticles (SLNs) are another lipoidal drug delivery technique that favors BCS class II therapeutics via topical administration, but they have significant drawbacks, including limited loading of drug and its leakage over time owing to solid lipid crystallization [89]. Surfactant stabilizes NLCs, which are a mixture of solid, lipid, and oil. Nanolipid carriers are industrially usable lipid NPs of the second generation, with an integrated matrix of liquid and solid lipids that favors high loading of drug and modification of desirable drug release profiles [90]. It overcome the problems associated with the delivery of lipophilic drug on the skin. The lipid core "hide" the lipophilic pharmaceuticals in these systems, while the lipid matrix aids in drug transport across the biological membrane [91]. NLCs, according to Iqbal and his coworkers, are superior to alternative lipid carrier systems in drug delivery to the dermis. These NLCs improve skin moisture, medication transport through the skin, and minimize skin irritation [92]. Chauhan and Sharma, developed and

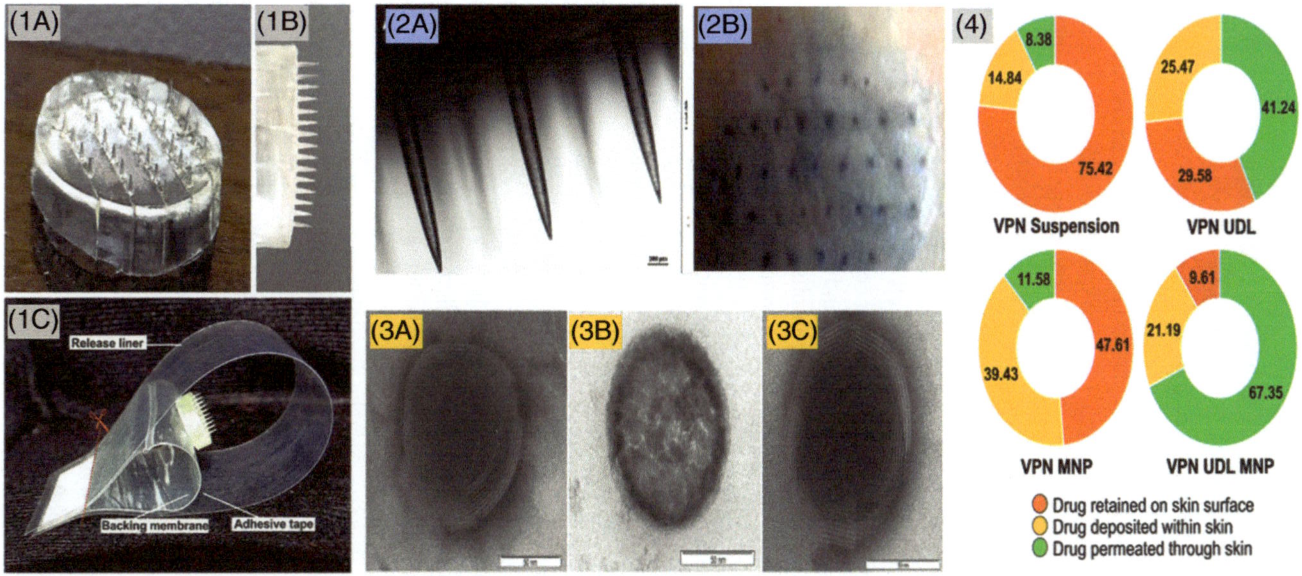

Fig. 10.3 Photographic view of drug-loaded ultradeformable liposomal microneedle patch 1(A) apex view, 1(B) edge view, and 1(C) its patch, 2(A) Microneedle, 2(B) VPN UDL MNP induced micropores stained on pig ear skin by trypan blue. 3(A–3C) are TEM images of VPN UDL MNP. (4) Deposition and permeation drug profile.

optimized NLC-laden rivastigmine. The formulation resulted small size (134.60 ± 15.10 nm) which ensures better permeation of rivastigmine resulting in increased pharmacological activity due to increased surface area and negative zeta potential (−11.8 ± 2.2 mV) indicated formation of the stable formulation. In vitro release of NLCs loaded transdermal patches offered sustained drug release in comparison to Exelon patch and was also found nonirritant to skin [93]. NLCs also derive an occlusive property, which improves drug penetration by reducing water loss from the skin and allowing for high permeability through the skin bilayer membranes. Transdermal patches being a noninvasive and self-administrable drug delivery system offers a higher and more consistent concentration of bioactive moiety over a longer period of time [94]. The epidemiology of dementia pain emphasizes its intensity, which is strongly related to the degree of dementia [95]. In Europe, only Risperidone is approved for demented patients with resistant aggressiveness, and it can be administered for up to 6 weeks, with a maximum of 12 [96]. Aromatherapy with Melissa and lavender has been shown to be effective in the management of agitation in dementia patients, although there is a lack of methodological consistency in clinical trials. However, the use of essential oils can provide analgesic relief [97]. Bergamot an essential oil (BEO) was used to control agitation in dementia by engineering it into solid lipid NPs. The delivery of BEO using nanotechnology odorless cream depicted reproducible and stable aromatic therapy effect with 10%–18 % degradation of active content up to 12 months. The incorporation of Nano drug delivery technique ensured a considerable reduction in total transepidermal water loss and a wide surface area of the SLN, allowing the loaded BEO to be exposed and in touch with the skin for longer periods of time, leading to more efficient release of BEO. The effectiveness and tolerability of an engineered essential oil with established significant analgesic qualities in acute and neuropathic pain on agitation will be further assessed in this double-blind clinical experiment [98]. Galantamine hydro bromide loaded HPMC-pectin-co-acrylic acid cross-linked hydrogels displayed pH-dependent response with a controlled drug release profile indicating decrease dosing frequency, which elevated patient compliance. Loading of drug into gel was confirmed by EDX whereas histomicrographs, blood samples revealed compatible, safer, and nontoxic to living organelles/tissues [99]. The drugs used in case of emergencies treatments, such as pain, centrally acting drugs, etc., transportation through nasal route for brain administration is significant because it delivers the drug faster and precisely with therapeutic impact. The formulation should pass through the olfactory membrane as well as the arachnoid membrane, which surrounds the arachnoid space, containing cerebrospinal fluid (CSF) to reach the CNS via the nasal cavity. The absorption of lipoidal NPs by the brain is a potential method. The olfactory route might be a way to deliver the small hydrophobic molecules either alone or combined with transcellular mechanisms. This encompasses transportation of drugs in a para cellular mode through interstitial space between cells, transcellular diffusion via a membrane or receptor-mediated endocytosis or transcytosis by vesicle carrier, and neuronal transport [100]. Telmisartan, an angiotensin receptor blocker was delivered intranasally using nanoemulgel mucoadhesive cargo. The size of the droplet was less than 200 nanometers with a change in zeta potential from negative (−26.1 ± 3.41 mV) to positive due to masking globules with chitosan in dispersed medium. The application of chitosan to encase nanoemulsion droplets strengthened their mucoadhesive properties, allowing for better absorption into goat nasal mucosa. The proposed nanoemulgel by Chin et al. was found to be promising platform for the administration of telmisartan through intranasal route, taking into account mucoadhesive properties, prolonged drug release, and increased ex vivo permeability [101]. Rivastigmine hydrogen tartrate incorporated NLC was prepared by modified solvent emulsification-diffusion method and was optimized by Box-Behnken design. In a *C. elegans* model, rivastigmine-loaded NLC showed 81.2 ± 2.1% drug diffusion in 12 hours via nasal mucosa of goat, expressing increased worm paralysis owing to higher accumulation of acetylcholine in synapses confirmed by aldicarb test. The use of ethanol lowers the dielectric constant (24.6) due to lower magnitude as compare to water (80.1) enables the hydrophilic compounds readily dissolvable by limiting leakage of drug. The integration of liquid lipids into solid lipids forms a blend that minimizes the crystalline nature of lipids and augments imperfections leading to the formation of oil-based nanopockets in the crystal lattice. It helps active molecules to entrap more results in increased entrapment efficiency thereby decreasing dose of drug. The elevated plus-maze test was used to examine memory-related responses, which revealed symbolic memory retention when compared to standard formulation, which could be due to the nanostructure and lipoidal nature of the delivery system, which could leads to drug accumulation in the brain, resulting in a better effect [102].

10.4.2 Nanocarriers approaches for Alzheimer

AD appears to be the most ubiquitous form of dementia globally, affecting more than 35 million people and anticipated to quadruple in the next 40 years as people live longer lives [103]. AD is a neurological disease that causes not only memory and cognitive impairment but also behavioral changes. Although the underlying processes of AD etiology are unknown [104]. Nanomedicine-based technologies or molecular strategies to overcome for AD and symptoms of dementia can be an alternative and effective therapeutic approach in place of conventional (nontargetable) drug delivery system [105]. During the treatment session of AD, liposomes have gained much attention because of being biocompatible, nontoxic, and amphipathic drug-delivery system for mobility of a variety of active molecules to the brain [106]. Incorporation of phospholipid (phosphatidylserine) improves neuronal signaling and deactivate microglia suggesting phosphatidylserine liposomes might be a suitable alternative for codelivery of drugs against AD [107]. Rivastigmine (a butyrylcholinesterase and acetyl cholinesterase inhibitor) was administered through noninvasive transdermal route using liposomal patches as cargo to prevent large plasma fluctuation after oral administration. Small unilamellar vesicles (50–150 nm) was reported by sonicated thin layer film hydration techniques. Because of the hydrophilic nature of rivastigmine, lipid bilayers acted as a barrier to rivastigmine release. As a result, liposomes can serve as long-acting drug repositories for rivastigmine. After 48 hours, liposomes showed a greater percentage of rivastigmine penetrating rat skin (91.5%) than the aqueous control rivastigmine (53%). This could be owing to the phospholipids utilized in liposomes having a permeation-enhancing effect which increases the activity of rivastigmine permeation 3-folds in pig skin by applying sonophoresis [108]. Long-term use of Huperzine A causes anorexia when administered orally and penetration of it via closely packed brick like stratum corneum was the major hurdle. Patel and his colleague performed a comparative in vitro/in vivo study on SLNs, NLCs, microemulsion and, these nanocarriers were converted to nano dispersed gel for transdermal administration. Permeation of drug via skin depends on lipophilicity, molecular mass, and solubility of drug with the excipients used in the formulation because only dissolved drug can penetrate easily. SLNs exhibited smaller size in comparison to microemulsion (ME) and NLCs. Increased globule size of ME was due to higher encapsulation of oil refers higher entrapment of drug in the nanocarrier. The larger globule size of ME could be due to the incorporation of the higher percentage of oil to encapsulate more HupA in the oil phase. In reference to PS, zeta potential also plays an important role in penetration of nanocarriers through skin. Highly negative zeta potential (NLCs and SLNs) exhibited poor skin permeation study in relation to ME with least zeta potential. Nanocarriers used for the delivery of HupaA were found to be an efficient promoter of drug through a rat skin and were also nonirritant for dermal application [109]. Intranasal administration is a viable alternative to oral and systemic delivery of therapeutics for the CNS, circumventing the BBB, and limiting systemic exposure [110]. Biodegradable polymeric NPs can be used to transfer therapeutics directly from nose to the brain by entering through nasal mucosal layer. NPs being 1–1000 nm in size, ultrafine particles made up of natural/synthetic polymer components [111]. The FDA-approved biodegradable copolymer poly (lactic-co-glycolic acid) (PLGA) has been widely employed in the synthesis of NPs and is currently being investigated for the construction of sustained/controlled drug delivery systems [112]. Erodible in situ gel using poloxamer 407 was created by Salatin and colleagues as a viable platform for extending rivastigmine hydrogen tartrate oozing from implanted PLGANPs. Nano precipitation methods-based NPs depicted negative zeta potential due to the presence of terminal carboxylic acid in PLGA and claimed an increase in PS and zeta potential on increasing the concentration of PLGA. Because of the biocompatible nature of formed NPs, the NPs' decreased cytotoxic impact on the A549 cell line demonstrated their eligibility for drug administration, and this attribute might potentially lessen the likelihood of negative consequences. The excellent findings of thorough in-vitro and ex-vivo experiments demonstrated the ability of such nanocomposites for intranasal medication delivery to the brain [113]. Herbal drugs are poor water-soluble constituents that limit their bioavailability and systemic clearance within the body while used in the treatment of cognitive disorders, such as dementia and AD [114]. Curcumin (Cur) loaded multistimuli-responsive self-assembled nanocargo was developed to improve the effectiveness of the herbal drug in brain inflammation shown in Fig. 10.4. Chitosan (CS) is a naturally occurring biodegradable polymer with cationic charges provoked by an abnormally acidic extracellular environment. This process is known as environmental triggering, like in a tumor. This is due to increased protonation of the amino groups in the CS in the acidic environment. Fucoidan (F), a sulfated amphiphilic marine polysaccharide, on the other hand, can target P-selectin, which is expressed by metastatic cancer cells. The combination of charged CS with F, as well as their respective properties of pH- and P-selectin responsiveness, allows for targeted administration of curcumin to inflammatory brain lesions, improving its distribution and accumulation. In vitro cellular absorption of validated the self-assembled nanocarrier's active targeting and nanodispersible characteristics, resulting in increased and effective accretion of the lipophilic bioactive Cur in inflammatory areas. The largest accumulation/absorption of Cur in the LPS-treated animal group delivered via the Cur-F/CS NCs showed the greatest inhibition of inflammatory responses compared to the other test groups in an in vivo evaluation of therapeutic benefits. This intriguing multifunctional nanocarrier with an unique drug delivery channel might have significant therapeutic applications for neurosurgeons in the future [115]. Elnaggar et al. were the first to develop ionically cross-linked CS/tripolyphosphate (TPP) NPs for nasal delivery to the brain. Ionic gelation was used to make pipeline-loaded chitosan NPs. The inclusion of a lipophilic drug in a hydrophilic carrier and the creation of monodisperse NPs of a natural polymer were the two biggest challenges in this formulation. Different drug loading procedures and loading concentrations were tested by adding to either CS solution during NPs synthesis (encapsulation method) or after NP formation (post-NP formation) to solve this issue (adsorption method). The ideal CS: TPP ratio was discovered to be 5:1, indicating a much smaller PS and greater zeta potential, indicating CS positive charge (60 mV). In comparison to nonstabilized NPs, the inclusion of poloxamer 188 (1%, w/v) as a stabilizer resulted in particles with a nonsignificant elevation in size but much reduced ZP and superior PDI. PS and ZP alterations were most likely induced by the adsorption of poloxamer on the surface of NPs, which reduced CS adherence and aggregation, resulting in lower particle polydispersity. Piperine is an insoluble drug that tends to clog the olfactory bulb, resulting in delivery failure. However, incorporating it into a nanocarrier eliminates olfactory bulb blockage and provides considerable cognitive boosting benefits [116]. GH (Galantamine hydro bromide) is a cholinesterase inhibitor with an inherent antioxidant potential. TNF-α is a critical mediator of immune-mediated brain inflammation. It has a role in the spread of inflammation by activating immune cells through TNF receptor-1. By activating the ROS-producing enzymes, this receptor can directly cause oxidative stress.

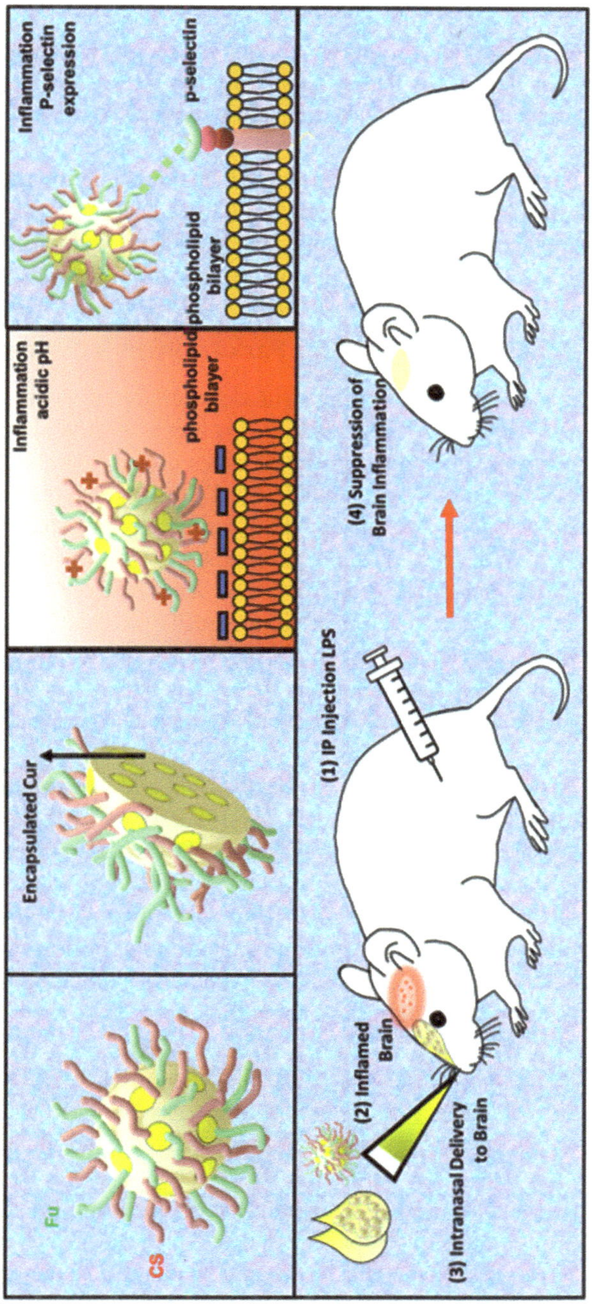

FIG. 10.4 Schematic representation of self-assembled pH-responsive Cur-loaded Chitosan nanocarrier by intranasal administration to the brain for suppression of brain inflammation.

When adequately blocked, TNF-α serves not only as a possible AD biomarker, but also as an AD treatment mechanism. The incorporation of GH in NPs was determined in rat brains for 1 hour after nasal injection and shown pharmacological efficacy over GH nasal solution without histological damage [117]. Pharmacokinetic behavior GH loaded in flexible liposomes was analyzed in rat model via nasal route in comparison to oral. Incorporation of cholinesterase inhibitor into nanocarrier revealed increased efficiency of the formulation, elevated level of C_{max} and area under curve was more than three times by nasal route as compare to oral. In vitro survival experiments on PC-12 cells revealed that the flexible liposome carrier is nontoxic to cultivated cells and loading of GH into flexible liposomes significantly reduces the cytotoxicity of GH to cells [118].

10.4.3 Nanocarriers approaches for Parkinsonism's disease

PD is an age-related, gradually elevating neurodegenerative disorder, making it the second most prevalent neurodegenerative disorder after Alzheimer [119]. The interplay of environmental and genetic variables causes sporadic PD. PD causes both motor and nonmotor symptoms [120]. Tremor at rest, bradykinesia, and muscular stiffness are the three most common motor symptoms caused by the loss of dopaminergic neurons. Psychiatric conditions (depression, anxiety), cognitive dysfunction (dementia), sleep disorder, and olfactory dysfunction (hyposmia/anosmia) dominate the clinical picture in PD patients. These motor and nonmotor symptoms together cause impairment and significantly affect PD patients' quality of life [121]. Dopamine entrapped NP comutated with borneol and lactoferrin (Lf-BNPs) was formulated in order to enhance permeability and specificity in striatum of brain *via* intranasal route. The cell viability studies revealed reduced toxicity in case of hybrid NP than NP with drug. In addition, Lf-BNPs show enhanced cellular uptake in SH-16HBE and SY5Y cells due to modifying its surface with lactoferrin and borneol. The delivery of NP via nasal route showed prominent absorption in pharmacokinetics studies and in pharmacodynamic research, dopamine Lf-BNPs reduced apomorphine-induced contralateral rotations, and elevated dopamine content in the lesioned striatum of 6-hydroxydopamine induced PD rats [122]. Ionic gelation method was used to prepare pramipexole-loaded chitosan nanoparticle (P-CNs) for an effective treatment via nasal route. The drug diffusion in in-vitro by dialysis membrane and ex-vivo on goat nasal mucosa was performed and showed complete release of the drug from C-NP suggesting benefits in in-vivo behavior. The photo actometer test was performed to assess the locomotor activity in rodents where, treating with the intranasal C-NPs shows improved locomotor activity than the pure drug [123]. Trapani et al. designed dopamine (DA) encapsulated liposomes and solid–lipid NP as innovative nose-to-brain noninvasive neurotransmitter delivery approach for PD. SLNs exhibited higher amount of dopamine accumulation on the surface than external side. In support SLNs, it resulted higher entrapment (81%) and highest mucoadhesive effect. Ex vivo study illustrated both the carrier as a safest nanocarrier for olfactory ensheathing cells and the uptake of SLNs was 100% to positive cells (dose-dependent manner) whereas, chitosan-glutathione-coated liposomes were internalized by 70% [124]. Buccal administration is also a noninvasive approach alternative to parenteral infusions for the delivery of apomorphine. The pH of the nanoscale lipospheres played an important role in the permeation. Dropping the pH of the formulation to 5.9 reduced the permeability rate by six times, while infusing an ethanol: propylene glycol solution boost it by four times [125]. The oral administration of levodopa increases a huge amount of homocysteine in the peripheral circulation, leading to the risk of cardiovascular disease, and restricting its therapeutic use. The delivery of L-DOPA laden sub-50 nm NPs via brain–lymphatic vasculature was developed as a noninvasive technique to administer levodopa to the brain. Using the flash nanocomplexation approach, the hydrophilic L-DOPA was effectively entrapped into tannic acid/polyvinyl alcohol NPs through hydrogen bonding, leading to a high L-DOPA loading strength and uniform size in a scalable way. Pharmacodynamics analysis revealed the levels of tyrosine hydroxylase and dopamine was elevated with reduced inflammation due to high degree of flexibility. The delivery of drug loaded NP via the brain–lymphatic vasculature has shown promising in the therapeutic response in the treatment of PD [126].

10.5 Clinical trial and future aspects

Immunotherapeutics targeting elimination and/or prevention of formation of Amyloid β have been allowed to proceed for clinical trials. They hold immense potential for becoming future cure for dementia. BAN-2401, aducanumab, gantenerumab, crenezumab, solanezumab, and intravenous immunoglobulin G (IVIG) are currently in the Phase III clinical trials. The research, as described previously in details, ushers new hope as the mechanism of the disease is now challenged and are addressed. The previous drawbacks of the therapies are getting eradicated strategically. Scientists have found ways to deliver drug straight to the brains by crossing the BBB, which was previously not possible properly, by employing nanocarriers and genetic carriers.

10.6 Conclusion

Dementia is a word that involves a large number of cognitive and behavioral symptoms that include memory lapses, inability to understand and communicating, mental confusion, and a decrease in a person's capacity to carry out everyday tasks. AD, parkinsonism, vascular dementia, and frontotemporal dementia are the most frequent kinds of dementia. It is a progressive disease, which means the symptoms will worsen over time. The delivery of anti-PD and anti-AD agents through the tight junction BBB, an impregnable fence that limits the effective management of the disease. Nanocarrier-based noninvasive techniques can circumvent the BBB and deliver the biologically active moiety to the specific regions in the brain to treat neurodegenerative illnesses. The use of intranasal and transdermal route by using penetration enhancer devices is gaining popularity for the direct delivery of drug to the brain. The immediate delivery of drug by encapsulating into nanocarriers guarantee's adequate drug loading in the brain and prolonged the release of drug. It is widely accepted that NPs in between 100 and 200 nanometers can be aimed for brain targeting as it is of nanometric in size. The preclinical investigations of nanocarriers such as lipid NPs, ME, liposomes, hydrogel, nanoemulgel, and SLNs have demonstrated their efficacy. The quick entrance and specific localization of the developed formulation can be considered safer whereas, systemic administration (IV, SC, and IM) and surgery (Invasive approach) increase the risk of side effects due to large dose or exposure of potent drug in the blood. As a result, the components of transdermal and intranasal nano formulations must be facile and at low concentrations to ensure their safety. Safety, toxicity, and efficacy of the nanocarrier-based formulation studies are necessary to confirm the preclinical results to gain further support for clinical trials. The formulation of novel devices using biodegradable polymers to conquer the anatomical barriers of the transdermal and nasal cavity. The issues concerning the complexity of the brain, the mechanisms of drug transport via both the route, and comprehensive neurotoxicological aspects need to be considered for nanotherapeutics to contribute in clinical practice. In conclusion, the application of nano-enabled carriers through the transdermal and intranasal route in the treatment of dementia could offer greater benefits in order to oral which prevents first-pass metabolism in a noninvasive nanocarrier-based drug delivery approach.

References

[1] Duong S, Patel T, Chang F. Dementia: what pharmacists need to know. Can Pharm J 2017;150(2):118–29.

[2] Nichols E, Steinmetz JD, Vollset SE, Fukutaki K, Chalek J, Abd-Allah F, et al. Estimation of the global prevalence of dementia in 2019 and forecasted prevalence in 2050: an analysis for the Global Burden of Disease Study 2019. Lancet Public Heal 2022;7(2):e105–25.

[3] Prince M, Bryce R, Albanese E, Wimo A, Ribeiro W, Ferri CP. The global prevalence of dementia: a systematic review and metaanalysis. Alzheimer's Dement [Internet] 2013;9(1):63–75.e2. http://dx.doi.org/10.1016/j.jalz.2012.11.007.

[4] Arvanitakis Z, Shah RC, Bennett DA. Diagnosis and management of dementia: review. J Am Med Assoc 2019;322(16):1589–99.

[5] Hugo J, Ganguli M. Dementia and cognitive impairment. Epidemiology, diagnosis, and treatment. Clin Geriatr Med [Internet] 2014;30(3):421–42. http://dx.doi.org/10.1016/j.cger.2014.04.001.

[6] Overshott R, Burns A. Treatment of dementia. Neurol Pract 2005;76(SUPPL. 5):53–59. doi:10.1136/jnnp.2005.082537.

[7] Schwarz S, Froelich L, Burns A. Pharmacological treatment of dementia. Curr Opin Psychiatry 2012;25(6):542–50.

[8] Oesterling BM, Gulati A, Joshi MD. Nanocarrier-based approaches for treatment and detection of Alzheimer's disease. J Nanosci Nanotechnol 2014;14(1):137–56.

[9] Chowdhury A, Kunjiappan S, Panneerselvam T, Somasundaram B, Bhattacharjee C. Nanotechnology and nanocarrier-based approaches on treatment of degenerative diseases. Int Nano Lett 2017;7(2):91–122.

[10] O'Brien JT, Holmes C, Jones M, Jones R, Livingston G, McKeith I, et al. Clinical practice with anti-dementia drugs: A revised (third) consensus statement from the British Association for Psychopharmacology. J Psychopharmacol 2017;31(2):147–68.

[11] Zucchella C, Sinforiani E, Tamburin S, Federico A, Mantovani E, Bernini S, et al. The multidisciplinary approach to Alzheimer's disease and dementia. A narrative review of non-pharmacological treatment. Front Neurol 2018;9(December):1–22.

[12] Bacskai BJ, Kajdasz ST, Mclellan ME, Games D, Seubert P, Schenk D, et al. Non-Fc-mediated mechanisms are involved in clearance of amyloid-β in vivo by immunotherapy. J Neurosci 2002;22(18):7873–8.

[13] Sengupta U, Nilson AN, Kayed R. The role of amyloid-β oligomers in toxicity, propagation, and immunotherapy. EBioMedicine 2016;6:42–9.

[14] Tabet N. Acetylcholinesterase inhibitors for Alzheimer's disease: anti-inflammatories in acetylcholine clothing!. Age Ageing 2006;35(4):336–8.

[15] Behrens S, Rattinger GB, Schwartz S, Matyi J, Sanders C, Deberard MS, et al. Use of FDA approved medications for Alzheimer's disease in mild dementia is associated with reduced informal costs of care. Int Psychogeriatrics 2018;30(10):1499–507.

[16] King E, O'Brien JT, Donaghy P, Morris C, Barnett N, Olsen K, et al. Peripheral inflammation in prodromal Alzheimer's and Lewy body dementias. J Neurol Neurosurg Psychiatry 2018;89(4):339–45.

[17] Cacabelos R. Pharmacogenetic considerations when prescribing cholinesterase inhibitors for the treatment of Alzheimer's disease. Expert Opin Drug Metab Toxicol 2020;16(8):673–701.

[18] Wolinsky D, Drake K, Bostwick J. Diagnosis and management of neuropsychiatric symptoms in Alzheimer's disease. Curr Psychiatry Rep 2018;20(12):1–13. doi:10.1007/s11920-018-0978-8.

[19] Singh M, Kaur M, Kukreja H, Chugh R, Silakari O, Singh D. Acetylcholinesterase inhibitors as Alzheimer therapy: from nerve toxins to neuroprotection. Eur J Med Chem 2013;70:165–88.

[20] Shi C, Liu J, Wu F, Yew DT. Ginkgo biloba extract in Alzheimer's disease: from action mechanisms to medical practice. Int J Mol Sci 2010;11(1):107–23.

[21] Rodda J, Carter J. Cholinesterase inhibitors and memantine for symptomatic treatment of dementia. BMJ 2012;344(7856):6–11.

[22] Cerejeira J, Lagarto L, Mukaetova-Ladinska EB. Behavioral and psychological symptoms of dementia. Front Neurol 2012(May):1–21.

[23] Ballard C, Kahn Z, Corbett A. Treatment of dementia with lewy bodies and Parkinson's disease dementia. Drugs and Aging 2011;28(10):769–77.

[24] O'Brien JT, Burns A. Clinical practice with anti-dementia drugs: A revised (second) consensus statement from the British Association for Psychopharmacology. J Psychopharmacol 2011;25(8):997–1019.

[25] Herrmann N, Gauthier S. Diagnosis and treatment of dementia: 6. Management of severe Alzheimer disease. CMAJ 2008;179(12):1279–87.

[26] Brambilla D, Le Droumaguet B, Nicolas J, Hashemi SH, Wu LP, Moghimi SM, et al. Nanotechnologies for Alzheimer's disease: diagnosis, therapy, and safety issues. Nanomedicine Nanotechnology, Biol Med 2011 Oct;7(5):521–40.

[27] Hamley IW. The amyloid beta peptide: a chemist's perspective. role in Alzheimer's and fibrillization. Chem Rev 2012;112(10):5147–92.

[28] Wolfe MS. Secretase targets for Alzheimer's disease: identification and therapeutic potential. J Med Chem 2001;44(13):2039–60.
[29] Dewachter I, Van Leuven F. Secretases as targets for the treatment of Alzheimer's disease: the prospects. Lancet Neurol 2002;1(7):409–16.
[30] Cui G, Shao S, Yang J, Liu J, Guo H. Designer self-assemble peptides maximize the therapeutic benefits of neural stem cell transplantation for Alzheimer's disease via enhancing neuron differentiation and paracrine action. Mol Neurobiol 2016;53(2):1108–23.
[31] Newcomb CJ, Moyer TJ, Lee SS, Stupp SI. Advances in cryogenic transmission electron microscopy for the characterization of dynamic self-assembling nanostructures. Curr Opin Colloid Interface Sci 2012;17(6):350–9.
[32] Bieschke J, Herbst M, Wiglenda T, Friedrich RP, Boeddrich A, Schiele F, et al. Small-molecule conversion of toxic oligomers to nontoxic β-sheet–rich amyloid fibrils. Nat Chem Biol 2012;8(1):93–101.
[33] Uddin MS, Kabir MT, Tewari D, Mathew B, Aleya L. Emerging signal regulating potential of small molecule biflavonoids to combat neuropathological insults of Alzheimer's disease. Sci Total Environ 2020;700:134836.
[34] Ghasemi F, Hormozi-Nezhad MR, Mahmoudi M. Label-free detection of β-amyloid peptides (Aβ40 and Aβ42): a colorimetric sensor array for plasma monitoring of Alzheimer's disease. Nanoscale 2018;10(14):6361–8.
[35] Lemere CA. Developing novel immunogens for a safe and effective Alzheimer's disease vaccine. Prog Brain Res 2009;175:83–93.
[36] Pandey G, Ramakrishnan V. Invasive and non-invasive therapies for Alzheimer's disease and other amyloidosis. Biophys Rev 2020;12(5):1175–86.
[37] Liu J, Yang B, Ke J, Li W, Suen WC. Antibody-based drugs and approaches against amyloid-β species for Alzheimer's disease immunotherapy. Drugs Aging 2016;33(10):685–97.
[38] Brown T. Deisign thinking. Harv Bus Rev 2008;86(6):84–92.
[39] Gentilucci L, De Marco R, Cerisoli L. Chemical Modifications designed to improve peptide stability: incorporation of non-natural amino acids, pseudo-peptide bonds, and cyclization. Curr Pharm Des 2010;16(28):3185–203.
[40] Pujals S, Giralt E. Proline-rich, amphipathic cell-penetrating peptides. Adv Drug Deliv Rev 2008;60(4–5):473–84.
[41] Consoli GML, Tosto R, Baglieri A, Petralia S, Campagna T, Di Natale G, et al. Novel peptide-Calix[4]arene conjugate inhibits Aβ aggregation and rescues neurons from Aβ's oligomers cytotoxicity in vitro. ACS Chem Neurosci 2021;12(8):1449–62.
[42] Di Natale G, Zimbone S, Bellia F, Tomasello MF, Giuffrida ML, Pappalardo G, et al. Potential therapeutics of Alzheimer's diseases: new insights into the neuroprotective role of trehalose-conjugated beta sheet breaker peptides. Pept Sci 2018;110(5):e24083.
[43] Kumar S, Henning-Knechtel A, Magzoub M, Hamilton AD. Peptidomimetic-based multidomain targeting offers critical evaluation of Aβ structure and toxic function. J Am Chem Soc 2018;140(21):6562–74.
[44] Derrick JS, Lim MH. Tools of the trade: investigations into design strategies of small molecules to target components in Alzheimer's disease. ChemBioChem 2015;16(6):887–98.
[45] Scott LE, Orvig C. Medicinal inorganic chemistry approaches to passivation and removal of aberrant metal ions in disease. Chem Rev 2009;109(10):4885–910.
[46] Chaudhuri TK, Paul S. Protein-misfolding diseases and chaperone-based therapeutic approaches. FEBS J 2006;273(7):1331–49.

[47] Koren J, Jinwal UK, Lee DC, Jones JR, Shults CL, Johnson AG, et al. Chaperone signalling complexes in Alzheimer's disease. J Cell Mol Med 2009;13(4):619–30.

[48] Wisniewski T, Frangione B. Immunological and anti-chaperone therapeutic approaches for Alzheimer disease. Brain Pathol 2005;15(1):72–7.

[49] Šimić G, Babić Leko M, Wray S, Harrington C, Delalle I, Jovanov-Milošević N, et al. Tau protein hyperphosphorylation and aggregation in alzheimer's disease and other tauopathies, and possible neuroprotective strategies. Biomolecules 2016;6(1):2–28.

[50] Ng PY, Chang IS, Koh RY, Chye SM. Recent advances in tau-directed immunotherapy against Alzheimer's disease: an overview of pre-clinical and clinical development. Metab Brain Dis 2020;35(7):1049–66.

[51] Panza F, Solfrizzi V, Seripa D, Imbimbo BP, Lozupone M, Santamato A, et al. Tau-centric targets and drugs in clinical development for the treatment of Alzheimer's disease. Biomed Res Int 2016;2016.

[52] Pedersen JT, Sigurdsson EM. Tau immunotherapy for Alzheimer's disease. Trends Mol Med 2015;21(6):394–402.

[53] Reddy VP, Aryal P, Robinson S, Rafiu R, Obrenovich M, Perry G. Polyphenols in alzheimer's disease and in the gut–brain axis. Microorganisms 2020;8(2):199.

[54] Weinreb O, Mandel S, Amit T, Youdim MBH. Neurological mechanisms of green tea polyphenols in Alzheimer's and Parkinson's diseases. J Nutr Biochem 2004;15(9):506–16.

[55] Colizzi C. The protective effects of polyphenols on Alzheimer's disease: a systematic review. Alzheimer's Dement Transl Res Clin Interv 2019;5(October):184–96.

[56] Gadhavi J, Shah S, Sinha T, Jain A, Gupta S. Charge neutralization of lysine via carbamylation reveals hidden aggregation hot-spots in tau protein flanking regions. FEBS J 2021(November).

[57] Nguyen P, Ramamoorthy A, Sahoo B, Zheng J, Straub J, Dominguez L, et al. Amyloid oligomers : a joint experimental /computational perspective on Alzheimer's disease, Parkinson's disease, Type II diabetes, and amyotrophic lateral sclerosis to cite this version : HAL Id : hal-03268585. 2021;

[58] Barghorn S, Zheng-Fischhofer Q, Ackmann M, Biernat J, Von Bergen M, Mandelkow EM, et al. Structure, microtubule interactions, and paired helical filament aggregation by tau mutants of frontotemporal dementias. Biochemistry 2000;39(38):11714–21.

[59] Hanford N, Figueiro M. Light therapy and Alzheimer's disease and related dementia: past, present, and future. J Alzheimer's Dis 2013;33(4):913–22.

[60] Burns A, Allen H, Tomenson B, Duignan D, Byrne J. Bright light therapy for agitation in dementia: a randomized controlled trial. Int Psychogeriatrics 2009;21(4):711–21.

[61] Forbes D, Culum I, Lischka A, Morgan D. Light therapy for managing cognitive, sleep, functional, behavioural, or psychiatric disturbances in dementia (Review). Cochrane Libr 2009(4):1–78.

[62] Gasca-Salas C, Fernández-Rodríguez B, Pineda-Pardo JA, Rodríguez-Rojas R, Obeso I, Hernández-Fernández F, et al. Blood-brain barrier opening with focused ultrasound in Parkinson's disease dementia. Nat Commun 2021;12(1):1–7.

[63] Nicodemus NE, Becerra S, Kuhn TP, Packham HR, Duncan J, Mahdavi K, et al. Focused transcranial ultrasound for treatment of neurodegenerative dementia. Alzheimer's Dement Transl Res Clin Interv 2019;5:374–81.

[64] Shin J, Kong C, Lee J, Choi BY, Sim J, Koh CS, et al. Focused ultrasound-induced blood-brain barrier opening improves adult hippocampal neurogenesis and cognitive function in a cholinergic degeneration dementia rat model. Alzheimer's Res Ther 2019;11(1):1–15.

[65] Saikia J, Pandey G, Sasidharan S, Antony F, Nemade HB, Kumar S, et al. Electric field disruption of amyloid aggregation: potential noninvasive therapy for Alzheimer's disease. ACS Chem Neurosci 2019;10(5):2250–62.

[66] Ohtsuki T, Nabeta T, Nakanishi H, Kawahata H, Ogihara T, Morishita R, et al. Electric field exposure improves subjective symptoms related to sleeplessness in college students: a pilot study of electric field therapy for sleep disorder. Immunol Endocr Metab Agents Med Chem 2017;17(1):37–48.

[67] Buss SS, Fried PJ, Pascual-Leone A. Therapeutic noninvasive brain stimulation in Alzheimer's disease and related dementias. Curr Opin Neurol 2019;32(2):292–304.

[68] Zemianek JM, Serra M, Guaraldi M, Shea TB. Stimulation with a low-amplitude, digitized synaptic signal to invoke robust activity within neuronal networks on multielectrode arrays. BioTechniques 2012;52(3):177–82.

[69] Brown P. 14 Pathological oscillatory activity in Parkinson's disease; what does it mean and how should we treat it? J Neurol Neurosurg Psychiatry 2020;91(8) e6.1-e6.

[70] Hescham S, Lim LW, Jahanshahi A, Blokland A, Temel Y. Deep brain stimulation in dementia-related disorders. Neurosci Biobehav Rev 2013;37(10):2666–75.

[71] Li Y, Zhang Y, Wang W, Zhang Y, Yu Y, Cheing GLY, et al. Effects of pulsed electromagnetic fields on learning and memory abilities of STZ-induced dementia rats. Electromagn Biol Med 2019;38(2):123–30.

[72] Thrasher AJ. A dose escalation study of cyclophosphamide (CTX) to enhance SB-728-T engraftment Dale Ando Sangamo BioSciences, Richmond CA, USA. Hum Gene Ther 2015;26:A2–36.

[73] Somani S, Robb G, Pickard BS, Dufès C. Enhanced gene expression in the brain following intravenous administration of lactoferrin-bearing polypropylenimine dendriplex. J Control Release 2015;217:235–42.

[74] Taliyan R, Kakoty V, Sarathlal KC, Kharavtekar SS, Karennanavar CR, Choudhary YK, et al. Nanocarrier mediated drug delivery as an impeccable therapeutic approach against Alzheimer's disease. J Control Release 2022.

[75] Kakoty V, Krishna KV, Dubey SK, Chitkara D, Taliyan R. Neuroprotective efficacy of co-encapsulated rosiglitazone and vorinostat nanoparticle on streptozotocin induced mice model of Alzheimer disease. ACS Chem Neurosci 2021;12(9):1528–41.

[76] Zeng H, Xu L, Zou Y, Wang S. Romidepsin and metformin nanomaterials delivery on streptozocin for the treatment of Alzheimer's disease in animal model. Biomed Pharmacother 2021;141(June):111864.

[77] Laher I. Systems biology of free radicals and antioxidantsSystems Biology of Free Radicals and AntioxidantsVol. 9783642300; 2014:1–4178.

[78] Horecký J, Bačiak L, Kašparová S, Pacheco G, Aliev G. Vančová O. Minimally invasive surgical approach for three-vessel occlusion as a model of vascular dementia in the rat-brain bioenergetics assay. J Neurol Sci 2009;283(1–2):178–81.

[79] Kalra J, Khan A. Eur J Pharmacol 2015;764:571–81.

[80] Lv L, Yang F, Li H, Yuan J. Brain-targeted co-delivery of β-amyloid converting enzyme 1 shRNA and epigallocatechin-3-gallate by multifunctional nanocarriers for Alzheimer's disease treatment. IUBMB Life 2020;72(8):1819–29.

[81] Sarathlal KCS, Kakoty V, Krishna KV, Dubey SK, Chitkara D, Taliyan R. Neuroprotective efficacy of co-encapsulated rosiglitazone and vorinostat nanoparticle on streptozotocin induced mice model of alzheimer disease. ACS Chem Neurosci 2021;12(9):1528–41.

[82] Fang F, Zou D, Wang W, Yin Y, Yin T, Hao S, et al. Non-invasive approaches for drug delivery to the brain based on the receptor mediated transport. Mater Sci Eng C [Internet] 2017;76:1316–27. http://dx.doi.org/10.1016/j.msec.2017.02.056.

[83] Zhao M, van Straten D, Broekman MLD, Préat V, Schiffelers RM. Nanocarrier-based drug combination therapy for glioblastoma. Theranostics 2020;10(3):1355–72.

[84] Tam VH, Sosa C, Liu R, Yao N, Priestley RD. Nanomedicine as a non-invasive strategy for drug delivery across the blood brain barrier. Int J Pharm [Internet] 2016;515(1–2):331–42. http://dx.doi.org/10.1016/j.ijpharm.2016.10.031.

[85] Sriramoju B, Kanwar R, Kanwar J. Nanomedicine based nanoparticles for neurological disorders. Curr Med Chem 2014;21(36):4154–68.

[86] Javed MN, Kohli K, Amin S. Risk assessment integrated qbd approach for development of optimized bicontinuous mucoadhesive limicubes for oral delivery of rosuvastatin. AAPS PharmSciTech 2018;19(3):1377–91.

[87] Srivastava PK, Thakkar HP. QbD-driven development of dissolving microneedle patch loaded with ultradeformable liposomes encapsulated Noopept: exploring a patient friendly, once-daily option to manage dementia. Eur J Pharm Sci [Internet] 2021;164(May):105909. https://doi.org/10.1016/j.ejps.2021.105909.

[88] Srivastava PK, Thakkar HP. Vinpocetine loaded ultradeformable liposomes as fast dissolving microneedle patch: tackling treatment challenges of dementia. Eur J Pharm Biopharm [Internet] 2020;156(April):176–90. https://doi.org/10.1016/j.ejpb.2020.09.006.

[89] Mishra V, Bansal KK, Verma A, Yadav N, Thakur S, Sudhakar K, et al. Solid lipid nanoparticles: emerging colloidal nano drug delivery systems. Pharmaceutics 2018;10(4):1–21.

[90] Makowski M, Silva ÍC, Do Amaral CP, Gonçalves S, Santos NC. Advances in lipid and metal nanoparticles for antimicrobial peptide delivery. Pharmaceutics 2019;11(11).

[91] Delshadi R, Bahrami A, McClements DJ, Moore MD, Williams L. Development of nanoparticle-delivery systems for antiviral agents: a review. J Control Release [Internet] 2021;331(October 2020):30–44. https://doi.org/10.1016/j.jconrel.2021.01.017.

[92] Iqbal B, Ali J, Baboota S. Silymarin loaded nanostructured lipid carrier: from design and dermatokinetic study to mechanistic analysis of epidermal drug deposition enhancement [Internet]. J Mol Liq 2018;255:513–29. Elsevier B.V. https://doi.org/10.1016/j.molliq.2018.01.141.

[93] Chauhan MK, Sharma PK. Optimization and characterization of rivastigmine nanolipid carrier loaded transdermal patches for the treatment of dementia. Chem Phys Lipids [Internet] 2019;224(July):104794. https://doi.org/10.1016/j.chemphyslip.2019.104794.

[94] Akhtar N, Singh V, Yusuf M, Khan RA. Non-invasive drug delivery technology: development and current status of transdermal drug delivery devices, techniques and biomedical applications. Biomed Tech 2020;65(3):243–72.

[95] Rajkumar AP, Ballard C, Fossey J, Orrell M, Moniz-Cook E, Woods RT, et al. Epidemiology of pain in people with dementia living in care homes: longitudinal course, prevalence, and treatment implications. J Am Med Dir Assoc 2017;18(5) 453.e1-453.e6.

[96] Ringman JM, Schneider L. Treatment options for agitation in dementia. Curr Treat Options Neurol 2019;21(7):1–14. doi:10.1007/s11940-019-0572-3.

[97] Watson K, Hatcher D, Good A. A randomised controlled trial of Lavender (Lavandula Angustifolia) and Lemon Balm (Melissa Officinalis) essential oils for the treatment of agitated behaviour in older people with and without dementia. Complement Ther Med [Internet] 2019;42:366–73. https://doi.org/10.1016/j.ctim.2018.12.016.

[98] Scuteri D, Cassano R, Trombino S, Russo R, Mizoguchi H, Watanabe C, et al. Development and translation of nanobeo, a nanotechnology-based delivery system of bergamot essential oil deprived of furocumarins, in the control of agitation in severe dementia. Pharmaceutics 2021;13(3,379):1–13. doi:10.3390/pharmaceutics13030379.

[99] Bashir S, Zafar N, Lebaz N, Mahmood A, Elaissari A. Hydroxypropyl methylcellulose-based hydrogel copolymeric for controlled delivery of galantamine hydrobromide in Dementia. Processes 2020;8(11):1–21.

[100] Keller LA, Merkel O, Popp A. Intranasal drug delivery: opportunities and toxicologic challenges during drug development. Drug Deliv Transl Res [Internet] 2022;12(4):735–57. https://doi.org/10.1007/s13346-020-00891-5.

[101] Chin LY, Tan JYP, Choudhury H, Pandey M, Sisinthy SP, Gorain B. Development and optimization of chitosan coated nanoemulgel of telmisartan for intranasal delivery: a comparative study. J Drug Deliv Sci Technol [Internet] 2021;62(December 2020):102341. https://doi.org/10.1016/j.jddst.2021.102341.

[102] Anand A, Arya M, Kaithwas G, Singh G, Saraf SA. Sucrose stearate as a biosurfactant for development of rivastigmine containing nanostructured lipid carriers and assessment of its activity against dementia in C. elegans model. J Drug Deliv Sci Technol [Internet] 2019;49(February 2018):219–26. https://doi.org/10.1016/j.jddst.2018.11.021.

[103] Zhang XX, Tian Y, Wang ZT, Ma YH, Tan L, Yu JT. The Epidemiology of Alzheimer's disease modifiable risk factors and prevention. J Prev Alzheimer's Dis 2021;8(3):313–21.

[104] Kumar B, Pathak R, Mary PB, Jha D, Sardana K, Gautam HK. New insights into acne pathogenesis: exploring the role of acne-associated microbial populations. Dermatologica Sin [Internet] 2016;34(2):67–73. http://dx.doi.org/10.1016/j.dsi.2015.12.004.

[105] Cano A, Turowski P, Ettcheto M, Duskey JT, Tosi G, Sánchez-López E, et al. Nanomedicine-based technologies and novel biomarkers for the diagnosis and treatment of Alzheimer's disease: from current to future challenges. J Nanobiotechnology [Internet] 2021;19(1):1–30. https://doi.org/10.1186/s12951-021-00864-x.

[106] Masoudi Asil S, Ahlawat J, Guillama Barroso G, Narayan M. Nanomaterial based drug delivery systems for the treatment of neurodegenerative diseases. Biomater Sci 2020;8(15):4088–107.

[107] Gupta A, Sharma R, Kuche K, Jain S. Exploring the therapeutic potential of the bioinspired reconstituted high density lipoprotein nanostructures. Int J Pharm [Internet] 2021;596(September 2020):120272. https://doi.org/10.1016/j.ijpharm.2021.120272.

[108] Salimi A, Gobadian H, Sharif Makhmalzadeh B. Dermal pharmacokinetics of rivastigmine-loaded liposomes: an ex vivo–in vivo correlation study. J Liposome Res [Internet] 2020:1–9. doi:10.1080/08982104.2020.1787440.

[109] Patel PA, Patil SC, Kalaria DR, Kalia YN, Patravale VB. Comparative in vitro and in vivo evaluation of lipid based nanocarriers of Huperzine A. Int J Pharm [Internet] 2013;446(1–2):16–23. http://dx.doi.org/10.1016/j.ijpharm.2013.02.014.

[110] Gallardo-Toledo E, Tapia-Arellano A, Celis F, Sinai T, Campos M, Kogan MJ, et al. Intranasal administration of gold nanoparticles designed to target the central nervous system: Fabrication and comparison between nanospheres and nanoprisms. Int J Pharm [Internet] 2020;590:119957. https://doi.org/10.1016/j.ijpharm.2020.119957.

[111] Patel RB, Rao HR, Thakkar DV, Patel MR. Comprehending the potential of metallic, lipid, and polymer-based nanocarriers for treatment and management of depression. Neurochem Int 2022;153:105259.

[112] Quarterman JC, Geary SM, Salem AK. Evolution of drug-eluting biomedical implants for sustained drug delivery. Eur J Pharm Biopharm 2021;159:21–35.

[113] Salatin S, Barar J, Barzegar-Jalali M, Adibkia K, Jelvehgari M. Thermosensitive in situ nanocomposite of rivastigmine hydrogen tartrate as an intranasal delivery system: Development, characterization, ex vivo permeation and cellular studies. Colloids Surfaces B Biointerfaces [Internet] 2017;159:629–38. http://dx.doi.org/10.1016/j.colsurfb.2017.08.031.

[114] Bhat A, Mahalakshmi AM, Ray B, Tuladhar S, Hediyal TA, Manthiannem E, et al. Benefits of curcumin in brain disorders. Biofactors 2019;45(5):666–89.

[115] Don TM, Chang WJ, Jheng PR, Huang YC, Chuang EY. Curcumin-laden dual-targeting fucoidan/chitosan nanocarriers for inhibiting brain inflammation via intranasal delivery. Int J Biol Macromol [Internet] 2021;181:835–46. https://doi.org/10.1016/j.ijbiomac.2021.04.045.

[116] Elnaggar YSR, Etman SM, Abdelmonsif DA, Abdallah OY. Intranasal piperine-loaded chitosan nanoparticles as brain-targeted therapy in Alzheimer's disease: optimization, biological efficacy, and potential toxicity. J Pharm Sci [Internet] 2015;104(10):3544–56. http://dx.doi.org/10.1002/jps.24557.

[117] Kandil LS, Farid RM, ElGamal SS, Hanafy AS. Intranasal galantamine/chitosan complex nanoparticles elicit neuroprotection potentials in rat brains via antioxidant effect. Drug Dev Ind Pharm [Internet] 2021;47(5):735–40. https://doi.org/10.1080/03639045.2021.1934861.

[118] Li W, Zhou Y, Zhao N, Hao B, Wang X, Kong P. Pharmacokinetic behavior and efficiency of acetylcholinesterase inhibition in rat brain after intranasal administration of galanthamine hydrobromide loaded flexible liposomes. Environ Toxicol Pharmacol [Internet] 2012;34(2):272–9. http://dx.doi.org/10.1016/j.etap.2012.04.012.

[119] Xue R, Qin N, Geng A Activated or impaired: an overview of DNA repair in neurodegenerative diseases. 2021;(February). 10.14336/AD.2021.1212

[120] Kuresan H, Samiappan D, Ghosh S, Sen GA. Early diagnosis of Parkinson's disease based on non-motor symptoms: a descriptive and factor analysis. J Ambient Intell Humaniz Comput [Internet] 2021(0123456789). doi:10.1007/s12652-021-02944-0.

[121] Md S, Bhattmisra SK, Zeeshan F, Shahzad N, Mujtaba MA, Srikanth Meka V, et al. Nanocarrier enabled drug delivery systems for nose to brain targeting for the treatment of neurodegenerative disorders. J Drug Deliv Sci Technol [Internet] 2018;43:295–310. https://doi.org/10.1016/j.jddst.2017.09.022.

[122] Tang S, Wang A, Yan X, Chu L, Yang X, Song Y, et al. Brain-targeted intranasal delivery of dopamine with borneol and lactoferrin co-modified nanoparticles for treating Parkinson's disease. Drug Deliv [Internet] 2019;26(1):700–7. https://doi.org/10.1080/10717544.2019.1636420.

[123] Raj R, Wairkar S, Sridhar V, Gaud R. Pramipexole dihydrochloride loaded chitosan nanoparticles for nose to brain delivery: development, characterization and in vivo anti-Parkinson activity. Int J Biol Macromol [Internet] 2018;109:27–35. http://dx.doi.org/10.1016/j.ijbiomac.2017.12.056.

[124] Trapani A, De Giglio E, Cometa S, Bonifacio MA, Dazzi L, Di Gioia S, et al. Dopamine-loaded lipid based nanocarriers for intranasal administration of the neurotransmitter: A comparative study. Eur J Pharm Biopharm 2021;167:189–200.

[125] Itin C, Komargodski R, Domb AJ, Hoffman A. Controlled delivery of apomorphine through buccal mucosa, towards a noninvasive administration method in Parkinson's disease: a preclinical mechanistic study. J Pharm Sci 2020;109(9):2729–34.

[126] Nie T, He Z, Zhu J, Chen K, Howard GP, Pacheco-Torres J, et al. Non-invasive delivery of levodopa-loaded nanoparticles to the brain via lymphatic vasculature to enhance treatment of Parkinson's disease. Nano Res 2021;14(8):2749–61.

Chapter 11

Futuristic aspect of nanocarriers on targeted delivery for dementia

Shobha Kumari[a], Jayant Singh Bhardwaj[a], Sanskruti Santosh Kharavtekar[a], Deepika Grewal[a], Shreyasi Ghosh Ray[a], Abhay Bhardwaj[b], Sunil Kumar Dubey[c], Prashant Kesharwani[d,e], Taruna Arora[f], Rajeev Taliyan[a]

[a]Neuropsychopharmacology Division, Department of Pharmacy, Birla Institute of Technology and Science-Pilani, Pilani, Rajasthan, India, [b]KIET School of Pharmacy, Ghaziabad, India, [c]Medical Research, R&D Healthcare Division, Emami Ltd, Belgharia, Kolkata, India, [d]Department of Pharmaceutics, School of Pharmaceutical Education and Research, Jamia Hamdard, New Delhi, India, [e]University Institute of Pharma Sciences, Chandigarh University, Mohali, Punjab, India, [f]Division of Reproductive Biology, Indian Council of Medical Research, Ansari Nagar, New Delhi, India

11.1 Introduction

Understanding the physiology of Alzheimer's disease (AD) may be further progress for medical researchers. Analysis conducted over the past 20 years has shown that macromolecules accumulating in the brain known as Amyloid-β (Aβ) are fundamentally responsible for the chronic effects of the disease [1–4]. However, there is still much to discover. It is thought that the buildup of Amyloid causes plaques and clumps to form, blocking neural signaling, and obliterating the connections between neurons [1–6]. Many researchers are investigating the role of a protein called tau (τ), which results in the formation of "neurofibrillary tangles (NFTs)" in the brain is another hallmark of subsequent neuronal death. Despite the fact that researchers have a limited grasp of tau's relevance and its connection with Aβ, previous studies have shown that the cognitive loss associated with AD is linked to the activities of those two proteins [1–4,7–9].

The detrimental effects of AD can be found in people all over the world. It is the most common cause of dementia, accounting for 60%–80% of all dementia cases [1,2,7,10]. The symptoms of dementia typically intensify over time as this disease progresses. During the early stages of Alzheimer's, memory loss is mild; nevertheless, persons with late-stage Alzheimer's lose the ability to maintain vocal communication and respond to their surroundings [2,3,11,12]. Over 5 million Americans, or one in nine, have AD stage referred to as dementia within the United States and over 30 million people worldwide. According to

Nanomedicine-Based Approaches for the Treatment of Dementia. https://doi.org/10.1016/B978-0-12-824331-2.00005-4
Copyright © 2023 Elsevier Inc. All rights reserved.

the forecast, the number of Alzheimer's patients will probably triple in the next 20–30 years as people are living longer lives [2,5,9,13].

Because advancing age is the most well-known risk factor, the majority of people with AD are 65 or older. Early onset AD affects up to 5% of people with the disease, and it is most common in adults in the 1940s and 1950s [1,2,8,10,13]. According to studies, persons aged 65 and up live for an average of 4–8 years after being diagnosed with AD. Some patients, on the other hand, live for 20 years or longer, reflecting the disease's slow and sneaky progression [1,8,14]. The prevalence of Alzheimer's continues to grow and poses a critical public health problem. All approved Alzheimer's treatments address symptoms alone and not the neurodegeneration of the disease. Accelerated clinical analysis is required for hopes of characteristic a self-made disease-modifying treatment option [5,7,9,15].

11.2 Pathophysiology of Alzheimer's disease

11.2.1 Amyloid-Beta (Aβ) and amyloid hypothesis

Aβ is a group of hydrophobic peptides with 39–43 amino acid residues, primarily A42 and A40, that result from improper processing of amyloid precursor protein (APP), a transmembrane protein that undergoes bifurcation by an enzyme called secretase. The result is two fragments: a large 100 kD hydrophilic fragment and an 11 kD membrane-associated protein. The cleavage of α-secretase does not result in the production of A peptides and has no pathogenic consequences. Instead, cleavage of APP by Alpha-secretase enzyme (BASE-1) followed by a β-secretase or presenilin enzyme results in Aβ [2,3,5,14,15,16–18]. With 40 and 42 amino acid residues, two isotypes of Aβ are generated. The Aβ42 peptide has two more hydrophobic residues as a result of this minor change [3,5,15]. As a result, aggregation of the Aβ42 form increases more than that of the more soluble Aβ40 form. A is produced at a rate of 7.6% per hour in humans, and it is eliminated at a rate of 8.3% per hour. Accumulation is caused by poor clearance rather than increased Aβ production, according to human evidence. Proteolytic degradation is the most common method of removing Aβ [13,19,20].

11.2.2 Tau protein

Tau is a protein that is connected with microtubules and acts to stabilize them. Because neurons have a long morphology, they have a well-established cytoskeleton that is stabilized by these tau proteins, that is why they occur most prominently in the axons of neurons. The phosphorylation of tau is mediated by kinases such as Cyclin-Dependent Kinase 5 (CDK5) and Glycogen Synthase Kinase 3 (GSK3β) [5,13,19–21]. Tau becomes destabilized when it is overphosphorylated or hyperphosphorylated, resulting in the creation of agglomerates known as NFTs. Some enzymes, like as phosphatase 2A and 2B, regulate this biologically by dephosphorylating p-tau and maintaining its right structure and functionality [5,19–23].

11.2.3 Link between Aβ and tau

The relationship between these two proteins is currently unknown. One of the interlinks to these molecules is the stress-inducible regulator of the calcineurin gene (RCAN1). Calcineurin is a serine/threonine phosphatase that dephosphorylates phosphorylated tau proteins. RCAN1 overexpression has been found in a few studies to cause GSK3β induction/activation, which is responsible for widespread tau phosphorylation [5,15,21,23–26].

Aβ42 has been demonstrated in parallel investigations to cause the production of reactive oxygen free radicals in both cells and mitochondria, which can lead to an increase in RCAN1 transcription (in vitro rats) [13,14,23,27].

The apolipoprotein E (apoE) e4 allele, which has been linked to an elevated incidence of sporadic AD type dementia in humans, has been identified as a risk factor. The e4 allele of apoE, unlike the e2 and e3 alleles, does not have a neuroprotective effect. Individuals with the apoE e4 allele have been reported to have higher amounts of RCAN1 and, as a result, more p-tau than noncarriers, according to studies. As a result, the possibility of a link between AD and RCAN1 is strengthened [13,23,27,28].

11.3 Protein degradation in Alzheimer's disease

Although Aβ is constantly digested and eliminated from the system, its total presence in the brain is the consequence of a balance between production and clearance rates. Aβ-degrading proteases (AβDP) are a group of peptidases and proteinases that alter Aβ levels [13]. The discovery that patients with sporadic AD had insufficient Aβ clearance in the CSF fluid supports the concept that increasing Aβ levels are caused not only by increased production but also by decreased clearance. Despite the fact that the AβDPs work together to degrade Aβ, their distinct regional and subcellular locations result in diverse peptide puddles, which may have varying pathogenicity [3,5,13]. Depending on their action under physiological or pathological settings, AβDPs can be classified as endogenous or pathogenic regulators. The ability of AβDPs to degrade Aβ fibrillar forms has opened up a world of possibilities for pharmacological and gene-therapy techniques [5,11,13,29].

11.3.1 Ubiquitination

Ubiquitination also known as ubiquitylation is a powerful mechanism that regulates most of the aspects of cell physiology, it is a process of attaching ubiquitin (a small protein) to the targeted protein which has to be degraded and mark it for degradation via proteasome.

Ubiquitination is classified into two forms based on the quantity of ubiquitin molecules attached to proteins:

1. Monoubiquitination.
2. Polyubiquitination.
   The ubiquitination process contains multiple enzymatic step.

11.3.1.1 Ubiquitin activation

The process is started by the ubiquitin-activating enzyme E1 establishing a covalent thioester link between the side chain of its own cysteine residues and the carboxyl group of the ubiquitin. The E1 enzymes for ubiquitin in humans are limited to only two [30,31].

11.3.1.2 Transfer of ubiquitin to an E2 enzyme

On the other hand, activated ubiquitin is later transported to a cysteine residue of an E2 ubiquitin-conjugating enzyme, which acts as a carrier. In humans, there are around 35 E2 enzymes [30–32].

11.3.1.3 Ubiquitylation of target proteins

The E3 ubiquitin ligase then recruits a preloaded E2-ubiquitin conjugate, detects the target protein substrate, and directly promotes or catalyzes the transfer of ubiquitin from the E2-ubiquitin conjugate to the target protein substrate. With the help of an E3-ubiquitin intermediate, this can be done immediately or in two phases. The c-terminus of ubiquitin is normally joined to the -amino group of lysine residues or the N-terminal amino group by an amide bond. In humans, there are around 600 E3 enzymes responsible for the selectivity of ubiquitylation processes [30–35].

11.4 Conventional treatment approached and their limitation

The conventional treatment for AD focuses solely on alleviating the disease's clinical symptoms. Many studies are being conducted in the scientific community in order to produce medications and their formulations for lasting cures. When the dosage of the medications is increased, the standard drug delivery system is least efficient to deliver the required dose of treatments to the targeted desirable site in the brain, resulting in either progression of the existing condition and in some cases leading to unexpected and undesired effects. In addition to this, there are various barriers that functions to protect the brain, but thus pose as a hurdle for achieving effective drug delivery in brain. These include the very selective blood–brain barrier (BBB), tight junctions, P-gp efflux pumps. For therapeutic approach for mild to severe AD patients, the USFDA has approved major two classes, acetylcholine esterase (AchE) inhibitors and NMDA receptor agonists. The former includes drugs such as rivastigmine, galantamine, donepezil, tacrine, and the later includes the drug memantine [37]. Recently, a monoclonal antibody, aducanumab (brand name Aduhelm) was approved under accelerated pathway by FDA for the treatment of AD [36]. Although these are currently being used, these are providing symptomatic relief and furthermore are linked to clinical toxicity. As a result, there is an unmet need for novel therapeutic strategies that provide superior therapeutic outcomes while causing the least amount of toxicity. It has been observed that many drug delivery systems have been unsuccessful in delivering required amount of drug directly to brain, via BBB, exception being nanoformulations [37]. Nanoformulations provide several advantages which make them more desirable to be explored, including delivery of lipophilic as well as hydrophilic drugs, delivery of drugs which has varied solubility issues across BBB, furthermore, they also offer properties like reduced toxicity, increased bioavailability, nonimmunogenicity [38–40]. Table 11.1 showed the most recent list of AD therapeutic drugs that have been approved.

Brain-targeted drug delivery systems can be investigated by encapsulating existing medicines in nanoparticles. Targeted drug delivery systems have potential to reduce the adverse effects of the existing medicines by improving their solubility permeability, biocompatibility, and having low toxicity, high bioavailability. Nanomedicines several have advantage that can deliver both hydrophobic and hydrophilic drug. They are superior to conventional drug delivery systems because they have improved medication distribution at the target site.

11.5 Traditional drug delivery technologies confront difficulties in targeting exact parts of the brain to treat the neurodegenerative disorders

The brain, as one of the body's most critical organs, has its own security mechanism to defend it. The CNS system, which covers the brain and spinal cord, is always shielded by its barrier system. The BBB, transporters, cerebrospinal fluid barrier (BCSFB) and tight junctions are the barrier system of the brain and play an essential role in the delivery of the drug to the brain [41–47].

11.5.1 Blood–brain barrier (BBB)

BBB permits simply necessary nourishment to enter, while it diffuses or effluxes harmful toxins. The brain's capillaries are not the same as the rest of the body's. The brain's microvascularization has several special qualities that enable it to operate as a barrier. The BBB maintains two distinct habitats for neurotransmitters to behave in central and peripheral. The primary function of brain capillaries is to regulate the flow of cellular materials between the brain and blood circulation [48–52]. The BBB's primary function is to keep a conducive environment for normal neural signaling. Because of these comprehensive barriers, the brain is protected from toxic component [53–55]. The BBB's primary function is to provide an appropriate atmosphere for neuron contact and function,

Table 11.1 Most recent list of approved Alzheimer's disease therapeutic drugs.

S. no.	Drug name	Type of targets	Type of therapy	Current status
1.	Donepezil	Cholinergic system	Minute particles	Approved
2.	Galantamine	Cholinergic system	Minute particles	Approved
3.	Rivastigmine	Cholinergic system	Minute particles	Approved
4.	Memantine	Glutaminergic system	Minute particles	Approved
5.	Riluzole	Glutaminergic system	Minute particles	Approved
6.	Semagacestat	γ-secretase inhibitor system	Minute particles	Discontinued
7.	Avagacestat	γ-secretase inhibitor system	Minute particles	Discontinued
8.	EVP-0962	γ-secretase inhibitor system	Minute particles	Discontinued
9.	BI 1181181	BACE inhibitor system	Minute particles	Discontinued
10.	RG7129	BACE inhibitor system	Minute particles	Discontinued
11.	LY2811376	BACE inhibitor system	Minute particles	Discontinued
12.	LY2886721	BACE inhibitor system	Minute particles	Discontinued
13.	E2609	BACE inhibitor system	Minute particles	Discontinued
14.	AZD3293	BACE inhibitor system	Minute particles	Discontinued
15.	CNP520	BACE inhibitor system	Minute particles	Discontinued
16.	JNJ-54861911	BACE inhibitor system	Minute particles	Discontinued
17.	Verubecestat	BACE inhibitor system	Minute particles	Discontinued
18.	AN-1792	Aβ clearance system	Immunotherapy (active) type	Discontinued

S. no.	Drug name	Type of targets	Type of therapy	Current status
19.	Bapineuzumab	Aβ clearance system	Immunotherapy (passive) type	Discontinued
20.	AAB-003	Aβ clearance system	Immunotherapy (passive) type	Discontinued
21.	GSK933776	Aβ clearance system	Immunotherapy (passive) type	Discontinued
22.	Solanezumab	Aβ clearance system	Immunotherapy (passive) type	Phase-III
23.	Crenezumab	Aβ clearance system	Immunotherapy (passive) type	Phase-II
24.	Gantenerumab	Aβ clearance system	Immunotherapy (passive) type	Phase-III
25.	BAN2401	Aβ clearance system	Immunotherapy (passive) type	Phase-III
26.	Aducanumab	Aβ clearance system	Immunotherapy (passive) type	Approved
27.	Epothilone D	Tau stabilization system	Minute particles	Discontinued
28.	Rember TM	Tau aggregation inhibitor system	Minute particles	Discontinued
29.	TRx0237	Tau aggregation inhibitor system	Minute particles	Phase-III
30.	AADvac-1	p-tau clearance system	Immunotherapy (active) type	Phase-II
31.	ACI-35	p-tau clearance system	Immunotherapy (active) type	Phase-II
32.	Alzhemed	Microglial activation inhibitor system	Minute particles	Discontinued
33.	Azeliragon	Microglial activation inhibitor system	Minute particles	Discontinued
34.	Ibuprofen	Microglial activation inhibitor system	Minute particles	Discontinued
35.	Flurizan	Microglial activation inhibitor system	Minute particles	Discontinued

which is essential to maintain equilibrium, manage efflux and influx, and protect the brain from toxic chemicals. BBB junctions significantly diminish gaps between endothelial spaces, preventing potentially toxic, or pathogenic particles from entering the brain through intracellular spaces. Because they continuously exhibit significant transendothelial resistance, tight junctions are the mainly key aspect of the BBB's composition. Occludin and claudins are transmembrane proteins that makeup TJs. The tight epithelial cells (EC) and mural cells primarily cover the capillaries in the brain. Pericytes, astrocytes, microglia, and neighboring neurons are the specialized cells present in the BBB [53]. ECs and tight junctions are surrounded by the base membrane. Mural cells are vascular smooth muscle cells that enclose well-built width blood arteries and pericytes. Mural cells are found distributed across the blood vessel wall lining. The pericytes live in the microvascular network's basement membrane (Fig. 11.1).

The term pericyte comes from its early anatomical interpretations ("peri-" around and "cyto-" cell) and corresponds to the abluminal side of microvessels' periendothelial genesis [56]. Pericytes cover the abluminal endothelial surface of approximately all arterioles, venules, and capillaries anatomically [57]. In response to brain impulses, pericytes are engaged in revascularization, reduce inflammation, cell growth, cytokine production trafficking, and blood flow control [58]. The another name of basement membrane is basal lamina composed of laminin, collagen type IV, nidogens, and heparan proteoglycans. Astrocytes are

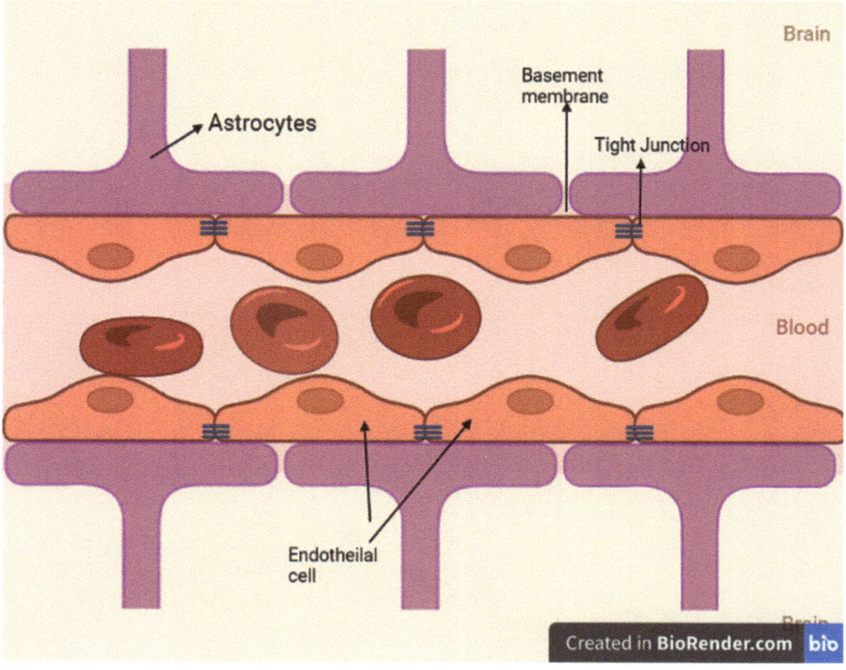

FIG. 11.1 Blood–brain barrier (BBB).

brain cells that enclose capillaries and are situated above the basement membrane. The astrocytes connect the brain cells with the blood arteries [59]. Astrocytes, which cover almost all of the cerebrovascular surface, regulate BBB integrity and cerebral blood flow. In the brain astrocytes contain gap junction proteins together with as connexin, aquaporin 4 (AQP4), and Kir4.1 channels are plentiful, making them particularly dynamic locations for regulating molecular ions and water flow, which is critical for BBB function [60]. Astrocytes are accountable for managing the tight junction at the BBB, transporter localization, and precise enzyme function, contributing to the improvement barrier activity [59,62].

The BBB is composed of a giant set of connections of endothelial cells (ECs), neurons, and glial cells, including microglia, forms the neurovascular unit [61]. Both exogenous and endogenous materials produced during pathogens infection, mainly exogenous produced that time as well as endogenous chemicals released by damaged native brain cells and activate microglia, astrocytes, neurons, ECs, and pericytes in the torn or infected brain. The microglial cells under physiological conditions express macrophage colony-stimulating factor (M-CSF)-1 receptor (CD115), the glycoproteins F4/80, the alpha-M integrin (CD11b), the fractalkine receptor (CX3CR1), the inhibitory immune receptor CD200R, and the intracellular calcium-binding protein Iba-1 [62]. During CNS disorders, the three different types of macrophages located in the CNS, perivascular, meningeal, and choroid plexus macrophages have the adaptability to modify fluidly to irregularities in the BBB, impacting their shape, activity, and engagement state, which changes microglia's influence on the BBB [63].

11.5.2 Efflux transporters

In the BBB of the brain, two types of membrane transporters are present which are uptake transporters and efflux transporters. The uptake transporters are in charge of transferring essential minerals and critical substances from the bloodstream to the brain cells via ECs and vascular tissue, while the down take transporters are in charge of transferring essential minerals and critical substances from the bloodstream to the brain cells via ECs and vascular tissue. Efflux transporters, on the other hand, act in the reverse direction of uptake transporters, pumping molecules from the brain to the vascular side. The efflux transporters are encoded by the ABC gene (ATP binding cassette) [64]. P-glycoprotein (Pgp) is a transporter protein found on the superheated plasma surfaces of vascular endothelium in the BBB that provide the protection to the brain by inhibiting the destructive substances from entering the bloodstream [65]. In humans, the Multidrug Resistance (MDR) gene encodes Pgp transpoters. Type I, also known as MDRI, is involved in resistance of drug and functions as an efflux pump at the barrier, whereas Type II, also known as MDRII, is present on hepatocytes and functions as a phosphatidyl translocator [64,67]. Pgp works as an efflux pump at the BBB, limiting the cellular absorption of drugs from the bloodstream into the brain. Its phrase is improved in several CNS disorders. Because of the increased density, certain pathologies may be more difficult to treat, even if new treatments are developed [66].

11.5.3 Blood cerebrospinal fluid barrier

The BBB and BCSFB form a tight barrier around the CNS. Choroid plexus epithelium constructs the BCSFB, while cerebral ECs focus the BBB. The BCSFB has multiple loci, it shows heterogeneity structurally and functionally. In both the inner and outer areas of the central nervous system, CSF encloses the vascular system at various epithelial locations of CNS. Two significant areas of the CNS where blood is near the CSF are the meningeal wall covering over the pleural cavity and the cerebral plex (CP) in folding of the ventricles [67] (Fig. 11.2).

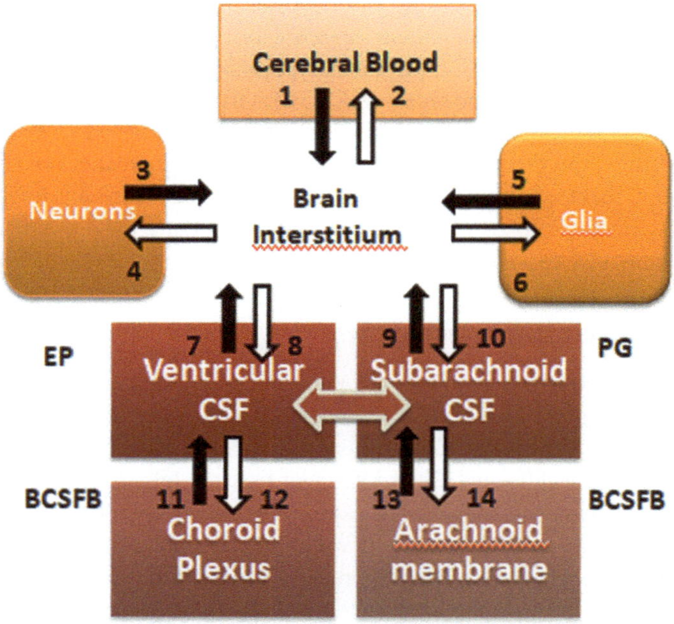

FIG. 11.2 The central nervous system's (CNS) key transport interfaces are depicted. Interstitial fluid (ISF) composition is influenced by several points where blood and CSF contact the brain. At all barrier locations of parenchymal cell membranes of neurons and glia, many secretory (outward full arrow) and resorptive (inward blank arrows) movements of water, ions, and molecules occur simultaneously (3–6). The aggregate of these several exchange activities determines the neural interstitial environment. Greater permeability between both the brain and the ventricular fluid and subarachnoid space CSF is possible due to the gap connections between CSF and the ependyma (EP) (7–10). Hydrostatic pressure gradient-driven bulk flow aids fluid transmission between the ISF and CSF compartments, promoting dispersion. At 2, 12, and 14, organic acid anions and amyloid peptide fragments, for example, undergo resorptive transport. Secretory transfer occurs frequently at 1, and it also occurs frequently at 11, but it occurs much less frequently at 13. Odd and even-numbered arrows show transport into and uptake from CNS extracellular fluid, respectively.

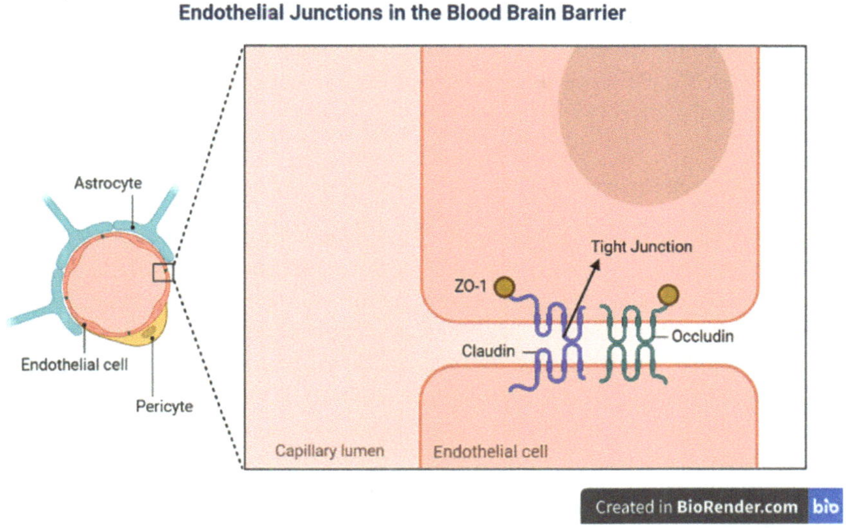

FIG. 11.3 Endothelial junctions in BBB.

11.5.4 Tight junctions (TJs)

TJs form lines of massive, repetitive occlusions among cerebral vascular endothelium at the BBB, decreasing transcellular migration of polar solvents, and biomolecules into the CNS dramatically. TJ dysfunction at the BBB could play a role in the pathogenesis of several neurological diseases and gaining a better understanding of the mechanisms involved could lead to more effective CNS medicine administration via the paracellular pathway. In the brain, it forms a protective wall among neighboring vascular ECs [68] (Fig. 11.3).

11.6 Novel drug delivery strategies for targeting brain to treat neurodegenerative disorders

11.6.1 Liposomes

The main aim of this novel drug delivery system to target the brain disease is to identify the specific target receptors and transporters that are highly expressed in BBB [69]. Liposomes are circular organic nanostructures with an aqueous core encased by a lipid bilayer and a lipid-soluble phospholipid layer on the exterior [70]. The hydrophobic membrane of a liposome traps an aqueous solution. Hydrophobic therapeutic agents rapidly diffuse across lipid bilayers, permitting these to transfer all hydrophilic or hydrophobic compounds [71]. Liposomes have several features, including nonimmunogenicity, nontoxicity, degradability, cytocompatibility, and versatility [72–74]. Liposomes can enhance the effectiveness, durability, and distribution of a drug, as well as allow for numerous routes of administration, targeted tissue action, and the avoidance of potential drug toxicity [70]. Liposomes could be assigned to a particular location through lipid-mediated passive diffusion or endocytosis, which together permits the passage through the BBB, or through the intranasal administration, which completely skips the BBB [75] (Fig. 11.4).

11.6.2 Dendrimers

The word "dendrimer" comes from the Greek words "dendron" (tree-like structure) and "meros" (fruit) (part). Dendrimers are long-chain 3D nanosized polymeric macromolecules composed of dendrons, which are monomeric units that are repeatedly branched. Dendrons are chemically distinct groups that are chemically linked to the dendrimer's core [76–83]. Dendrimers are polymers molecules consisting of multiple surface functional molecules that are symmetrical and monodispersed [84]. Dendrimers have a basic structure in which so many diverging cycles, sometimes called generations, are added. Each generation is given a number that indicates how often branching processes were conducted on the core molecule [76]. Dendrimers are nanoscale macromolecules with a hyperbranched globular shape that are commonly employed for medication delivery. Dendrimers, in contrast to typical polymer nano vehicles, are monodisperse and have well-defined chemical structures. Dendrimers have a special structure that enables them to store therapeutic drugs via a covalent coupling or electrically charged adsorption [85]. Dendrimers are nanoscale compounds having excellent structural uniformity, ability to dissolve, bioactivity, nonimmunogenicity, great dispersion, specific shape and texture, and fully efficient ending edges [86–89].

11.6.3 Antibody-coated nanoparticles

One of the most well-known explanations for the pathogenesis of AD is the amyloid hypothesis, which explains the formation and deposition of the amyloid–peptide, which could also lead to neuronal loss, neurotoxicity, and a range of other symptoms, including dementia. Currently, numerous medications are being developed with the goal of altering the condition rather than just treating the symptoms. Aβ aggregation inhibitors and beta-secretase inhibitors are medications that target the start of Aβ formation. Immunotherapy is one of the therapeutic strategies available. Antibodies against Aβ are used in this case as a targeted approach. The usage of antibodies, or passive immunization, aids in the maintenance of antibody in the body. Antibodies already have a high level of specificity when it comes to hitting the target. The properties of nanoparticles are merged with the specificity of antibodies when these antibodies are mixed with nanocarriers. The cellular absorption and intracellular stability are both improved as a result of this conjugation. These are the key advantages of using information from nanocarriers for coupled antibodies nanomaterials to connect antibodies. These antibody-conjugated nanoparticles are useful for

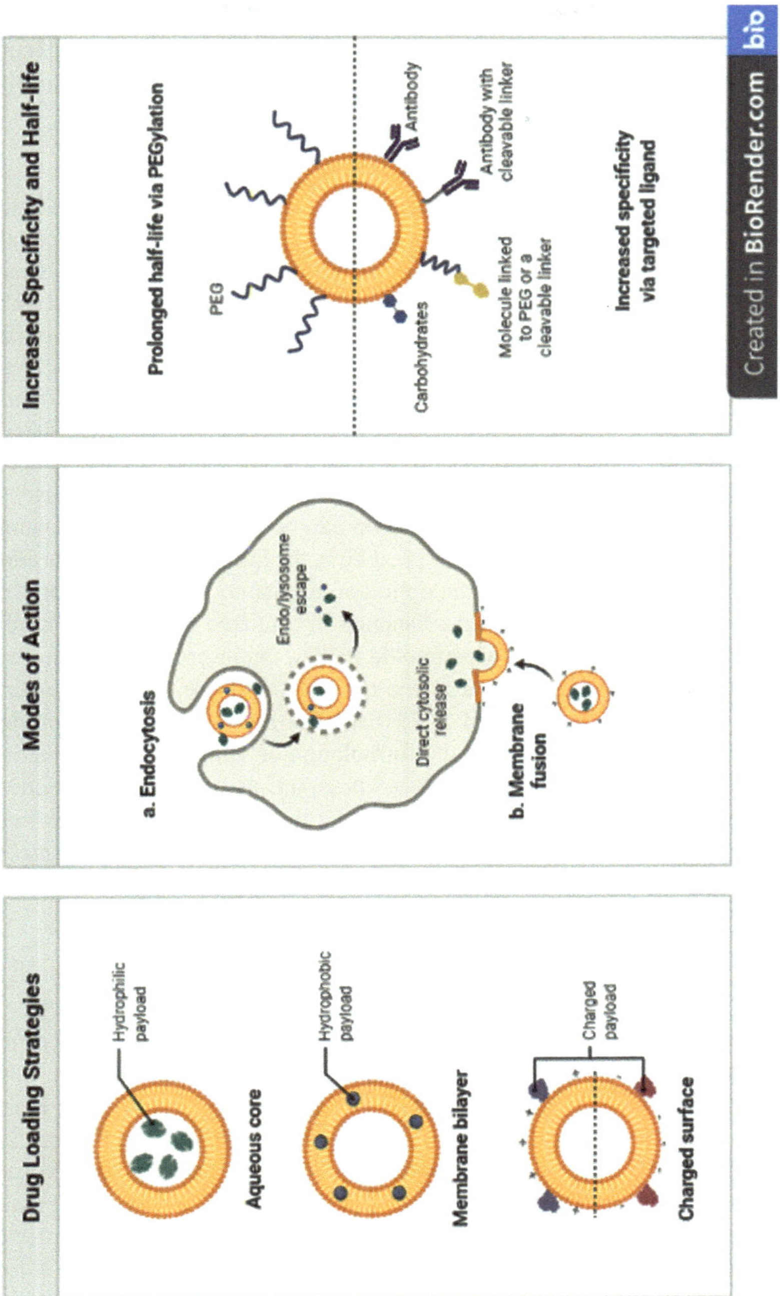

FIG. 11.4 Liposomes-based drug delivery system.

both medicinal and diagnostic reasons. With enhanced cellular and molecular level of coupled nanomaterials, the coupled nanoparticles provide the essential specificity for therapeutic application. In vitro or in vivo diagnostic purposes are both possible. Various researchers are currently investigating the use of conjugated antibodies to target amyloids in Alzheimer's and dementia patients [90].

11.6.4 Polymeric micelles

Polymeric micelles are self-assembling core/shell structures, whose base is the created from amphiphilic copolymers in aqueous medium. There are certain physical and inherent properties of polymeric micelles which makes it a desirable option to explore for, in the treatment of neurodegenerative disease. The physical properties include association, which involves the process of micellization, a transformation of unimers into nanoscopic supramolecular structures, well known as micelles [91–93]. Other physical properties of polymeric micelles which needs to be highlighted includes formation of spherical shaped structure, the size ranging from 10 to 100 nm and physical stability which is the ability of the polymeric micelles to withstand dilution [94–96]. This property of polymeric micelles to withstand the dilution can be termed as thermodynamic stability, which is a crucial property especially in the intravenous administration [91,94]. In an attempt to explore the option of polymeric nanoparticle for drug delivery in brain, C. Scialabba and colleagues, formulated a novel amphiphilic graft copolymer using the polyaspartamide PHEA, via insertion of polysorbate as well as C17- squalenyl chains in the polymer structure, thus formulating a novel copolymer system called as PHEA-EDA-Sq17-PS80. This modified polymeric structure, converts into the formulation of micelle core via interactions of Sq17 alkyl chains. Thus, in other words, self-assembling itself forming into a micelle structure in aqueous medium. Furthermore, these micelles were loaded with hydrophobic drug substance, Riv. In addition to this, the researchers observed the successful internalization of these loaded micelles by the neuroblastoma cell-line [97].

11.6.5 Polymeric nanoparticles

Polymeric nanoparticles are diverse nanoparticles, which can be modified into distinct shapes and has various physiochemical properties, which tends to make them a favorable option to be explored for drug delivery in brain. These polymeric nanoparticles can be manufactured with much ease, are efficiently scaled up, highly stable in in vivo environment, and can be used successfully to achieve sustained drug delivery. These properties together make these polymeric nanoparticles, as one of the advantageous option in order to explore for achieving drug delivery to brain [98,99]. The crucial point in formulation of polymeric nanoparticle is appropriate selection of polymer, which is sufficiently nontoxic and efficacious. Mainly, the following properties need to be ascertained prior to opting a polymer for polymeric nanoparticles formulation, these are, nontoxicity, nonimmunogenic, biocompatibility, and biodegradability [102]. There are many polymers that are commonly explored for targeting brain delivery, these include, poly-alkyl-cyanoacrylate, polylactide-co-glycolide (PLGA), PEG, poly-ε-caprolactone (PCL), PLA, and chitosan [100–102]. Chitosan has properties like increased bioadhesivity and biocompatibility. Furthermore, chitosan can be modified using the ligands which can in turn enhance the cellular uptake of polymeric nanoparticles via the mechanism of receptor mediated endocytosis [103]. The chitosan has the groups of amine and hydroxyl group present as its active site. If the chitosan has the positively charged groups which leads to bond formation with the membrane, as it has negative charge, thus enhance the drug release [104]. PLGA is another polymer which is biodegarable and nontoxic. It also holds certain other properties which help in penetration through BBB and sustained drug delivery. A modified polymer comprising of PLGA-PEG-PLGA polymers using polysorbate 80 coatings were formulated to target drug delivery [105]. Although this is the case, there are few limitations for the use of polymeric nanoparticles which mainly include, maintenance of safety, efficacy, and tolerability. Furthermore, the maintenance of size is another crucial concern to be paid attention to whilst formulating polymeric nanoparticles [106,107].

11.6.6 Gold nanoparticles

Generally size range of these gold nanoparticles lies within 10 to 100 nm. These are a form of colloidal dispersions involving gold molecules. They have wide applications in the field of science, including imaging studies, detection of tumors, gene therapies, as well as in various drug delivery systems. The primary advantages of using these gold nanoparticles in the treatment of neurodegenerative disorders are its comparatively decreased toxicities, nonimmunogenicity, and biocompatible properties [108,109]. In neurodegenerative disorders, gold nanoparticles can be used for detection of amyloid-beta oligomers that are associated with the pathophysiology of AD [110]. The gold nanoparticles formulated by Hou et al. were stabilized with D-glutathione as well as L-glutathione. The stabilizing compound, glutathione, acts as an antioxidant naturally available in human body, which has a primary action of reducing oxidative stress on different cells present in body [111,112]. Hou et al. observed that upon parenteral (intravenous) administration of the glutathione-modified gold nanoparticles decreased the formations of amyloid-beta 42 aggregates in AD-induced C57BL/6. Furthermore, even an enhancement in cognitive and memory functions was observed, thus can validate a possible use of glutathione stabilized gold nanoparticles as a therapeutic in AD [112]. Muller et al. concluded that the gold nanoparticles which he formulated were effective in reducing the inflammation of neuronal cells as well as in reducing the oxidative stress in AD rat models (Streptozotocin-induced AD) [113].

11.6.7 Quantum dot

QD which is also known as C-dots or carbon quantum dots is carbon-based particles of size 1–20 nm. The main properties of these QD include, fluorescence, optical absorptivity, stability, and improved aqueous solubility [114]. As a result of the favorable properties like super penetration through BBB, high biocompatible nature, convenient production process, and least toxic properties, these are widely considered in therapeutic care of neurodegenerative disorders [117–119]. The graphene quantum dots formulated by Liu et al, via heating of graphene sheet with water or ethanol at 200°C for the duration of 10 hours, were anticipated for a possible use of the formulation as therapeutic strategy for AD. This conclusion was based on the thioflavin fluorescence assay which revealed that the formulated graphene rods significantly hampered the production of aggregates of amyloid-beta [120]. Another study observed the possible use of quantum dots as nanocarriers, specifically via a formulation of iron oxide bounded carbon dots, playing the role of the nanocarrier for the active ingredient curcumin. The formulation was effective in inhibiting the aggregation of amyloid-beta 1–42 as well as the synthesis of amyloid beta fibril-induced reactive oxygen species in PC_{12}cells [115]. A study by Nair et al. highlights the use of quantum dots in combination with silver nanoparticles in blocking the formation of Amyloid beta 1–42 aggregates, confirmed via thioflavin fluorescence assay [122].

11.6.8 Carbon nanotubes

Carbon nanotubes are basically allotropes of carbon. These are formed of base material graphite and then engineered into cylindrical tubes which are in the nano-size range [116,117]. The advantageous part of these nanotubes is the customized structural properties, as well as its mechanical and electronic properties. These properties are attributed to their nano size, mass, and the enhanced mechanical strength [118,119]. The structure mainly constitutes of aligned carbon atoms in a pattern to form a cylindrical structure. Single-walled carbon nanotubes and multiwalled carbon nanotubes are two different types based on the count of carbon layers. These carbon nanotubes are widely being explored for the treatments of neurodegenerative diseases. The nanoscale size of these tubes enables their transport through the BBB, leading to effective drug delivery in the brain [120]. Yang and colleagues observed the potential use of single-walled carbon nanotubes for delivering acetylcholine in AD mice brains [121]. Carbon nanorods can be used as therapeutic tool for targeting various drugs for neurological diseases. The characteristic properties of these carbon nanotubes enable their increased potential in the field of neuroscience [122]. Xue et al. observed the potential use of single-walled carbon nanotubes as a novel tool with neuroprotection against AD. In the study, it was demonstrated that the modified single-walled carbon nanotubes were efficient in restoring the functional autophagy via reversing the abnormal mTOR signaling activation [123].

11.6.9 Viral carrier

For insertion of a desired functional gene which can be an addition or act as a replacement in the genome, so as to correct the defaulted function of the gene, is gene therapy in general. This transfer is carried out with the help of the gene transporters which are widely known as viral vector or viral carriers [124,125]. The expected outcome from the gene therapy involved in the field of neuroscience is achievement of genetic material delivery passing through the BBB, to its exact site [126]. Although the viral vectors seem to be interesting tool, it has faced several setbacks in the past. However, the current researchers are keen on exploring the viral vectors for its safe and efficient use in the field of neuroscience [126]. For targeting AD, the researchers have mainly focused on two viral carriers, namely, lentivirus and adeno associated virus [127]. The viral carrier system mainly utilizes the properties of virus to infect and replicate in the host cell, as a tool in delivery of desired gene in the host cell. However, viral vectors initially should be validated based on specific criteria prior to its use, these include pathogenicity, tissue specificity, and identification [6]. Lentiviral vectors are often associated with numerous advantages, including delivery of transgene into nondividing cells. These nondividing cells include neurons too, thus making Lenti virus as a high potential carrier for targeting brain delivery. Furthermore, it offers robustness in in vivo conditions, stability, and high efficiency [128]. Hence, due to these properties, lentiviral carrier system can be considered amongst desirable vectors for therapeutic care in AD. Another type of vector which is widely being used is adeno-associated virus. These vectors' transduction of neurons, long-term gene expression, and low immunogenicity AD outweigh their risks [127,129]. Sehera et al. studied the property of long-term transgene expression via observing the 1-methyl-4-phenyl-1,2,3,6-tetrahydropyridine lesioned nonhuman-primate model of PD expressing an enzyme responsible for synthesis of dopamine, even later to 15 years of administration Adeno-associated virus (AAV) vector [129,130]. This suggests the property of adeno-associated vectors of long-lasting expression can be utilized for gene therapy in the AD.

11.6.10 Nanocrystals

Nanocrystals are crystalline drug particles with a size range of nanometers that can be manufactured using both top-down and bottom-up methods. In the bottom-up method, the nanoparticles are created from the drug molecules in solution, such as precipitation. Top-down ways entail reducing bigger size particles to the nanometer range by milling. Furthermore, in some procedures, two or more technologies are used in succession, for example, the combination of microprecipitation and high-pressure homogenization. To stabilize the nanoparticles in some conditions, drying is used. This ensures higher physical stability and also prevents aggregation, sedimentation, and creaming [109].

A distinct advantage of nanocrystals (nanosuspension) is that they can be injected intravenously with 100% bioavailability [110]. Nanocrystals with diameters ranging from 100 to 300 nm may be administered intravenously without causing any adverse effects, such as capillary occlusion. Because of this, the nanocrystals circulate in the bloodstream and get dissolved depending on the dissolving qualities, allowing them to reach the target region. Further, certain fluorescent molecules are also being combined with the nanocrystals in order to produce hybrid formulations that can be utilized for treatment as well as diagnostic purposes. For creating a tumor targeting and imaging hybrid nanosystem, Zhao et al. incorporated a guest fluorescent material into the crystal lattice of paclitaxel which is a weakly soluble anticancer medication [111]. When compared to traditional formulations, nanocrystals provide a universal approach or delivering poorly soluble medicines and provide greater therapeutic results. The present uses of nanocrystal methods, however, are quite restricted. The goal for the future is to broaden its therapeutic use to serve a greater number of people. Because the great majority of oncology medications are insoluble in water, injectable nanocrystals offer an option for cancer treatment. Because of their capacity to improve the permeability of pharmacological molecules, nanocrystals offer the potential for parenteral administration. This process is related to nanocrystals' higher solubility in forming a high concentration gradient, which promotes drug molecule penetration through barriers such as the stratum corneum, cornea, and lung mucosa. Furthermore, the enhanced adhesivity generated from the higher specific surface area of nanocrystals extends the period of nanocrystals at the administering site, hence maintaining a large concentration gradient [112].

11.6.11 Microneedles

Microneedles (MNs) are an innovative strategy for transdermal drug delivery. It can be described as a combination of a hypodermic needle and a transdermal patch. The base plate has MN arrays attached perpendicular to it. The length of each MN ranges from 0.25 to 1 mm. Materials like metal, ceramic, glass, silicon, and polymers are used for making MNs [131]. Skin is an absorptive organ and its structure can be divided into three layers—epidermis, dermis, and subcutis. It contains various cells such as T lymphocytes, Langerhans cells, mast cells, keratinocytes, macrophages, and dendritic cells—all of which are important for the immune system [131]. Langerhans cells are antigen-presenting cells (APCs) that take up antigens, transporting them to the draining lymph nodes. Mast cells can act as APCs themselves or transmit signals that can mobilize dendritic cells in the skin toward the drainage of lymph nodes. Capillary permeability and leukocyte diapedesis into the skin get increased when ECs are activated by proinflammatory mediators. The responses of CD4+ and CD8+ T cells in the draining lymph nodes are directly or indirectly induced by dendritic cells, leading to the preparation and expansion of adaptive immunity. The primed and expanded B and T cells can supply systemic protection by occupying the skin and other distal epithelial tissues. Transdermal drug delivery can bypass the first-pass effect and lead to sustained drug release. However, the stratum corneum which is the outermost layer of skin, acts as a barrier to effective drug delivery [139]

Topical creams have poor bioavailability as only 10%–20% of the loaded drug is able to cross the skin barrier. Hypodermic needles have high bioavailability and fast onset of action but poor patient compliance due to the pain caused. Further, skilled professionals are needed to administer the drug as patients do not have the expertise to inject it themselves. Transdermal patches are painless, but their bioavailability is low as the molecules need to cross the stratum corneum [132]. Since the superficial dermis contains a capillary bed and accompanying lymphatic capillaries, the onset of action is quick with MNs. Due to the number of immune cells in the dermis, it is an ideal delivery method for vaccine administration. There is higher control with MN compositions which leads to accurate doses [133].

Due to their small size and length, MNs are painless and safe to use. The patch application does not require professional knowledge. The overall size of the medication package is reduced as MN patches combine the functioning of the drug formulation, needle, and syringe. This also results in an overall reduction or elimination of sharps waste. The MN's enhanced solid-state formulation eliminates the requirement for a cold-chain system. Costs are also saved in terms of manufacturing, logistics, and dose sparing.

The drug is delivered via the topical route through diffusion. The skin is briefly disturbed in MN delivery. The device is manufactured by assembling hundreds of MNs in arrays on a small patch—similar to a commercially available transdermal patch. This enables it to administer enough drug to provide the desired therapeutic response. The device can go around the barrier layer by piercing the stratum corneum. The medicine is inserted directly into the epidermis or higher dermis layer, which subsequently goes into the systemic circulation and brings about a healing effect once it makes it to the target region [132].

Skin permeability has been examined using a variety of chemical, biological, and physical approaches. Chemical and biochemical approaches do not appear to be particularly effective for delivering biotherapeutics and vaccines across the skin. While physical approaches hold more potential for macromolecule distribution, they often entail the use of specialized machines that are bulky, expensive, and require training to operate. MNs, on the other hand, can be made into a low-cost patch that patients can easily apply for biomacromolecule distribution. The use of MNs to deliver vaccines to APCs in the skin is also being considered [134]. Proteins like insulin, vaccines, antibodies, and drugs for skin diseases have been well-researched as potential candidates for MNs.

11.7 Novel proteolytic therapies for Alzheimer's disease

11.7.1 Small-molecule PROTACs peptide

Proteolysis targeting chimaera (PROTAC) is a new technique for selectively triggering protein degradation in cells. There have been numerous studies in which various peptides have been synthesized based on previously gained knowledge about ubiquitylation and the related potency of protein targeting chimaeras (PROTAC). Because tau is an unstructured, flexible protein, a variety of multifunctional chimeric molecules including three sections were created to aid in the detection and degradation of p-tau [16,17]:

1. A moiety capable of recognizing tau.
2. An E3 ligase-binding moiety.
3. A peptide that penetrates cells.

As candidates for inducing tau degradation, a number of multifunctional compounds were created. TH006 appeared to be the most promising of the different compounds synthesized, resulting in the greatest reduction in EGFP fluorescence intensity [16,17,19,26].

11.7.2 TH006

The binding affinity of TH006 with tau in vitro was determined using a fluorescence polarization test. Increased recombinant hTau40 protein was treated with 0.1 mM CF-TH006 (TH006 labeled with 5(6)-carboxyfluorescein [CF]). The fluorescence polarization measurements were used to calculate the affinity between CF-TH006 and tau. The KD was around 0.3944 0.1589 mM [19–21,25]. The tau-binding specificity of TH006 was also confirmed by synthesizing CF-CP1, a CF-labeled control peptide with four mutant residues in the tau-binding domain. The binding capacity with tau was tested using the control peptides CF-CP1 and CF, respectively. CF-CP1 and CF had no interaction with tau, according to the findings [21,22,27,135].

11.7.2.1 TH006 can induce tau degradation

For 2 hours, neuronal N2a cells with tau-EGFP overexpression were pretreated with cycloheximide (CHX; 20 mg/mL), a protein production inhibitor. The cells were then treated for 24 hours with various doses of TH006. The intensity of intracellular fluorescence was lowered in a dose-dependent manner, according to flow cytometry studies. The TH006-induced tau degradation was further demonstrated in dose- and time-dependent manners using a western blotting experiment probed with antitau (human) antibody [21].

11.7.2.2 TH006 can increase polyubiquitination of tau depending on VHL E3 ligase

MG132 and bafilomycin A1, an autophagy inhibitor, were utilized in a study to disrupt the two primary protein breakdown pathways: the proteasome and the autophagy pathway. After 24 hours of treatment with 200 mMTH006, the tau level in tau-overexpressed N2a cells was found to be lower [21].

11.7.3 The role of neprilysin-2 (NEP-2) in amyloid-beta clearance

Furthermore, NEP inhibitors greatly increased Aβ levels in the rat's brain, resulting in the formation of senile plaques. In mice, this effect was independently replicated [136–138]. Neprilysin (NEP) is one of the most significant enzymes that regulate the amount of Aβ in the brain. NEP is a zinc-dependent metalloprotease that is responsible for bisecting peptides at the amino position of hydrophobic residues, inactivating a variety of peptides including enkephalins, glucagon, substance P, bradykinin, and many more. This is a cell surface-associated enzyme that has been found to digest short peptides in the peripheral and central nervous systems. Aβ was radiolabeled in an in-vivo investigation, and it was discovered that NEP was the primary degrader of Aβ [136,138,139]. Furthermore, NEP inhibitors greatly increased Aβ levels in the rat's brain, resulting in the formation of senile plaques. This effect was replicated in mice on its own [140,141]. A study showing that overexpression of NEP results in a considerable reduction of senile plaque in APP-transgenic mice further supports NEP's critical role as an A-degrading enzyme. There is a decrease in NEP mRNA and protein expression, which is linked to being older or having AD [137,142,143]. Although NEP expression is varied in most brain regions, it is predominantly expressed in the brain stem, hypothalamus, and pituitary, according to various rat studies. A involvement in the hypothalamus-pituitary axis has been hypothesized based on the neuropeptide's location and metabolism [140,142–145].

11.8 Conclusion and prospects for the future

Nanotechnology has paved the way for a slew of new possibilities, allowing for a more focused and targeted treatment approach. It has the potential to overcome such obstacles in the delivery of targeted drugs to the brain. Nanotechnology has a wide range of applications in improved therapies for AD. Microencapsulation is now being studied to enable the less destructive, therapeutically efficient, targeted medication delivery with minimal cytotoxicity for the treatment of long-term neurological disorders like AD and dementia. Continued work could lead to newer options, opening the door for a very effective treatment method using nanotechnology to treat AD.

References

[1] Alzheimer's Association. Alzheimer's disease facts and figures. Alzheimer's Dement 2015;11(2015):332–84. https://doi.org/10.1016/j.jalz.2015.02.003.

[2] Swerdlow RH. Pathogenesis of Alzheimer's disease. Clin Interv Aging 2007;2:347–59.

[3] Tiwari S, Atluri V, Kaushik A, Yndart A, Nair M Alzheimer's disease: pathogenesis, diagnostics, and therapeutics. International journal of nanomedicine 2019;14:5541.

[4] Components C. Processing and degradation of cellular components. Cell Biol 2017:393–405. https://doi.org/10.1016/b978-0-323-34126-4.00023-2.

[5] Wang DS, Dickson DW, Malter JS. β-Amyloid degradation and Alzheimer's disease. J Biomed Biotechnol 2006(2006):1–12. https://doi.org/10.1155/JBB/2006/58406.

[6] Taliyan R, Kakoty V, Sarathlal KC, Kharavtekar SS, Karennanavar CR, Choudhary YK, Singhvi G, Riadi Y, Dubey SK, Kesharwani P. Nanocarrier mediated drug delivery as an impeccable therapeutic approach against Alzheimer's disease. J Control Release 2022;343:528–50. https://doi.org/10.1016/j.jconrel.2022.01.044.

[7] Burns A, Iliffe S. Alzheimer's disease. BMJ 2009;338:467–71. https://doi.org/10.1136/bmj.b158.

[8] Chen YG. Research progress in the pathogenesis of Alzheimer's Disease. Chin Med J (Engl) 2018;131:1618–24. https://doi.org/10.4103/0366-6999.235112.

[9] Agrawal M, Prathyusha E, Ahmed H, Dubey SK, Kesharwani P, Singhvi G, Naidu VGM, Alexander A. Biomaterials in treatment of Alzheimer's disease. Neurochem Int 2021;145:105008. https://doi.org/10.1016/J.NEUINT.2021.105008.

[10] Henry W, Querfurth HW, LaFerla FM Mechanisms of disease Alzheimer's disease. New Engl J Med 2010;362:329–344.

[11] Lendon CL, Ashall F, Goate AM. Exploring the etiology of Alzheimer disease using molecular genetics. J Am Med Assoc 1997;277:825–31. https://doi.org/10.1001/jama.277.10.825.

[12] Smith DG, Cappai R, Barnham KJ. The redox chemistry of the Alzheimer's disease amyloid β peptide. Biochim Biophys Acta - Biomembr 2007;1768:1976–90. https://doi.org/10.1016/j.bbamem.2007.02.002.

[13] Graham WV, Bonito-Oliva A, Sakmar TP. Update on Alzheimer's disease therapy and prevention strategies. Annu Rev Med 2017;68:413–30. https://doi.org/10.1146/annurev-med-042915-103753.

[14] Ballard C, Gauthier S, Corbett A, Brayne C, Aarsland D, Jones E. Alzheimer's disease. Lancet 2011;377:1019–31. https://doi.org/10.1016/S0140-6736(10)61349-9.

[15] Marr R, Hafez D. Amyloid beta and Alzheimer's disease: the role of neprilysin-2 in amyloid-beta clearance. Front Aging Neurosci 2014;6:1–7. https://doi.org/10.3389/fnagi.2014.00187.

[16] Kargbo RB. Treatment of cancer and Alzheimer's disease by PROTAC degradation of EGFR. ACS Med Chem Lett 2019;10:1098–9. https://doi.org/10.1021/acsmedchemlett.9b00283.

[17] Wang W, Zhou Q, Jiang T, Li S, Ye J, Zheng J, Wang X, Liu Y, Deng M, Ke D, Wang Q, Wang Y, Wang JZ. A novel small-molecule PROTAC selectively promotes tau clearance to improve cognitive functions in Alzheimer-like models. Theranostics 2021;11:5279–95. https://doi.org/10.7150/thno.55680.

[18] Saido T, Leissring MA. Proteolytic degradation of amyloid β-protein. Cold Spring Harb Perspect Med 2012;2 http://doi.org/10.1101/cshperspect.a006379.

[19] Wang C, Zhang Y, Xing D, Zhang R. PROTACs technology for targeting non-oncoproteins: advances and perspectives. Bioorg Chem 2021;114:105109. https://doi.org/10.1016/j.bioorg.2021.105109.

[20] Bonet-Costa V, Pomatto LCD, Davies KJA. The proteasome and oxidative stress in Alzheimer's disease. Antioxidants Redox Signal 2016;25:886–901. https://doi.org/10.1089/ars.2016.6802.

[21] Chu TT, Gao N, Li QQ, Chen PG, Yang XF, Chen YX, Zhao YF, Li YM. Specific knockdown of endogenous tau protein by peptide-directed ubiquitin-proteasome degradation. Cell Chem Biol 2016;23:453–61. https://doi.org/10.1016/j.chembiol.2016.02.016.

[22] Stewart MD, Ritterhoff T, Klevit RE, Brzovic PS. E2 enzymes: more than just middle men. Cell Res 2016;26:423–40. https://doi.org/10.1038/cr.2016.35.

[23] Gao N, Chen YX, Zhao YF, Li YM. Chemical methods to knock down the amyloid proteins. Molecules 2017;22:1–9. https://doi.org/10.3390/molecules22060916.

[24] Gould TD, Dao DT, Kovacsics CE. Mood and Anxiety Related Phenotypes in Mice. Neuromethods 2009;42:1–20. https://doi.org/10.1007/978-1-60761-303-9.

[25] Tomasi TB, Magner WJ, Khan ANH. Epigenetic regulation of immune escape genes in cancer. Cancer Immunol Immunother 2006;55:1159–84. https://doi.org/10.1007/s00262-006-0164-4.

[26] Tonali N, Nencetti S, Orlandini E, Ciccone L. Application of PROTAC strategy to TTR-Aβ protein-protein interaction for the development of Alzheimer's disease drugs. Neural Regen Res 2021;16:1554–5. https://doi.org/10.4103/1673-5374.303017.

[27] de Tullio MB, Morelli L, Castaño EM. The irreversible binding of amyloid peptide substrates to insulin-degrading enzyme: a biological perspective. Prion 2008;2:51–6. https://doi.org/10.4161/pri.2.2.6710.

[28] Kurochkin IV, Guarnera E, Berezovsky IN. Insulin-degrading enzyme in the fight against Alzheimer's disease. Trends Pharmacol Sci 2018;39:49–58. https://doi.org/10.1016/j.tips.2017.10.008.

[29] Ciechanover A, a. Kwon YT. Degradation of misfolded proteins in neurodegenerative diseases: therapeutic targets and strategies. Exp Mol Med 2015;47:e147. https://doi.org/10.1038/emm.2014.117.

[30] Protacs | Cambridge MedChem Consulting, (n.d.).

[31] Pettersson M, Crews CM. PROteolysis targeting chimeras (PROTACs)—past, present and future. Drug Discov Today Technol 2019;31:15–27. https://doi.org/10.1016/J.DDTEC.2019.01.002.

[32] Schneider M, Radoux CJ, Hercules A, Ochoa D, Dunham I, Zalmas LP, Hessler G, Ruf S, Shanmugasundaram V, Hann MM, Thomas PJ, Queisser MA, Benowitz AB, Brown K, Leach AR. The protactable genome. Nat Rev Drug Discov 2021;20:789–97. https://doi.org/10.1038/S41573-021-00245-X.

[33] Tinworth CP, Lithgow H, Dittus L, Bassi ZI, Hughes SE, Muelbaier M, Dai H, Smith IED, Kerr WJ, Burley GA, Bantscheff M, Harling JD. PROTAC-Mediated Degradation of Bruton's tyrosine kinase is inhibited by covalent binding. ACS Chem Biol 2019;14:342–7. https://doi.org/10.1021/ACSCHEMBIO.8B01094.

[34] Churcher I. Protac-induced protein degradation in drug discovery: breaking the rules or just making new ones?. J Med Chem 2018;61:444–52. https://doi.org/10.1021/ACS.JMEDCHEM.7B01272.

[35] Bondeson DP, Mares A, Smith IED, Ko E, Campos S, Miah AH, Mulholland KE, Routly N, Buckley DL, Gustafson JL, Zinn N, Grandi P, Shimamura S, Bergamini G, Faelth-Savitski M, Bantscheff M, Cox C, Gordon DA, Willard RR, Flanagan JJ, Casillas LN, Votta BJ, Den Besten W, Famm K, Kruidenier L, Carter PS, Harling JD, Churcher I, Crews CM. Catalytic in vivo protein knockdown by small-molecule PROTACs. Nat Chem Biol 2015;11:611–7. https://doi.org/10.1038/NCHEMBIO.1858.

[36] Tampi RR, Forester BP, Agronin M. Aducanumab: evidence from clinical trial data and controversies. Drugs Context 2021;10:2021–3. https://doi.org/10.7573/dic.2021-7-3.

[37] Karthivashan G, Ganesan P, Park S-Y, Kim J-S, Choi D-K. Therapeutic strategies and nano-drug delivery applications in management of ageing Alzheimer's disease. Drug Deliv 2018;25:307–20. https://doi.org/10.1080/10717544.2018.1428243.

[38] Mirza AZ, Siddiqui FA. Nanomedicine and drug delivery: a mini review. Int Nano Lett 2014;4:94. https://doi.org/10.1007/s40089-014-0094-7.

[39] Patra JK, Das G, Fraceto LF, Campos EVR, Rodriguez-Torres MDP, Acosta-Torres LS, Diaz-Torres LA, Grillo R, Swamy MK, Sharma S, Habtemariam S, Shin HS. Nano based drug delivery systems: recent developments and future prospects. J Nanobiotechnol 2018;16 http://doi.org/10.1186/s12951-018-0392-8.

[40] Singh AP, Biswas A, Shukla A, Maiti P. Targeted therapy in chronic diseases using nanomaterial-based drug delivery vehicles. Signal Transduct Target Ther 2019;4:33. https://doi.org/10.1038/s41392-019-0068-3.

[41] Choudhari M, Hejmady S, Saha RN, Damle S, Singhvi G, Alexander A, Kesharwani P, Dubey SK. Evolving new-age strategies to transport therapeutics across the blood-brain barrier. Int J Pharm 2021:120351. https://doi.org/10.1016/j.ijpharm.2021.120351.

[42] Kakoty V, S. KC, Dubey SK, Yang CH, Kesharwani P, Taliyan R. The gut-brain connection in the pathogenicity of Parkinson disease: putative role of autophagy. Neurosci Lett 2021;753:135865. https://doi.org/10.1016/j.neulet.2021.135865.

[43] Agrawal M, Saraf S, Saraf S, Dubey SK, Puri A, Gupta U, Kesharwani P, Ravichandiran V, Kumar P, Naidu VGM, Murty US, Ajazuddin AA. Stimuli-responsive In situ gelling system for nose-to-brain drug delivery. J Control Release 2020;327:235–65. https://doi.org/10.1016/j.jconrel.2020.07.044.

[44] Gorain B, Rajeswary DC, Pandey M, Kesharwani P, Kumbhar SA, Choudhury H. Nose to brain delivery of nanocarriers towards attenuation of demented condition. Curr Pharm Des 2020;26 http://doi.org/10.2174/1381612826666200313125613.

[45] Zeeshan F, Mishra DK, Kesharwani P. From the nose to the brain, nanomedicine drug delivery. In: Theory and Applications of Nonparenteral Nanomedicines. Academic Press-Cambridge, Massachusetts: Elsevier; 2021. p. 153–80. https://doi.org/10.1016/b978-0-12-820466-5.00008-9.

[46] Choudhury H, Pandey M, Chin PX, Phang YL, Cheah JY, Ooi SC, Mak K-K, Pichika MR, Kesharwani P, Hussain Z, Gorain B. Transferrin receptors-targeting nanocarriers for efficient targeted delivery and transcytosis of drugs into the brain tumors: a review of recent advancements and emerging trends. Drug Deliv Transl Res 2018;8:1545–63. https://doi.org/10.1007/s13346-018-0552-2.

[47] Md S, Bhattmisra SK, Zeeshan F, Shahzad N, Mujtaba MA, Srikanth Meka V, Radhakrishnan A, Kesharwani P, Baboota S, Ali J. Nano-carrier enabled drug delivery systems for nose to brain targeting for the treatment of neurodegenerative disorders. J Drug Deliv Sci Technol 2018;43:295–310. https://doi.org/10.1016/j.jddst.2017.09.022.

[48] Zlokovic BV. The blood-brain barrier in health and chronic neurodegenerative disorders. Neuron 2008;57:178–201. https://doi.org/10.1016/j.neuron.2008.01.003.

[49] Gothwal A, Khan I, Kesharwani P, Chourasia MK, Gupta U. Micelle-based drug delivery for brain tumors. In: Nanotechnology-Based Targeted Drug Delivery Systems for Brain Tumors. Academic Press-Cambridge, Massachusetts: Elsevier; 2018. p. 307–26. https://doi.org/10.1016/B978-0-12-812218-1.00011-7.

[50] Gorain B, Choudhury H, Pandey M, Amin M, Singh B, Gupta U, Kesharwani P. Dendrimers as effective carriers for the treatment of brain tumor. In: Nanotechnology-Based Targeted Drug Delivery Systems for Brain Tumors. Academic Press- Cambridge, Massachusetts: Elsevier; 2018. p. 267–305. https://doi.org/10.1016/B978-0-12-812218-1.00010-5.

[51] Meher JG, Chaurasia M, Singh A, Chourasia MK. Carbon nanotubes (CNTs): a novel drug delivery tool in brain tumor treatment, nanotechnology-based target. Drug Deliv Syst Brain Tumors 2018:375–96. https://doi.org/10.1016/B978-0-12-812218-1.00014-2.

[52] Patel HK, Gajbhiye V, Kesharwani P, Jain NK. Ligand anchored poly(propyleneimine) dendrimers for brain targeting: comparative in vitro and in vivo assessment. J Colloid Interface Sci 2016;482:142–50. https://doi.org/10.1016/j.jcis.2016.07.047.
[53] Barchet TM, Amiji MM. Challenges and opportunities in CNS delivery of therapeutics for neurodegenerative diseases. Expert Opin Drug Deliv 2009;6:211–25. https://doi.org/10.1517/17425240902758188.
[54] Dwivedi N, Shah J, Mishra V, Mohd Amin MCI, Iyer AK, Tekade RK, Kesharwani P, Dendrimer-mediated approaches for the treatment of brain tumor, 27 (2016) 557–580. https://doi.org/10.1080/09205063.2015.1133155.
[55] Mishra V, Kesharwani P. Dendrimer technologies for brain tumor. Drug Discov Today 2016;21. https://doi.org/10.1016/j.drudis.2016.02.006.
[56] Balabanov R, Dore-Duffy P. Role of the CNS microvascular pericyte in the blood-brain barrier. J Neurosci Res 1998;53:637–44. https://doi.org/10.1002/(SICI)1097-4547(19980915)53:6<637::AID-JNR1>3.0.CO;2-6.
[57] Lai CH, Kuo KH. The critical component to establish in vitro BBB model: Pericyte. Brain Res Rev 2005;50:258–65. https://doi.org/10.1016/j.brainresrev.2005.07.004.
[58] Armulik A, Genové G, Mäe M, Nisancioglu MH, Wallgard E, Niaudet C, He L, Norlin J, Lindblom P, Strittmatter K, Johansson BR, Betsholtz C. Pericytes regulate the blood-brain barrier. Nature 2010;468:557–61. https://doi.org/10.1038/nature09522.
[59] Mathiisen TM, Lehre KP, Danbolt NC, Ottersen OP. The perivascular astroglial sheath provides a complete covering of the brain microvessels: an electron microscopic 3D reconstruction. Glia 2010;58:1094–103. https://doi.org/10.1002/glia.20990.
[60] Song S, Huang H, Guan X, Fiesler V, Bhuiyan MIH, Liu R, Jalali S, Hasan MN, Tai AK, Chattopadhyay A, Chaparala S, Sun M, Stolz DB, He P, Agalliu D, Sun D, Begum G. Activation of endothelial Wnt/β-catenin signaling by protective astrocytes repairs BBB damage in ischemic stroke. Prog Neurobiol 2021;199:101963. https://doi.org/10.1016/j.pneurobio.2020.101963.
[61] da Fonseca ACC, Matias D, Garcia C, Amaral R, Geraldo LH, Freitas C, Lima FRS. The impact of microglial activation on blood-brain barrier in brain diseases. Front Cell Neurosci 2014;8:1–13. https://doi.org/10.3389/fncel.2014.00362.
[62] Thurgur H, Pinteaux E. Microglia in the neurovascular unit: blood–brain barrier–microglia interactions after central nervous system disorders. Neuroscience 2019;405:55–67. https://doi.org/10.1016/j.neuroscience.2018.06.046.
[63] Lassmann H, Zimprich F, Vass K, Hickey WF. Microglial cells are a component of the perivascular glia limitans. J Neurosci Res 1991;28:236–43. https://doi.org/10.1002/jnr.490280211.
[64] Demeule M, Régina A, Jodoin J, Laplante A, Dagenais C, Berthelet F, Moghrabi A, Béliveau R. Drug transport to the brain: key roles for the efflux pump P-glycoprotein in the blood-brain barrier. Vascul Pharmacol 2002;38:339–48. https://doi.org/10.1016/s1537-1891(02)00201-x.
[65] Aryal M, Fischer K, Gentile C, Gitto S, Zhang YZ, McDannold N. Effects on P-glycoprotein expression after blood-brain barrier disruption using focused ultrasound and microbubbles. PLoS One 2017;12:1–15. https://doi.org/10.1371/journal.pone.0166061.
[66] Schinkel AH, Jonker JW. Mammalian drug efflux transporters of the ATP binding cassette (ABC) family: an overview. Adv Drug Deliv Rev 2012;64:138–53. https://doi.org/10.1016/j.addr.2012.09.027.
[67] Engelhardt B, Sorokin L. The blood-brain and the blood-cerebrospinal fluid barriers: function and dysfunction. Semin Immunopathol 2009;31:497–511. https://doi.org/10.1007/s00281-009-0177-0.

[68] Lochhead JJ, Yang J, Ronaldson PT, Davis TP. Structure, function, and regulation of the blood-brain barrier tight junction in central nervous system disorders. Front Physiol 2020;11. https://doi.org/10.3389/fphys.2020.00914.

[69] Ross C, Taylor M, Fullwood N, Allsop D. Liposome delivery systems for the treatment of Alzheimer's disease. Int J Nanomedicine 2018;13:8507–22. https://doi.org/10.2147/IJN.S183117.

[70] Hernandez C, Shukla S. Liposome based drug delivery as a potential treatment option for Alzheimer's disease. Neural Regen Res 2022;17:1190–8. https://doi.org/10.4103/1673-5374.327328.

[71] Zahin N, Anwar R, Tewari D, Kabir MT, Sajid A, Mathew B, Uddin MS, Aleya L, Abdel-Daim MM. Nanoparticles and its biomedical applications in health and diseases: special focus on drug delivery. Environ Sci Pollut Res Int 2020;27:19151–68. https://doi.org/10.1007/s11356-019-05211-0.

[72] Harilal S, Jose J, Parambi DGT, Kumar R, Mathew GE, Uddin MS, Kim H, Mathew B. Advancements in nanotherapeutics for Alzheimer's disease: current perspectives. J Pharm Pharmacol 2019;71:1370–83. https://doi.org/10.1111/jphp.13132.

[73] G. B, A.-D. BE, N. A, K. P, P. M, C. H, liposome M. A lipid-based drug delivery system for efficient drug delivery. Curr Pharm Des 2021;27. https://doi.org/10.2174/1381612827666210830095941.

[74] Sheikh A, Alhakamy NA, Md S, Kesharwani P. Recent progress of RGD modified liposomes as multistage rocket against cancer. Front Pharmacol 2022;12:4024. https://doi.org/10.3389/FPHAR.2021.803304/BIBTEX.

[75] Kratz F. Albumin as a drug carrier: design of prodrugs, drug conjugates and nanoparticles. J Control Release 2008;132:171–83. https://doi.org/10.1016/j.jconrel.2008.05.010.

[76] Sasi S, Joseph SK, Arian AM, Thomas S, Amrutha VU, Arya GK, Nair SC. An updated review on the application of dendrimers as successful nanocarriers for brain delivery of therapeutic moieties. Int J Appl Pharm 2021;13:1–9. https://doi.org/10.22159/ijap.2021v13i1.39812.

[77] Kokare CR, Khot SV, Gorain B, Kesharwani P. Characterization of dendrimers. In: Dendrimer-Based Nanotherapeutics. Academic Press- Cambridge, Massachusetts: Elsevier; 2021. p. 125–41. https://doi.org/10.1016/B978-0-12-821250-9.00006-8.

[78] Gawande V, Choudhury H, Kesharwani P. Dendrimer nomenclature and synthesis methods. In: Dendrimer-Based Nanotherapeutics. Academic Press- Cambridge, Massachusetts: Elsevier; 2021. p. 75–94. https://doi.org/10.1016/B978-0-12-821250-9.00009-3.

[79] Singh S, Singh G, Sehrawat S, Rawat P, Molugulu N, Singh V, Ahmed FJ, Kesharwani P. Conclusion and future considerations of dendrimers. In: Dendrimer-Based Nanotherapeutics. Academic Press- Cambridge, Massachusetts: Elsevier; 2021. p. 449–58. https://doi.org/10.1016/B978-0-12-821250-9.00005-6.

[80] Choudhury H, Sisinthy SP, Gorain B, Kesharwani P. History and introduction of dendrimers. In: Dendrimer-Based Nanotherapeutics. Academic Press- Cambridge, Massachusetts: Elsevier; 2021. p. 1–14. https://doi.org/10.1016/B978-0-12-821250-9.00014-7.

[81] Jain K, Jain NK, Kesharwani P. Types of dendrimers. In: Dendrimer-Based Nanotherapeutics. Academic Press- Cambridge, Massachusetts: Elsevier; 2021. p. 95–123. https://doi.org/10.1016/B978-0-12-821250-9.00007-X.

[82] Bandaru R, Sanket AS, Ṛekha S, Kamble O, Dewangan RP, Kesharwani P, Samal SK, Dandela R. Biological interaction of dendrimers. In: Dendrimer-Based Nanotherapeutics. Academic Press- Cambridge, Massachusetts: Elsevier; 2021. p. 63–74. https://doi.org/10.1016/B978-0-12-821250-9.00023-8.

[83] Gorain B, Pandey M, Choudhury H, Jain GK, Kesharwani P. Dendrimer for solubility enhancement. In: Dendrimer-Based Nanotherapeutics. Academic Press- Cambridge, Massachusetts: Elsevier; 2021. p. 273–83. https://doi.org/10.1016/B978-0-12-821250-9.00025-1.

[84] Gauro R, Nandave M, Jain VK, Jain K. Advances in dendrimer-mediated targeted drug delivery to the brain. J Nanoparticle Res 2021;23:1–20. https://doi.org/10.1007/s11051-021-05175-8.

[85] Zhu Y, Liu C, Pang Z biomolecules dendrimer-based drug delivery systems for brain targeting, Mdpi.Com. https://doi.org/10.3390/biom9120790.

[86] Islam Y, Leach AG, Smith J, Pluchino S, Coxonl CR, Sivakumaran M, Downing J, Fatokun AA, Teixidò M, Ehtezazi T. Peptide based drug delivery systems to the brain. Nano Express 2020;1:012002. https://doi.org/10.1088/2632-959x/ab9008.

[87] Kesharwani P, Choudhury H, Meher JG, Pandey M, Gorain B. Dendrimer-entrapped gold nanoparticles as promising nanocarriers for anticancer therapeutics and imaging. Prog Mater Sci 2019;103:484–508. https://doi.org/10.1016/j.pmatsci.2019.03.003.

[88] Kesharwani P, Jain K, Jain NK. Dendrimer as nanocarrier for drug delivery. Prog Polym Sci 2014;39:268–307.

[89] Kesharwani P, Iyer AK. Recent advances in dendrimer-based nanovectors for tumor-targeted drug and gene delivery. Drug Discov Today 2015;20:536–47. https://doi.org/10.1016/j.drudis.2014.12.012.

[90] Sun Z, Ma C, Li G, Zheng X, Hao Y, Yang Y, Application of antibody fragments against A β with emphasis on combined application with nanoparticles in Alzheimer's disease, 12 (2021) 1–11. https://doi.org/10.3389/fphar.2021.654611.

[91] Croy SR, Kwon GS. Polymeric micelles for drug delivery. Curr Pharm Des 2006;12:4669–84. https://doi.org/10.2174/138161206779026245.

[92] Modi D, Mohammad MHW, Garg V, Bhatia M, Kesharwani P, Jain GK. Formulation development, optimization, and in vitro assessment of thermoresponsive ophthalmic pluronic F127-chitosan in situ tacrolimus gel. J Biomater Sci Polym Ed 2021. https://doi.org/10.1080/09205063.2021.1932359.

[93] Patnaik S, Gorain B, Padhi S, Choudhury H, Gabr GA, Md S, Kumar Mishra D, Kesharwani P. Recent update of toxicity aspects of nanoparticulate systems for drug delivery. Eur J Pharm Biopharm 2021;161:100–19. https://doi.org/10.1016/j.ejpb.2021.02.010.

[94] Kwon GS. Polymeric micelles for delivery of poorly water-soluble compounds. Crit Rev Ther Drug Carrier Syst 2003;20:357–403. https://doi.org/10.1615/critrevtherdrugcarriersyst.v20.i5.20.

[95] Nagarajan R. Solubilization of hydrocarbons and resulting aggregate shape transitions in aqueous solutions of Pluronic (R) (PEO-PPO-PEO) block copolymers. Colloids Surfaces B Biointerfaces 1999;16:55–72.

[96] Meher JG, Dixit S, Pathan DK, Singh Y, Chandasana H, Pawar VK, Sharma M, Bhatta RS, Konwar R, Kesharwani P. Chourasia MK. Paclitaxel-loaded TPGS enriched self-emulsifying carrier causes apoptosis by modulating survivin expression and inhibits tumour growth in syngeneic mammary tumours. Artif Cells, Nanomedicine, Biotechnol 2018:1–15. https://doi.org/10.1080/21691401.2018.1492933.

[97] Scialabba C, Rocco F, Licciardi M, Pitarresi G, Ceruti M, Giammona G. Amphiphilic polyaspartamide copolymer-based micelles for rivastigmine delivery to neuronal cells. Drug Deliv 2012;19:307–16. https://doi.org/10.3109/10717544.2012.714813.

[98] Martin-Banderas L, a Holgado M, Venero JL, Alvarez-Fuentes J, Fernández-Arévalo M. Nanostructures for drug delivery to the brain. Curr Med Chem 2011;18:5303–21.

[99] Zhong Y, Meng F, Deng C, Zhong Z. Ligand-directed active tumor-targeting polymeric nanoparticles for cancer chemotherapy. Biomacromolecules 2014;15:1955–69 https://doi.org/10.1021/bm5003009.

[100] Tosi G, Costantino L, Ruozi B, Forni F, Vandelli MA. Polymeric nanoparticles for the drug delivery to the central nervous system. Expert Opin Drug Deliv 2008;5:155–74. https://doi.org/10.1517/17425247.5.2.155.

[101] Severino P, da Silva CF, Andrade LN, de Lima Oliveira D, Campos J, Souto EB. Alginate nanoparticles for drug delivery and targeting. Curr Pharm Des 2019;25:1312–34. https://doi.org/10.2174/1381612825666190425163424.

[102] Zhao Y, Xiong S, Liu P, Liu W, Wang Q, Liu Y, Tan H, Chen X, Shi X, Wang Q, Chen T. Polymeric nanoparticles-based brain delivery with improved therapeutic efficacy of ginkgolide B in Parkinson's disease. Int J Nanomed 2020;15:10453–67. https://doi.org/10.2147/IJN.S272831.

[103] Peniche H, Peniche C. Chitosan nanoparticles: a contribution to nanomedicine. Polym Int 2011;60:883–9.

[104] Mohammed MA, Syeda JTM, Wasan KM, Wasan EK. An overview of chitosan nanoparticles and its application in non-parenteral drug delivery. Pharmaceutics 2017;9. https://doi.org/10.3390/pharmaceutics9040053.

[105] Sardoiwala MN, Kaundal B, Choudhury SR. Development of engineered nanoparticles expediting diagnostic and therapeutic applications across blood–brain barrier. In: Handbook of Nanomaterials for Industrial Applications. Elsevier; 2018:696–709.

[106] Shakeri S, Ashrafizadeh M, Zarrabi A, Roghanian R, Afshar EG, Pardakhty A, Mohammadinejad R, Kumar A, Thakur VK. Multifunctional polymeric nanoplatforms for brain diseases diagnosis, therapy and theranostics. Biomedicines 2020;8. https://doi.org/10.3390/biomedicines8010013.

[107] Cano A, Sánchez-López E, Ettcheto M, López-Machado A, Espina M, Souto EB, Galindo R, Camins A, García ML, Turowski P. Current advances in the development of novel polymeric nanoparticles for the treatment of neurodegenerativediseases. Nanomedicine (Lond) 2020;15:1239–61. https://doi.org/10.2217/nnm-2019-0443.

[108] Yeh YC, Creran B, Rotello VM. Gold nanoparticles: Preparation, properties, and applications in bionanotechnology. Nanoscale 2012;4:1871–80. https://doi.org/10.1039/c1nr11188d.

[109] Rai M, Yadav A. Nanobiotechnology in Neurodegenerative Diseases. Springer International Publishing; 2019. 1st ed. https://doi.org/10.1007/978-3-030-30930-5.

[110] Elbassal EA, Morris C, Kent TW, Lantz R, Ojha B, Wojcikiewicz EP, Du D. Gold nanoparticles as a probe for Amyloid-β oligomer and amyloid formation. J Phys Chem C Nanomater Interfaces 2017;121:20007–15. https://doi.org/10.1021/acs.jpcc.7b05169.

[111] Pocernich CB, Butterfield DA. Elevation of glutathione as a therapeutic strategy in Alzheimer disease. Biochim Biophys Acta 2012;1822:625–30. https://doi.org/10.1016/j.bbadis.2011.10.003.

[112] Hou K, Zhao J, Wang H, Li B, Li K, Shi X, Wan K, Ai J, Lv J, Wang D, Huang Q, Wang H, Cao Q, Liu S, Tang Z. Chiral gold nanoparticles enantioselectively rescue memory deficits in a mouse model of Alzheimer's disease. Nat Commun 2020;11:4790. https://doi.org/10.1038/s41467-020-18525-2.

[113] Muller AP, Ferreira GK, Pires AJ, de Bem Silveira G, de Souza DL, de A. Brandolfi J, de Souza CT, Paula MMS, Silveira PCL. Gold nanoparticles prevent cognitive deficits, oxidative stress and inflammation in a rat model of sporadic dementia of Alzheimer's type. Mater Sci Eng C Mater Biol Appl 2017;77:476–83. https://doi.org/10.1016/j.msec.2017.03.283.

[114] Barman MK, Patra A. Current status and prospects on chemical structure driven photoluminescence behaviour of carbon dots. J Photochem Photobiol C Photochem Rev 2018;37:1–22. https://doi.org/10.1016/j.jphotochemrev.2018.08.001.
[115] Kuang Y, Zhang J, Xiong M, Zeng W, Lin X, Yi X, Luo Y, Yang M, Li F, Huang Q. A novel nanosystem realizing curcumin delivery based on Fe(3)O(4)@Carbon Dots nanocomposite for Alzheimer's disease therapy. Front Bioeng Biotechnol 2020;8:614906. https://doi.org/10.3389/fbioe.2020.614906.
[116] Hirlekar R, Yamagar M, Garse H, Vij M, Kadam V. Carbon nanotubes and its applications: a review. Asian J Pharm Clin Res 2009;2:17–27.
[117] Singh BGP, Baburao C, Pispati V, Pathipati H, Muthy N, Prassana SRV, Rathode BG. Carbon nanotubes. A novel drug delivery system. Int J Res Pharm Chem 2012;2:523–32.
[118] Zhang Y, Bai Y, Yan B. Functionalized carbon nanotubes for potential medicinal applications. Drug Discov Today 2010;15:428–35.
[119] Usui Y, Haniu H, Tsuruoka S, Saito N. Carbon nanotubes innovate on medical technology. Med Chem 2012;2:1–6.
[120] He H, Pham-Huy LA, Dramou P, Xiao D, Zuo P, Pham-Huy C. Carbon nanotubes: applications in pharmacy and medicine. Biomed Res Int 2013;2013. https://doi.org/10.1155/2013/578290.
[121] Yang Z, Zhang Y, Yang Y, Sun L, Han D, Li H, Wang C. Pharmacological and toxicological target organelles and safe use of single-walled carbon nanotubes as drug carriers in treating Alzheimer disease. Nanomed Nanotechnol, Biol Med 2010;6:427–41. https://doi.org/10.1016/j.nano.2009.11.007.
[122] Xiang C, Zhang Y, Guo W, Liang X-J. Biomimetic carbon nanotubes for neurological disease therapeutics as inherent medication. Acta Pharm Sin B 2020;10:239–48. https://doi.org/10.1016/j.apsb.2019.11.003.
[123] Xue X, Wang L-R, Sato Y, Jiang Y, Berg M, Yang D-S, Nixon RA, Liang X-J. Single-walled carbon nanotubes alleviate autophagic/lysosomal defects in primary glia from a mouse model of Alzheimer's disease. Nano Lett 2014;14:5110–7. https://doi.org/10.1021/nl501839q.
[124] Baum C, Schambach A, Modlich U, Thrasher A. [Gene therapy of SCID-X1]. Bundesgesundheitsblatt Gesundheitsforschung Gesundheitsschutz 2007;50:1507–17. https://doi.org/10.1007/s00103-007-0385-5.
[125] Wirth T, Parker N, Ylä-Herttuala S. History of gene therapy. Gene 2013;525:162–9. https://doi.org/10.1016/j.gene.2013.03.137.
[126] Choudhury SR, Hudry E, Maguire CA, Sena-Esteves M, Breakefield XO, Grandi P. Viral vectors for therapy of neurologic diseases. Neuropharmacology 2017;120:63–80. https://doi.org/10.1016/j.neuropharm.2016.02.013.
[127] Sasmita AO. Current viral-mediated gene transfer research for treatment of Alzheimer's disease. Biotechnol Genet Eng Rev 2019;35:26–45. https://doi.org/10.1080/02648725.2018.1523521.
[128] Connolly JB. Lentiviruses in gene therapy clinical research. Gene Ther 2002;9:1730–4. https://doi.org/10.1038/sj.gt.3301893.
[129] Ittner LM, Klugmann M, Ke YD. Adeno-associated virus-based Alzheimer's disease mouse models and potential new therapeutic avenues. Br J Pharmacol 2019;176:3649–65. https://doi.org/10.1111/bph.14637.
[130] Sehara Y, Fujimoto K-I, Ikeguchi K, Katakai Y, Ono F, Takino N, Ito M, Ozawa K, Muramatsu S-I. Persistent expression of dopamine-synthesizing enzymes 15 years After gene transfer in a primate model of parkinson's disease. Hum Gene Ther Clin Dev 2017;28:74–9. https://doi.org/10.1089/humc.2017.010.

[131] McAlister E, Kirkby M, Donnelly RF Microneedles for drug delivery and monitoring. InMicrofluidic Devices for. Biomedical Applications, 1. Woodhead Publishing; 2021 Jan. p. 225–260.

[132] Waghule T, Singhvi G, Dubey SK, Pandey MM, Gupta G, Singh M, Dua K. Microneedles: A smart approach and increasing potential for transdermal drug delivery system. Biomed Pharmacother. 2019 Jan;109:1249-1258. doi: 10.1016/j.biopha.2018.10.078. Epub 2018 Nov 9. PMID: 30551375.

[133] Waghule T, Singhvi G, Kumar S, Monohar M. Biomedicine & pharmacotherapy microneedles : a smart approach and increasing potential for transdermal drug delivery system. Biomed Pharmacother 2019;109:1249–58. https://doi.org/10.1016/j.biopha.2018.10.078.

[134] Kim Y, Park J, Prausnitz MR. Microneedles for drug and vaccine delivery ☆. Adv Drug Deliv Rev 2012;64:1547–68. https://doi.org/10.1016/j.addr.2012.04.005.

[135] Muñoz-Torrero D, Mangoni AA, Liu H, Hulme C, Rautio J, Karaman R, De Sousa ME, Prokai-Tatrai K, Sabatier JM, Siciliano C, Luque FJ, Kokotos G, Ragno R, Collina S, Guillou C, Tschow MG, Agrofoglio LA. Breakthroughs in medicinal chemistry: new targets and mechanisms, new drugs, new hopes–2. Molecules 2018;23:1–9. https://doi.org/10.3390/molecules23010065.

[136] Bonvouloir N, Crine P, Boileau G, DesGroseillers L, Lemieux N, Molecular cloning, tissue distribution, and chromosomal localization of MMEL2, a gene coding for a novel human member of the neutral endopeptidase-24.11 family, 20 (2004) 493–498. http://doi.org/10.1089/104454901316976127.

[137] Iwata N, Tsubuki S, Takaki Y, Shirotani K, Lu B, Gerard NP, Gerard C, Hama E, Lee HJ, Saido TC. Metabolic regulation of brain Aβ by Neprilysin. Science (80-) 2001;292:1550–2. https://doi.org/10.1126/SCIENCE.1059946.

[138] Ghaddar G, Ruchon AF, Carpentier M, Marcinkiewicz M, Seidah NG, Crine P, Desgroseillers L, Boileau G. Molecular cloning and biochemical characterization of a new mouse testis soluble-zinc-metallopeptidase of the neprilysin family. Biochem J 2000;347:419–29. https://doi.org/10.1042/BJ3470419.

[139] Iwata N, Tsubuki S, Takaki Y, Watanabe K, Sekiguchi M, Hosoki E, Kawashima-Morishima M, Lee HJ, Hama E, Sekine-Aizawa Y, Saido TC. Identification of the major Aβ1–42-degrading catabolic pathway in brain parenchyma: suppression leads to biochemical and pathological deposition. Nat Med 2000;62(6):143–50. 2000. https://doi.org/10.1038/72237.

[140] Nisemblat Y, Belinson H, Dolev I, Michaelson DM. Activation of the amyloid cascade by intracerebroventricular injection of the protease inhibitor phosphoramidon. Neurodegener Dis 2008;5:166–9. https://doi.org/10.1159/000113692.

[141] Dolev I, Michaelson DM. A nontransgenic mouse model shows inducible amyloid-β (Aβ) peptide deposition and elucidates the role of apolipoprotein E in the amyloid cascade. Proc Natl Acad Sci U S A 2004;101:13909–14. https://doi.org/10.1073/PNAS.0404458101.

[142] Yasojima K, Akiyama H, McGeer EG, McGeer PL. Reduced neprilysin in high plaque areas of Alzheimer brain: a possible relationship to deficient degradation of β-amyloid peptide. Neurosci Lett 2001;297:97–100. https://doi.org/10.1016/S0304-3940(00)01675-X.

[143] Hartlage-Rübsamen M, Zeitschel U, Apelt J, Gärtner U, Franke H, Stahl T, Günther A, Schliebs R, Penkowa M, Bigl V, Roßner S. Astrocytic expression of the Alzheimer's disease β-secretase (BACE1) is stimulus-dependent. Glia 2003;41:169–79. https://doi.org/10.1002/GLIA.10178.

[144] Caccamo A, Oddo S, Sugarman MC, Akbari Y, LaFerla FM. Age- and region-dependent alterations in Aβ-degrading enzymes: implications for Aβ-induced disorders. Neurobiol Aging 2005;26:645–54. https://doi.org/10.1016/J.NEUROBIOLAGING.2004.06.013.

[145] Marr RA, Spencer BJ. Diabetes NEP-Like Endopeptidases and Alzheimers Disease. Curr Alzheimer Res 2010;7:223–9. https://doi.org/10.2174/156720510791050849.

Index

Page numbers followed by "*f*" and "*t*" indicate, figures and tables respectively.

FSC
www.fsc.org
MIX
Papier | Fördert
gute Waldnutzung
FSC® C083411

Kolibri 360 GmbH
Ferdinand-Jühlke-Straße 7
99095 Erfurt, Deutschland
produktsicherheit@kolibri360.de